MW00844898

PRACTICAL MATHEMATICS IN NUCLEAR MEDICINE TECHNOLOGY

Second Edition

Patricia Wells, MAE, CNMT

Former Program Director

Muhlenberg Regional Medical Center
Schools of Nursing, Medical Imaging and Therapeutic Science
Plainfield, New Jersey

&

Overlook School of Nuclear Medicine Technology
Summit, New Jersey

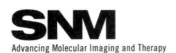
Advancing Molecular Imaging and Therapy

Published by
THE SOCIETY OF NUCLEAR MEDICINE
1850 Samuel Morse Drive, Reston, VA 20190
www.snm.org

Society of Nuclear Medicine Inc.
1850 Samuel Morse Drive, Reston, VA 20190-5316

© 2011 Society of Nuclear Medicine, Inc. All rights reserved

All rights reserved. No part of this book may be reproduced or utilized in any form or by any means, electronic or mechanical, including photocopying, recording, or by any information storage or retrieval system, without permission in writing from the publisher. Inquiries should be addressed in writing to Publications, Society of Nuclear Medicine, 1850 Samuel Morse Drive, Reston, Virginia 20190-5316.

Printed in the United States of America.

Library of Congress Cataloging-in-Publication Data

Wells, Patricia, 1950-
  Practical mathematics in nuclear medicine technology / Patricia Wells. -- 2nd ed.
      p. ; cm.
  Includes bibliographical references and index.
  Summary: "Simplifies the mathematics that technologists and students are likely to encounter in the practice of clinical nuclear medicine technology"--Provided by publisher.
  ISBN 978-0-932004-86-4 (softcover)
 1. Nuclear medicine--Mathematics. 2. Nuclear medicine--Mathematics--Problems, exercises, etc. I. Society of Nuclear Medicine (1953-) II. Title.
  [DNLM: 1. Mathematical Concepts. 2. Nuclear Medicine. WN 25]
  R905.W44 2010
  616.07'5750151--dc22

                                                                            2010043614

Preface to First Edition

Math does not come easily to me, so I have always been a bit chagrined when put in the position to teach it to others. Because I have repeatedly found myself in that position, I have had to work out simple methods to explain math to myself, so I could, in turn, explain it to my students. This book is a product of that process.

This book is intended as a supplemental textbook for students and on-the-job trainees, and as a reference book for practicing technologists. The purpose of the book is to simplify the mathematics that technologists and students are likely to encounter in the practice of clinical nuclear medicine technology. I have purposely left theories and most derivations to those much more adept at explaining them.

I have included a review of some math basics that have frequently posed problems for my own students over the years.

Because demonstration and practice are essential aspects of learning, I have provided many solved examples and more than 1,000 practice problems. The answers to all problems will be found in Appendix C, with many expanded to demonstrate the step-by-step process.

Throughout the book, I have interspersed * **Notes.** These are useful insights, helpful hints, or special reminders that have seemed to help my students understand concepts and avoid particular mistakes.

I am greatly indebted to all the students I have had the pleasure to teach throughout the years, as they have taught me as much as I have taught them. They have especially taught me the value of simplicity and clarity. I thank them all.

I also want to thank the friends, colleagues and students who took time out of their busy lives to review, correct, and comment on this manuscript.

Jan Alexander	Tracey Johnson	Martha Pickett
Brian Barnes ✚	Sonja Joyner	John Reed
James Bellamy	Anthony Knight	Mark Richard ✚
Al Broscius	Daniel Leahey	Raymond Robinson
James Donlan	Vivian Loveless	Nancy Sawyer ✚
Dionne Duval	David Luckenbach	Jerry Stewart
Gladys Figaro	Patrick McClaughrey	Paul Thaxton
John Findlay	Miriam Miller	Jonathan Walker
Cecilia Gomes	Banjo Olowe	Martha Wells
Mary Hesselgrave	Karim Paez	Valerie Whitehead

I owe them a great debt.

Patricia Wells
1999

✚ Deceased

Preface to Second Edition

I give my sincere thanks to the kind people who reviewed and critiqued the new parts of this book.

James Bellamy
Carla Coley
Martha Pickett
Paul Thaxton

I also give endless thanks to Arthur Maune, who patiently reviewed and revised the whole book again and again. This new volume would not exist without his efforts.

In the ten years since the first edition of this book was published, nuclear medicine has become more and more computerized. Many of the mathematical computations technologist performed 10, 20, and 30 years ago are now being done for us. But the need to understand the mathematics behind the numbers we are handed is still paramount. Without this understanding we are mere technicians, rather than the expert technologists we strive to be.

I hope all who use this book, students, educators, and practicing technologists, will find it a simple route to comprehending the essential mathematics of nuclear medicine.

Patricia Wells
2011

Introduction

> * **Note:** A **scientific calculator** is an essential tool for people using this text. Because individual calculator design varies, specific instructions for calculator use have not been included. Refer to the instruction booklet provided by the manufacturer to determine the order in which keys are used for various functions.

This book is designed as a workbook.

The chapters of the book are divided into sections with each section dealing with a particular process or procedure. Each section is divided into several parts:

1. The **Principles** portion gives a description of the process or procedure. Where necessary it includes background information important to understanding the process.

2. The **How to** section contains the step-by-step method used to solve the problems. This portion is enclosed in a shadowbox. Each shadowbox has a reference number, such as I-4. The I designates chapter I and the -4 designates the fourth equation presented in that chapter.

3. **Examples** with step-by-step solutions are provided for each mathematical process.

4. Numerous practice **Problems** are given. Because repetition is so important to learning math, you are encouraged to work all the problems. Solutions to all problems will be found in Appendix C.

5. **Additional Applications** follow the problems in many sections. These problems require manipulation of the equation, combining of processes, or the application of the process to a more complicated situation. Solutions to these problems are also found in Appendix C.

    6. A list of **References** is included at the end of each section. The references are listed by author, page and edition, with the full bibliographic information listed in the **References Section** at the end of the book. These references may provide a more detailed description of a process or the derivation of an equation.

7. * **Note:** Throughout the book special notes have been included which I have found to be useful for understanding a process or for preventing common mistakes. These notes are highlighted as you see here or may be included in a "How to" shadowbox.

8. ➢ **Regulations:** NRC and DOT regulations are highlighted within sections of the book as demonstrated here. They are included in any section that covers a procedure that is affected by or involves NRC regulations.

9. **Decay Charts** for many of the radionuclides used in clinical nuclear medicine are found in Appendix A. Pre-calibration factors are included in some charts.

10. The **Solutions to the Problems** are found in Appendix C. Several problems for each section are expanded in the answer section to show the step-by-step process used to solve them. Other solutions are expanded when manipulation of the equation is required or when processes are combined.

Important note concerning abbreviations and decimal formats

The Joint Commission and the Institute for Safe Medication Practices have published guidelines to help prevent medical errors. Because some symbols can be mistaken for similar symbols when handwritten, it is recommended that these symbols should not be used.

When it is not written clearly, the symbol for micro, μ, can be look like the symbol for milli, m. The Joint Commission has recommended that the abbreviation for microgram, μg, be replaced with mcg or that the word be written out. The mcg abbreviation is used in this book.

Neither the Joint Commission nor the Nuclear Regulatory Commission have addressed the issue of μCi, which when poorly written, can look like mCi. Because an alternative abbreviation has not yet been recommended by these agencies, this book uses the μCi. **However, the author strongly recommends that students and technologists write out the word "microcuries" when referring to dosages that are being ordered or administered to patients, in order to prevent errors.**

The Joint Commission and the Institute for Safe Medication Practices have also noted the potential for errors when decimal points are used. A "naked" decimal point that does not have an integer or a 0 to the left can easily be overlooked. **Therefore ".X" should always be written as "0.X".** A "trailing" zero after a decimal point can also be missed, so decimal places should only be used when that level of accuracy is required. Typically, in nuclear medicine, decimal places are not needed when ordering dosages. However, when recording dose calibrator readings, decimal places are used. For example, a 20-mCi unit dose is ordered. When the unit dosage is measured in the dose calibrator, a reading of 20.3 mCi would be recorded as such.

References:

The Joint Commission. *The Official "Do Not Use" List of Abbreviations*. December 29, 2009. http://www.jointcommission.org/PatientSafety/DoNotUseList/. Accessed March 13, 2010.

Institute for Safe Medication Practices. *List of Error-Prone Abbreviations, Symbols, and Dose Designations*. 2010. https://www.ismp.org/tools/abbreviations/. Accessed March 13, 2010.

Table of Contents

Chapter I. Basics Math Skills for Nuclear Medicine Technology $\quad$ 1

Chapter II. Statistics $\quad$ 51

Chapter III. Radiation Protection $\quad$ 81

Chapter IV. Instrumentation   101

Chapter V. Radiopharmacy   151

Chapter VI. Clinical Procedures   211

Appendices   255

Reference List   325

Index   327

Chapter I. Basic Math Skills for Nuclear Medicine Technology

1. Significant figures and rounding of numbers

Principles:

Significant figures are units that reflect the accuracy of a number. For example, if a box contains exactly 92 syringes, the number 92 has two significant figures. If you say the box has about 90 syringes, this number has one significant figure. It is an estimate that is accurate to only the tens place. As a second example, your department does about 450 bone scans a year. This number has two significant figures. If you count the exact number of bone scans that were performed and report it as 434, this number has three significant figures. In each case, only the units that reflect accuracy are counted as significant figures.

When you can count something, such as objects or procedures, and obtain an exact count, you are finding an absolute value. Most numbers used in nuclear medicine are NOT absolute values. They are measurements, such as the number of photons detected by a camera or the time required for half the radioactivity to leave an organ. These numbers contain an element of inaccuracy, because every measurement is rounded at some point. We measure to the point of accuracy needed for any particular situation and ignore the insignificant figures that could, in actuality, be measured.

The last significant figure, or digit, in a number representing any measurement is an approximation, because every measurement is rounded. If a dose calibrator is set to read doses to a single decimal place, it will round each measurement to that point. In reality each dose can be measured to many decimal places. Such a high degree of accuracy, however, is unnecessary in clinical nuclear medicine, so the dose activity is rounded to a single decimal place, and the number in that place is considered significant.

The last significant figure, or digit, in any number that has been rounded always has a degree of inherent error. For example, if you divide 17,358 counts by 1,672 seconds, the answer is 10.38157895 counts per second (cps). Although the answer appears to have 10 significant figures, it does not. Because there are only 4 digits in 1 of the 2 elements of the problem, the answer is not reliable beyond 4 significant figures. We must therefore, round to 4 significant figures. The answer would now be 10.38 cps. The last retained digit, the 8, is not a truly accurate number because it is produced by rounding. However, it is sufficiently accurate to be considered a significant figure.

I-1 How to determine how many significant figures are present in a number:

1. Integers from 1 through 9 are always significant.
2. If a 0 is simply a space holder, as in 5,000 or 0.02, then it is NOT a significant figure.
3. When a 0 is sandwiched between other integers, as in 407, then it IS a significant figure.
4. When a 0 is the last digit of an accurate measurement, such as a dose calibrator readout of 18.0 mCi, then it IS a significant figure. In this case the machine is providing an accurate reading to the tenth of a mCi; the tenths place happens to be a zero.
5. To avoid confusion over the significance of a 0, it is usually dropped from a decimal place if a number is rounded to 0. For example, when rounding 56.99 to two significant figures, it is rounded to 57, not 57.0.

* **Note:** It can sometimes be difficult to determine if a zero at the end of a number is actually significant. The number 500 could be an accurate measurement, just as it could be a rounded estimate. The context of a problem is usually a good indicator for the level of accuracy used in a measurement. In nuclear medicine a whole number ending in multiple zeros is usually an estimate.

Examples:

A. The number 5,000,000 has only 1 significant figure. The zeros denote unmeasured   units.

B. The number 0.002 has only 1 significant figure. The two zeros preceding the 2 are unmeasured place holders.

C.

Actual Number	Number of Significant Figures
25,600	3
56.89	4
0.28946	5
0.0009538	4
20,456	5

I-2 How to determine how many significant figures should be used:

There are three factors that need to be considered.

1. How much accuracy can actually be achieved?
2. How much accuracy is actually required, either by necessity or regulation?
3. How much error can be introduced without affecting the quality of the results?

Examples:

A. When drawing up a dose of radiopharmaceutical, you will measure the volume to the tenth of a milliliter (ml), because this is the smallest unit that can be accurately measured with a 3- or 5-ml syringe. Therefore if a dose volume calculation gives an answer of 0.77 ml, you must round up to 0.8 ml, because the calibration marks on your syringe do not permit the measurement of 0.77 ml.

Does it matter that you draw up 0.8 ml instead of 0.77 ml of radiopharmaceutical? No, because the activity in a dose must fall within a range, such as 20–23 mCi. It does not have to be an exact number such as 20.0 or 22.4 mCi. Why? Because the small difference in administered radioactivity, usually plus or minus 10% of the prescribed dose, will not change the quality of the study, nor will it significantly affect the patient's radiation dose.

B. A radiologist determines the standard dose for Tc99m HDP will be 23 mCi. When a dose is prepared, it is not necessary to draw up exactly 23.0 mCi. The institution's license will specify an acceptable dose range, usually plus or minus 10% of the prescribed dose. Therefore, any dose of Tc99m HDP falling between 20.7 mCi and 25.3 mCi will be acceptable. When the dose is measured in the dose calibrator, the actual activity should be recorded to the tenths place, such as 23.3 mCi, because the dose calibrator provides a reasonably accurate digital readout to this level.

C. Tc99m MAA, which is used for lung perfusion imaging, consists of minute particles. Manufacturers recommend that patients receive between 800,000 and 1,200,000 particles per dose. If a kit containing an average of 5 million particles is diluted to 6 ml, will each milliliter contain 833,333 particles?

$$\frac{5{,}000{,}000 \text{ particles}}{6 \text{ ml}} = 833{,}333 \text{ particles / ml}$$

Although this appears mathematically correct, it is highly unlikely that each milliliter contains this exact number of particles. Why? Because the number of particles actually contained in the MAA kit is an estimate, not an exact number. The answer to the above equation cannot have a greater degree of accuracy than the original measurement on which it is based. The answer is therefore rounded to one significant figure: 800,000.

Does it matter? In this case failure to achieve such accuracy doesn't matter. If the acceptable range of particles per dose is 800,000 to 1,200,000, how much difference do 33,333 particles make? Very little. They constitute only 4% of the estimated dose. Since most measurements in nuclear medicine accept a 10% error, this level of accuracy is well within acceptable limits.

I-3 How to round numbers:

1. Select the digits to be retained based on the potential for accuracy.
2. Examine the first digit to be dropped. This is the first number to the right of the retained number.
3. If the first digit to be dropped is less than 5, the retained number is left unchanged. If 1.3826 is to be rounded to three significant figures, the 1.38 is retained and the 2 and 6 are dropped. The first number dropped is a 2, so the retained number is unchanged.
4. If the first digit to be dropped is greater than 5, increase the retained number by one unit. If 1.3826 is to be rounded to two significant figures, the retained number would be increased by 1 unit to 1.4, because the first digit to be dropped is an 8.
5. If the first digit to be dropped is a 5, round down when the retained number is even and round up if the retained number is odd. Round 3.325 to 3.32, and 6.735 to 6.74. In other words, the resulting number will always become an even number when the first number dropped is a 5.
6. If a decimal place is rounded up to a 0, drop the 0. For example, 56.99 is rounded to 57, not 57.0. If the last digit retained is a 0, keep it. For example, 25.02 would be rounded to 25.0.

* Note: Some references recommend rounding up one unit whenever the first digit to be dropped is 5 or greater. This is simply another school of thought. The method listed above, however, will be used throughout this book.

Examples:

A. Round 1.9582 to 4 significant figures.

The answer is 1.958 because the 2 that was dropped is less than 5.

B. Round 9.351 to 2 significant figures.

The answer is 9.4 because the first digit dropped is a 5 and the retained number is odd. The retained number is therefore increased by 1 unit.

C. Round 8.057 to 2 significant figures.

The answer is 8.0 because the first digit dropped is a 5 and the retained number is even. The retained number therefore remains unchanged.

D. Round 0.06895 to 2 significant figures.

Since the 0 to the right of the decimal is merely a place holder, you drop the 9 and the 5 to produce a number with 2 significant figures. The retained number is rounded up because the first digit dropped, the 9, is greater than 5. Answer = 0.069.

E. Round 0.00197 to 2 significant figures.

The answer is 0.002. Although the number was rounded to 0.0020, the 0 is dropped when a number is rounded up to a zero.

Problems:

How many significant figures appear in each of the following numbers?

1. 49.06
2. 0.000385
3. 2.0003
4. 8,000,000,000
5. 0.0020

Round each number to 2 significant figures.

6. 24,756
7. 7,923
8. 85.7
9. 9,954
10. 0.0758
11. 0.000436
12. 0.8254
13. 0.33062

Round each number to 3 significant figures.

14. 8.744
15. 2,359
16. 1,233,728
17. 0.046859
18. 0.000137289
19. 1.6488
20. 18.52

References:

Christian & Waterstram-Rich (6th Ed.), p. 9–10.

2. Significant figures and mathematical operations

Principles:

Each rounding operation adds a small element of error or inaccuracy. You must, therefore, decide if rounding off numbers as you proceed through multiple mathematical operations will add significant error to the results. The more steps in the operation, the more error if rounding is used at every step.

I-4 How to minimize error when rounding numbers during multiple mathematical steps.

Round each intermediate answer so it retains at least one more significant figure than the final answer will contain.

Example:

A. Perform the following operation without rounding until the final answer.

$$\frac{(123.7)(35)}{(1,395)(82)} = \frac{4,329.5}{114,390} = 0.038$$

Perform the same operation and round the intermediate answers to 2 significant figures, which is the number of significant figures that should appear in the final answer.

$$\frac{(123.7)(35)}{(1,395)(82)} = \frac{4,300}{110,000} = 0.039$$

Perform the same operation and round the intermediate answers to 3 significant figures, which is 1 more than the final answer should contain.

$$\frac{(123.7)(35)}{(1,395)(82)} = \frac{4,330}{114,000} = 0.038$$

The same level of accuracy was achieved with the first and third methods. The second method introduced a small error that is probably not important in this case. However, if this small error is introduced in every step of a long operation, the error would accumulate and eventually become significant.

I-5 How to determine the number of significant figures in a product or quotient:

The product or quotient of an operation can only have as many significant figures as the least accurate number in the equation. If any number in the equation has only 1 significant figure, then so must the answer. If the least accurate number contains 3 significant figures, then so must the answer.

Examples:

A. Determine the product of 6.31 × 2.223 to the appropriate significant figure.

6.31 × 2.223 = 14.02713

Since 6.31 is the least accurate number, with only 3 significant figures, then the product of the operation can only assure accuracy to 3 significant figures. The answer should therefore be recorded as 14.0. In this case the zero is a significant figure.

Therefore 6.31 × 2.223 = 14.0

B. Determine the quotient of 124 ÷ 19 to the appropriate significant figure.

124 ÷ 19 = 6.5263

Since 19 is the least accurate number with only 2 significant figures, the quotient should be 6.5.

Therefore 124 ÷ 19 = 6.5

I-6 How to determine the number of significant figures in a sum or difference:

The sum or the difference of a mathematical operation must have the <u>same number of significant</u> *decimal* places as the least accurate number in the operation (i.e., the number with the fewest decimal places).

If there are no decimal places the answer is rounded to the number of significant figures in the least accurate number.

* Note: Why use significant decimal places instead of significant figures? Add 0.00342 to 0.00007. If rounded to significant figures the answer becomes 0.003, thereby losing its accuracy. By using significant decimals instead, the answer is left at 0.00349 because both numbers in the problem have 5 decimal places.

Examples:

A. Add 9.392 + 1.2 + 4.001 + 5.8240 and record the sum with the appropriate number of significant decimal places.

    The sum is 20.417. The number with the fewest decimal places is 1.2, so the sum must be expressed as 20.4.

B. Subtract 8.246 from 9.88 and record the answer with the appropriate number of significant decimal places.

    9.88 − 8.246 = 1.634

    However, only 2 significant decimal places occur in the least accurate number, so the answer must be recorded with only two decimal places. Therefore the appropriate answer is 1.63.

C. Subtract 2,200 from 7,630 and record the answer with the appropriate number of significant figures.

    7,630 − 2,200 = 5,430

    Since there are no decimals in the problem, the answer is rounded to the number of significant figures in the least accurate number. The answer should therefore contain 2 significant figures: 5,400.

Problems:

Perform the designated calculations, rounding the final answer to the appropriate number of significant figures.

1. 2.45×251
2. 0.005×21.9
3. 0.0125×316.9
4. 75.5×123
5. 4.69×0.00532
6. $41.5 \div 0.575$
7. $1.16 \div 0.00355$
8. $6.19 \div 6147$
9. $1.33 \div 3.92$
10. $3924 \div 11$

11. $35.64 + 74,406$
12. $2.706325 + 3.7100$
13. $4.2 + 1.0521$
14. $1.107 + 23.1403$
15. $100.1 + 140.02$
16. $6,157.9 - 3.04$
17. $120.21 - 1.136$
18. $4,549.3 - 255.62$
19. $5,594.6 - 17.70$
20. $27.356 - 5.58$

References:

Christian & Waterstram-Rich (6th Ed.), p. 9–10.

3. Powers and exponents

Principles:

When a number is multiplied by itself one or more times, it is said to be raised to a given power. If 4 is multiplied by 4, then 4 has been raised to the second power, or squared. When 4 is raised to the third power, or cubed, then 4 is multiplied three times: $4 \times 4 \times 4$.

The power is expressed as an exponent or index. It is written as a superscript to the right of the number: 4^2, 4^3, 4^4, etc.

---

* Note: 4^3 signifies that 4 is multiplied three times, $4 \times 4 \times 4$, NOT that 4 is multiplied by 3. 5^6 signifies that 5 is multiplied 6 times, $5 \times 5 \times 5 \times 5 \times 5 \times 5$, NOT 5×6.

I-7 How to convert exponential numbers to whole numbers:

Refer to the instruction booklet that came with your scientific calculator to determine how to utilize the exponent functions (x^2 and y^x) on your instrument.

Examples:

A. Convert 6^2 to a whole number.

   Answer: 36

B. Convert 5^4 to a whole number.

   Answer: 625

C. Convert 3^9 to a whole number.

   Answer: 19,683

Problems:

Convert each of the following to a whole number.

1. 2^5
2. 10^6
3. 9^2
4. 18^3
5. 25^4
6. 5^0
7. 79^3
8. 15^5
9. 10^8

10. 2^{10}

References:

Christian & Waterstram-Rich (6th Ed.), p. 9–10.

4. Roots

Principles:

The square root of a value is the number that was raised to the power of two to create the value, in other words, $\sqrt[2]{x^2} = x$. The $\sqrt{}$ sign is the symbol of a root. The small number to the left of the sign is the index. It designates the power to which a number was raised to produce the value written within the sign.

The cube root, 4th root, 5th root, etc., can also be written using this method. They would appear as $\sqrt[3]{x}, \sqrt[4]{x},$ and $\sqrt[5]{x}$, respectively. The cube root gives the value that was raised to the third power to produce the number that appears within the sign; in other words, $\sqrt[3]{x^3} = x$. Other roots would be expressed in the same way: $\sqrt[4]{x^4} = x$, etc.

---

* Note: $\sqrt[2]{}$ is often written simply as $\sqrt{}$. If no index is indicated, a square root is implied.

A scientific calculator will have a $\sqrt{x}$ and a $\sqrt[x]{y}$ function. The $\sqrt{x}$ function allows you to calculate the square root, while the $\sqrt[x]{y}$ function allows you to calculate any root. The $\sqrt[x]{y}$ function may be accessed by an inverse (INV) or second (2nd) key. For example, the $\sqrt[x]{y}$ function may be written above the y^x key. In order to utilize the $\sqrt[x]{y}$ function, you press the INV or 2nd key, then the y^x key.

I-8 How to calculate the root of a number:

Refer to the instruction booklet that came with your scientific calculator to determine how to utilize the root functions ($\sqrt{x}$ and $\sqrt[x]{y}$) on your instrument.

Examples:

A.   Calculate the square root of 64.

   Answer: $\sqrt{64} = 8$, because $8^2 = 64$.

B.   Convert $\sqrt{506}$ to a simple number.

   Answer: $\sqrt{506} = 22.5$, because $22.5^2 = 506$.

C.   Calculate the cube root of 729.

   Answer: $\sqrt[3]{729} = 9$, because $9^3 = 729$.

D. Calculate the 4th root of 10,000.

Answer: $\sqrt[4]{10,000} = 10$, because $10^4 = 10,000$.

Problems:

Convert each of the following to a whole number.

1. $\sqrt{144}$
2. $\sqrt[3]{3,375}$
3. $\sqrt[5]{7,776}$
4. $\sqrt[3]{24}$
5. $\sqrt{100,000}$
6. $\sqrt{129,600}$
7. $\sqrt[3]{57,070}$
8. $\sqrt[6]{1,260,000}$
9. $\sqrt[4]{8,400}$
10. $\sqrt[3]{25,000}$

References:

Christian & Waterstram-Rich (6th Ed.), p. 7–8.

5. Scientific notation

Principles:

Scientific notation uses exponents to make the recording and manipulation of very large and very small numbers more convenient. Typically, the number is expressed as a single digit to the left of the decimal and 1 or more digits to the right, followed by 10 raised to the appropriate power.

Examples:

A. $8,210,000 = 8.21 \times 10^6$

> * **Note:** In some cases, it is more convenient to adjust the decimal so more digits are placed to the left. This may be done for adding and subtracting numbers, or for expressing them in certain commonly accepted forms.

B. $8,210,000$ also equals 82.1×10^5 or 821×10^4

> * **Note:** It is reasonable to assume that you are being asked for the standard scientific notation format used in example A, useless otherwise specified.

> **I-9 How to convert a whole number to scientific notation:**
>
> 1. Move the decimal point to the left until a single digit lies to the left of the decimal point.
> 2. Count the number of places the decimal was moved.
> 3. Use the number of places as the exponent of 10.
> 4. Rewrite the number.

> * **Note:** With a whole number, the decimal point is not written, but in reality it exists at the end of the number. For example, the number "821" could be written as "821.".

Examples:

A. Convert 8,210,000 to standard scientific notation.

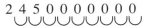

   2. The decimal is moved 6 places to left.
   3. The exponential notation becomes 10^6.
   4. Rewrite the number as 8.21×10^6.

B. Express 2,450,000,000 in standard scientific notation.

   2 4 5 0 0 0 0 0 0

   The decimal is moved 9 spaces to the left, so 2,450,000,000 equals 2.45×10^9·

I-10 How to convert a number in scientific notation to a whole number:

1. Move the decimal to the right the number of places to which 10 has been raised.
2. Add zeros if necessary.

Examples:

A. Convert 4.37×10^{12} to a whole number.

The decimal must be moved 12 places to the right, which is the opposite direction the decimal is moved in order to create the scientific notation. A sufficient number of zeros is added to the number to accomplish this.

4 3 7 0 0 0 0 0 0 0 0 0 0, so 4.37×10^{12} equals 4,370,000,000,000.

B. Convert 3.11×10^5 to a simple whole number.

3 1 1 0 0 0

The decimal is moved 5 places to the right, requiring the addition of 3 zeros, so 3.11×10^5 equals 311,000.

I-11 How to convert a decimal to scientific notation:

1. Move the decimal point to the right until a single digit lies to the left of the decimal point.
2. Count the number of places the decimal was moved.
3. Use the number of places as the negative exponent of 10. The negative denotes that the number was created by moving the decimal to the right.
4. Rewrite the number.

Examples:

A. Convert 0.00000075 to scientific notation.

0 . 0 0 0 0 0 0 7 5

The decimal point is moved 7 places to the right, so 0.00000075 equals 7.5×10^{-7}.

B. Convert 0.00236 to scientific notation.

0 . 0 0 2 3 6

The decimal point is moved 3 places to the right, so 0.00236 equals 2.36×10^{-3}.

I-12 How to convert a number in scientific notation to its simple decimal form:

1. Move the decimal to the left the number of places to which ten has been raised.
2. Add zeros between the decimal point and the first digit if necessary.

Examples:

A. Convert 5.9×10^{-6} to a simple decimal.

The decimal must be moved 6 places to the left, which is the opposite direction the decimal was moved in order to create the scientific notation. A sufficient number of zeros is added to the number to accomplish this.

0 0 0 0 0 5 9

Therefore 5.9×10^{-6} equals 0.0000059.

* Note: Good practice dictates that a zero is always placed on the left side of a decimal point if no other digit is present in that position. Copying machines frequently produce pages with black flecks. A number such as .5 could be mistaken for 5 if the decimal point is thought to be a fleck on the paper. However, 0.5 leaves no doubt as to the true number intended.

* Note: When working in scientific notation, the exponential component becomes larger as the decimal is moved to the left. (Larger & left go together.)

For example, if you move the decimal in 23.45×10^{2} one place to the left, it becomes 2.345×10^{3}. 10^{3} (or 1,000) is larger than 10^{2} (or 100). If you move the decimal in 23.45×10^{-3} one place to the left, it becomes 2.345×10^{-2}. 10^{-2} (or 0.01) is larger than 10^{-3} (or 0.001).

Problems:

Express the following numbers in standard scientific notation; e.g., $897 = 8.97 \times 10^{2}$.

1.	3,564	6.	45,493.1
2.	6,157.9	7.	110.7
3.	120.3	8.	1,001,924
4.	2,706,325	9.	5,594.6
5.	426	10.	27,359.8

Convert the following to whole numbers; e.g., $8.97 \times 10^{2} = 897$.

11.	7.44×10^{5}	16.	2.55×10^{3}
12.	3.04×10^{2}	17.	2.314×10^{5}
13.	11.33×10^{1}	18.	1.4002×10^{4}
14.	3.71×10^{4}	19.	1.77×10^{3}
15.	1.052×10^{6}	20.	5.5740×10^{6}

Express the following numbers in standard scientific notation.

21. 16.3×10^4
22. 234.8×10^3
23. 879.02×10^8
24. 77.4×10^{14}
25. $190,674.27 \times 10^{18}$

Convert the following to scientific notation; e.g., $0.897 = 8.97 \times 10^{-2}$.

26. 0.25
27. 0.0050
28. 0.0125
29. 0.000575
30. 0.0075419

31. 0.0469
32. 0.0000355
33. 0.000295
34. 0.606
35. 0.00001125

Convert the following to decimals; e.g., $8.97 \times 10^{-2} = 0.0897$.

36. 2.45×10^{-1}
37. 2.19×10^{-8}
38. 3.08×10^{-5}
39. 1.20×10^{-3}
40. 5.32×10^{-2}

41. 4.15×10^{-4}
42. 1.16×10^{-1}
43. 1.68×10^{-3}
44. 1.33×10^{-2}
45. 3.92×10^{-6}

Convert the following to standard scientific notation.

46. 0.253×10^{-2}
47. 0.00971×10^{-6}
48. $0.0000854 \times 10^{-15}$
49. 0.01548×10^{-5}
50. $0.00000841 \times 10^{-12}$

51. 0.0799×10^{-4}
52. 0.372×10^{-3}
53. 0.002844×10^{-24}
54. 0.00176×10^{-7}
55. $0.00000849 \times 10^{-11}$

References:

Christian & Waterstram-Rich (6th Ed.), p. 2–3, 34.

6. Mathematical operations using exponential numbers

Principles:

---

* Note: Numbers written in scientific notation are NOT treated as decimals when rounding. They are numbers that have been rearranged to contain decimals. Instead they are treated as whole numbers and answers are rounded to the number of significant figures in the least accurate number.

The following rules apply to exponential numbers.

$$\left(a^m\right)\left(a^n\right)=a^{m+n} \qquad \frac{a^m}{a^n}=a^{m-n} \qquad a^1=a \qquad a^0=1$$

I-13 How to multiply exponential numbers:

1. Apply the rules of exponents: $\left(a^m\right)\left(a^n\right)=a^{m+n}$
2. Group the whole numbers together and the exponents together.
3. Multiply whole number by whole numbers.
4. Add the exponents.
5. Round off to the appropriate significant figures. (See Basic Math Skills Section 1.)
6. Reformat the answer into standard scientific notation. (See Basic Math Skills Section 5.)

A. Multiply 3.75×10^2 by 8.904×10^5 by 1.67×10^{-4}.

Regroup as $(3.75 \times 8.904 \times 1.67)\ (10^2 \times 10^5 \times 10^{-4})$.
Multiply whole numbers and add exponents: $\left(55.7613\right)\left(10^{2+5+(-4)}\right)=55.7613\times10^3$.
Round to significant figures and reformat into standard scientific notation:
$55.8 \times 10^3 = 5.58 \times 10^4$

I-14 How to divide exponential numbers:

1. Apply the rules of exponents: $\frac{a^m}{a^n}=a^{m-n}$
2. Group the whole numbers together and the exponents together.
3. Divide whole numbers by whole numbers.
4. Subtract the exponents.
5. Round off to the appropriate significant figures. (See Basic Math Skills Section 1.)
6. Reformat the answer into standard scientific notation. (See Basic Math Skills Section 5.)

Examples:

A. Divide 8.63×10^7 by 4.61×10^5.

$$\frac{8.63 \times 10^7}{4.61 \times 10^5} = \frac{8.63}{4.61} \times \frac{10^7}{10^5} = 1.872 \times 10^{7-5} = 1.872 \times 10^2$$

The answer is rounded to 3 significant figures: 1.87×10^2.

B. Divide 3.84×10^2 by 8.96×10^5.

$$\frac{3.84 \times 10^2}{8.96 \times 10^5} = \frac{3.84}{8.96} \times \frac{10^2}{10^5} = 0.42857 \times 10^{2-5} = 0.42857 \times 10^{-3}$$

Round to significant figures and reformat into standard scientific notation:
$0.428 \times 10^{-3} = 4.28 \times 10^{-4}$.

I-15 How to add or subtract exponential numbers:

1. Reformat the numbers so the exponents are identical.
2. Add or subtract.
3. Round off to the appropriate significant figures. (See Basic Math Skills Section 1.)
4. Reformat the answer into standard scientific notation. (See Basic Math Skills Section 5.)

Examples:

A. Add 8.273×10^5 and 5.821×10^4.

Reformat one of the numbers: $8.273 \times 10^5 = 82.73 \times 10^4$

Add: 82.73×10^4
     $+\ \ 5.821 \times 10^4$
         88.551×10^4

Reformat the answer into standard scientific notation and round to 4 significant figures: 8.855×10^5. A maximum of 4 significant numbers is used in the answer because both numbers in the problem have only 4 significant figures.

B.   Subtract 2.61×10^3 from 8.486×10^4.

Reformat one of the numbers: $2.61 \times 10^3 = 0.261 \times 10^4$

Subtract: 8.486×10^4
        $- \ \underline{0.261 \times 10^4}$
           8.225×10^4

Reformat the answer. The answer is already in standard scientific notation, but needs to be rounded to 3 significant figures: 8.22×10^4

Problems:

Perform the designated calculations, round to the appropriate number of significant figures, and record the answer in the standard scientific notation format.

1. $(2.5 \times 10^{-1})(5.0 \times 10^{-3})$
2. $(1.25 \times 10^2)(4.69 \times 10^{-2})$
3. $(7.5419 \times 10^{-3})(5.75 \times 10^{-4})$
4. $(3.55 \times 10^5)(2.95 \times 10^4)$
5. $(6.06 \times 10^{-1})(1.125 \times 10^{-5})$
6. $(7.44 \times 10^5) \div (3.04 \times 10^2)$
7. $(3.71 \times 10^4) \div (11.33 \times 10^1)$
8. $(1.052 \times 10^6) \div (2.55 \times 10^3)$
9. $(2.314 \times 10^5) \div (1.4002 \times 10^4)$
10. $(1.77 \times 10^{-3}) \div (5.574 \times 10^{-6})$
11. $(3.564 \times 10^1) + (6.1579 \times 10^3)$
12. $(1.202 \times 10^2) + (2.706325 \times 10^6)$
13. $(4.2 \times 10^1) + (4.593 \times 10^4)$
14. $(1.107 \times 10^2) + (1.001924 \times 10^6)$
15. $(5.5946 \times 10^3) + (2.70544 \times 10^4)$
16. $(7.44 \times 10^5) - (3.04 \times 10^2)$
17. $(3.71 \times 10^4) - (11.33 \times 10^3)$
18. $(1.052 \times 10^6) - (2.55 \times 10^3)$
19. $(2.314 \times 10^5) - (1.4002 \times 10^4)$
20. $(5.5740 \times 10^6) - (1.77 \times 10^3)$

References:

Christian & Waterstram-Rich (6th Ed.), p. 7–8.

7. Direct and inverse proportions

Principles:

Direct proportions:

When a ratio $\dfrac{x_1}{y_1}$ equals a ratio of $\dfrac{x_2}{y_2}$ the relationship is called a direct proportion. In other words, the ratios vary directly with one another. As x_1 becomes larger, x_2 also increases. When x_1 becomes smaller, x_2 decreases. The same holds true for y_1 and y_2: as one varies, so does the other.

This relationship can be expressed in several ways. In each of the following equations, any element can be the unknown (X).

1. $\dfrac{x_1}{y_1} = \dfrac{x_2}{y_2}$ To solve this equation, cross-multiply, isolate X, and solve for X.

2. $x_1 y_2 = x_2 y_1$ This equation is also produced when you cross-multiply to solve equation 1.

3. $x_1 : y_1 :: x_2 : y_2$ Read: x_1 is to y_1 as x_2 is to y_2. To solve this equation, the product of the extremes (x_1 and y_2) equals the product of the means (x_2 and y_1). This also results in equation 2.

Regardless of the equation you chose to utilize, you will obtain the same answer. Equations 1 and 3 will be used in this book. You will see that equation 2 will appear in the process of solving each equation.

I-16 How to solve a direct proportion:

Using $\dfrac{x_1}{y_1} = \dfrac{x_2}{y_2}$

1. Cross multiply to give: $x_1 y_2 = x_2 y_1$.
2. Isolate the unknown (X), which can be any element in the equation.
3. Solve for X.

Using $x_1 : y_1 :: x_2 : y_2$

1. Rearrange the equation so the product to the extremes ($x_1 y_2$) equals the product of the means ($x_2 y_1$). $x_1 y_2 = x_2 y_1$.
2. Isolate the unknown (X), which can be any element in the equation.
3. Solve for X.

Examples:

A. If a 200-μCi point source produces 6,000 cps, how many cps will be produced by a 500-μCi source?

$$\frac{200\ \mu Ci}{6,000\ cps} = \frac{500\ \mu Ci}{X\ cps}$$

Cross-multiply: $(200\ \mu Ci)(X\ cps) = (500\ \mu Ci)(6,000\ cps)$

Isolate and solve for X: $X = \dfrac{(500\ \mu Ci)(6,000\ cps)}{200\ \mu Ci} = 15,000\ cps$

OR

200 μCi : 6,000 cpm :: 500 μCi : X cpm

Multiply the means and the extremes: $(500\ \mu Ci)(6,000\ cps) = (200\ \mu Ci)(X\ cps)$

Isolate and solve for X: $X = \dfrac{(500\ \mu Ci)(6,000\ cps)}{200\ \mu Ci} = 15,000\ cps$

B. If 150,000 counts are acquired in 120 seconds, how many counts will be acquired when the source is counted for 15 minutes?

Convert 120 seconds to minutes: $\dfrac{120\ s}{60\ s/min} = 2\ min$

Set up the proportion: $\dfrac{150,000\ counts}{2\ min} = \dfrac{X\ counts}{15\ min}$

Cross-multiply: $(150,000\ counts)(15\ min) = (X\ counts)(2\ min)$

Isolate and solve for X: $X = \dfrac{(150,000\ counts)(15\ min)}{2\ min} = 1,125,000\ counts$

---

* Note: Identical units must be used for $x_1\ and\ x_2$, and for $y_1\ and\ y_2$. In Example A, x represents activity. Note that μCi is used throughout the equation. In Example B, y represents time. The problem presents y in both seconds and in minutes; therefore, one of them must be changed before the problem can be solved.

Principles:

Inverse proportions:

Proportions do not always vary directly. In some instances, one element decreases as the other increases and vice versa. This is an inverse proportion.

This relationship can be expressed by two equations. Any element in the equation can be the unknown (X).

1. $\dfrac{x_1}{x_2} = \dfrac{y_2}{y_1}$ To solve this equation, cross-multiply, isolate X, and solve for X.

2. $x_1 y_1 = x_2 y_2$ This equation is produced when you cross-multiply to solve equation 4. To solve, isolate and solve for X.

Both equations will produce the same answer. This author prefers the second equation and will use it here, because there is less likelihood of arranging the elements incorrectly.

I-17 How to solve an inverse proportion:

Using $x_1 y_1 = x_2 y_2$

1.   Isolate the unknown (X), which can be any element in the equation.
2.   Solve for X.

---

*   **Note:** Compare the equations for direct and inverse proportions.

I.16   Direct: $\dfrac{x_1}{y_1} = \dfrac{x_2}{y_2}$ OR $x_1 y_2 = x_2 y_1$

I.17   Inverse: $\dfrac{x_1}{x_2} = \dfrac{y_2}{y_1}$ OR $x_1 y_1 = x_2 y_2$

Examples:

A.   Two milliliters of solution of 20% HCl are placed in a volumetric flask and diluted to 100 ml. What is the percent concentration of the diluted solution?

$(20\%)(2\ ml) = (X\ \%)(100\ ml)$.

Isolate and solve for X: $X = \dfrac{(20\%)(2\ ml)}{100\ ml} = 0.4\%$

* **Note:** What would have happened if a direct proportion equation had been used to solve Example A?

$$\frac{20\%}{2\,\text{ml}} = \frac{X\,\%}{100\,\text{ml}} \qquad X = \frac{(20\%)(100\,\text{ml})}{2\,\text{ml}} = 1{,}000\%$$

The answer, 1,000%, is obviously impossible. You cannot have a higher concentration in the diluted solution than in the original. Therefore an inverse relationship exists: as you add volume, you decrease the concentration.

B. A laboratory procedure requires blood to be centrifuged at 1,500 rpm for 10 minutes. If the maximum speed for a particular centrifuge is only 1,000 rpm, how long must the sample be spun to achieve the same effect?

This is an inverse proportion because the slower the centrifuge spins, the longer the sample must be centrifuged.

(1,500 rpm)(10 min) = (1,000 rpm)(X s)

Isolate and solve for X: $X = \dfrac{(1{,}500\,\text{rpm})(10\,\text{min})}{1{,}000\,\text{rpm}} = 15\,\text{min}$

Problems:

* **Note:** Before setting up a ratio for a proportion, determine if the numbers vary directly or inversely. Then apply the appropriate equation.

Solve the following direct proportions.

1. $\dfrac{45\,\text{mCi}}{2.3\,\text{ml}} = \dfrac{X\,\text{mCi}}{0.8\,\text{ml}}$

2. $\dfrac{12{,}500\,\text{cpm}}{0.51\,\text{mCi}} = \dfrac{500{,}000\,\text{cpm}}{X\,\text{mCi}}$

3. $\dfrac{0.6\,\text{mrem}}{60\,\text{min}} = \dfrac{X\,\text{mrem}}{22\,\text{min}}$

4. You have a radioactive source that produces 20,000 counts in 3 minutes. You need to acquire 50,000 counts. How long will the acquisition take?

5. If a 10-μCi source will produce 35,000 cps, how many cps will a 4-μCi source produce?

6. The exposure rate one meter from a patient is 1000 mR/h. If the technologist stands at this point for 20 minutes, what is the total exposure to the technologist? (See Radiation Protection Section 3.)

7.   Furosemide is administered to adult patients at a rate of 0.50 mg/kg of body weight. How much furosemide should be given to an adult who weighs 85 kg? (See Radiopharmacy Section 8.)

8.   If a radioactive source produces 5,000 cps, how many counts would be produced in 2 minutes' time?

9.   The doctor has ordered 20 mg of Zantac® for a patient. If the pharmaceutical comes in a vial that has a concentration of 25 mg/ml, what volume will be needed to meet the prescription? (See Radiopharmacy Section 5.)

10. You are to prepare a dose of 20 mCi of a radiopharmaceutical that has a concentration of 50 mCi/ml. What volume of the radiopharmaceutical must be administered?

11. If 5 µCi of radionuclide produce 1,500 cpm, how many µCi will be needed to spike a phantom so it will provide 30,000 cpm?

Solve the following inverse proportions.

Problems 12–14 demonstrate dilutions.

12. $(12 \text{ µCi})(5.0 \text{ ml}) = (X \text{ µCi})(100 \text{ ml})$ or $\dfrac{12 \text{µCi}}{X \text{ µCi}} = \dfrac{100 \text{ ml}}{5.0 \text{ ml}}$

13. $(65{,}000 \text{ cpm})(2.0 \text{ ml}) = (420 \text{ cpm})(X \text{ ml})$ or $\dfrac{65{,}000 \text{ cpm}}{420 \text{ cpm}} = \dfrac{X \text{ ml}}{2.0 \text{ ml}}$

14. $(984{,}000 \text{ cpm})(1.0 \text{ ml}) = (11{,}000 \text{ cpm})(X \text{ ml})$

15. A 4.0-ml aliquot of 15% NaCl is put in a flask and diluted to 50 ml. What is the percent concentration of the diluted solution? (See Clinical Procedures Section 11.)

16. To adequately separate white blood cells from plasma, the technologist is required to spin the plasma in a centrifuge at a rate of $2{,}000 \times g$ for 5 minutes. The centrifuge can only attain $1{,}000 \times g$. How long should the plasma be centrifuged to provide the same result?

17. A B12 radioassay requires centrifugation of test samples for 15 minutes at $1{,}500 \times g$. The centrifuge speed is set at $2{,}000 \times g$. How long should the test tubes be spun at this rate to achieve the same degree of separation?

18. A 1.0-ml aliquot of Cr51 was measured in a well counter, giving a reading of 12,600 counts. The aliquot is then placed in a flask of water. If a 1.0-ml sample of the diluted solution produces 63 counts, how many ml are there in the diluted solution?

19. A radiopharmaceutical kit has been prepared with 75 mCi in 1.0 ml of solution (in other words, 75 mCi/ml). The technologist diluted the kit by adding 4.0 ml of saline for a total volume of 5 ml. What is the concentration, in mCi/ml, of the diluted solution? (See Clinical Procedures, Sections 10 and 11.)

20. A radiopharmaceutical kit was prepared with 2.0 ml of generator eluate containing 130 mCi, resulting in a concentration of 65 mCi/ml. The kit was then diluted with an additional 1.0 ml of saline for a total volume of 3.0 ml. What is the concentration of the final solution?

References:

Christian & Waterstram-Rich (6th Ed.), p. 3–5.

8.   Converting within the metric system

Principles:

Nuclear medicine utilizes the metric system for all measurements. The technologist needs to be able to convert numbers within the metric system. A large number with small units, such as 40,000 μCi, is better expressed and more easily manipulated as a smaller number with larger units, such as 40 mCi. You can also convert from large units to smaller ones when appropriate; for example, 0.002 Ci can be changed to 2 mCi.

unit	symbol	measurement
meter	m	length
gram	g	weight
liter	l *	volume
curie	Ci •	radioactivity
becquerel	Bq •	radioactivity

* When liter stands alone it is often abbreviated with the capital L, instead of the small l used in the combination form, which can be confused with the number 1.

•   Both curie and becquerel are used to measure radioactivity. (See Basic Math Skills Section 9.)

Metric prefixes commonly used in nuclear medicine:

prefix	symbol	exponential form	simple number form
giga	G	10^9	1,000,000,000
mega	M	10^6	1,000,000
kilo	k	10^3	1000
deca	da	10^1	10
deci	d	10^{-1}	0.1
centi	c	10^{-2}	0.01
milli	m	10^{-3}	0.001
micro	μ	10^{-6}	0.000001
nano	n	10^{-9}	0.000000001
pico	p	10^{-12}	0.000000000001

***Note**: See Important Note Concerning Abbreviations and Decimal Formats on page vii concerning the use of the μ symbol.

***Note**: As the units become smaller, you will need more of them (i.e., a larger number). As the units become larger, you will have fewer of them (i.e., a smaller number). An easy reference to help keep this straight comes from the familiar:
    1 yard = 3 feet = 36 inches
When converting from yards to inches, the units become smaller, so the number must become larger.

I-18 How to convert numbers in scientific notation between units of measurement:

Either of the following processes can be used. The same answer will be obtained.

Using the inverse proportion method:

1. Identify the powers of the units of measurement (10^x).
2. Apply the inverse proportion equation. (See Basic Math Skills Section 7.)

$$x_1 y_1 = x_2 y_2 \quad \text{or} \quad \frac{x_1}{x_2} = \frac{y_2}{y_1}$$

Where x_1 = original number

x_2 = unknown (X)

y_1 = original units expressed as an exponential number

y_2 = desired units expressed as an exponential number

3. Isolate and solve for X. (See Basic Math Skills Section 6.)
4. Reformat the answer into standard scientific notation.

Using the quick method:

1. Calculate the change in power (Δ) from the original unit to the new unit.
Δ = original − new
2. Add or subtract Δ from the original exponent as designated by the sign. The final number should become larger if the new units are smaller, as more of them are needed. The final number should become smaller if the new units are larger, as fewer of them are needed.
3. If necessary, reformat the answer into standard scientific notation.

Examples:

A. Convert 3.6×10^{11} cm to μm.

Inverse proportion method:

1. Identify the powers of the units of measurement. $\quad$ cm $= 10^{-2}$ $\qquad$ μm $= 10^{-6}$
2. Apply the inverse proportion equation and solve.

$$\left(3.6 \times 10^{11}\right)\left(10^{-2}\right) = \left(X\right)\left(10^{-6}\right)$$

$$X = \frac{\left(3.6 \times 10^{11}\right)\left(10^{-2}\right)}{10^{-6}} = \frac{3.6 \times 10^{11+(-2)}}{10^{-6}} = 3.6 \times 10^{9-(-6)}$$

$$X = 3.6 \times 10^{15} \, \mu m$$

3. The answer is already in standard scientific notation.

Quick method:

1. Calculate the change in power (Δ).

   original: cm = 10^{-2}
   new: μm = 10^{-6}
   $\Delta = (-2) - (-6) = 4$ (The + sign in the answer is assumed.)

2. Add or subtract Δ from the original exponent as designated by the sign.

   $$3.6 \times 10^{11+4} = 3.6 \times 10^{15}$$

B. Convert 8.5×10^{35} μCi to MCi (megacuries)

Inverse proportion method:

1. Identify the powers of the units of measurement. μCi = 10^{-6} MCi = 10^{6}

2. Apply the inverse proportion equation and solve.

$$\left(8.5 \times 10^{35}\right)\left(10^{-6}\right) = \left(X\right)\left(10^{6}\right)$$
$$X = \frac{\left(8.5 \times 10^{35}\right)\left(10^{-6}\right)}{10^{6}} = \frac{8.5 \times 10^{35+(-6)}}{10^{6}} = 8.5 \times 10^{29-6}$$
$$X = 8.5 \times 10^{23}$$

3. The number is already in standard scientific notation.

Quick method:

1. Calculate Δ.

   original: μCi = 10^{-6}
   new: MCi = 10^{6}
   $\Delta = (-6) - (6) = -12$

2. Add or subtract Δ from the original exponent as designated by the sign.

   $$8.5 \times 10^{35-12} = 8.5 \times 10^{23} \text{ MCi}$$

C.   Convert 500 µCi to mCi.

Inverse proportion method:

1.   Identify the powers of the units of measurement.   µCi = 10^{-6} mCi = 10^{-3}

2.   Apply the inverse proportion equation and solve.

$$(500)(10^{-6}) = (X)(10^{-3})$$

$$X = \frac{(500)(10^{-6})}{10^{-3}} = (500\mu Ci)(10^{-6-(-3)})$$

$$X = 500 \times 10^{-3} \text{ mCi}$$

3.   In nuclear medicine, small numbers such as this are not usually expressed in scientific notation. Instead it would be written as 0.5 mCi.

Quick method:

1.   Calculate Δ.

original: µCi = 10^{-6}
new: mCi = 10^{-3}
Δ = (−6) − (−3) = −3

2.   Add or subtract Δ from the original exponent as designated by the sign.

500 is actually 500 × 10^{0}, because 10^{0} = 1.
$500 \times 10^{0-3} = 500 \times 10^{-3}$ mCi

Principles:

A shortcut for commonly used units of radioactivity:

Conversions between Ci, mCi, and µCi are probably the most common metric conversions in nuclear medicine. The international units for measuring radioactivity, GBq, MBq, and kBq, are being used more and more frequently. (See Basic Math Skills Section 9.) Note that each unit in the series is three units or decimal places different from the other.

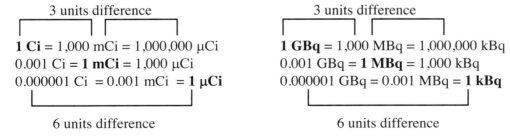

3 units difference

1 Ci = 1,000 mCi = 1,000,000 µCi
0.001 Ci = 1 mCi = 1,000 µCi
0.000001 Ci = 0.001 mCi = 1 µCi

6 units difference

3 units difference

1 GBq = 1,000 MBq = 1,000,000 kBq
0.001 GBq = 1 MBq = 1,000 kBq
0.000001 GBq = 0.001 MBq = 1 kBq

6 units difference

I-19 How to convert between commonly used units of radioactivity (Ci to mCi to μCi or GBq to MBq to kBq):

Increase or decrease the number of decimal places to the right, or the number of zeros to the left by 3 or 6, depending on the change in units.

---

* Note: A common error made when converting between units is moving the decimal in the wrong direction. Use the previously mentioned "yards-feet-inches" guideline to keep the directions straight.

Examples:

A. Convert 500 μCi to mCi.

  When converting from a small unit to a larger one, the number decreases, so the decimal is moved to the left 3 places.

  5 0 0 μCi = 0.500 mCi

B. Convert 0.085 mCi to μCi.

  When converting from a large unit to a smaller one, the number increases, so the decimal is moved to the right 3 places.

  0 .0 8 5 mCi = 85 μCi

C. Convert 423,000 μCi to Ci.

  The number must become smaller, so the decimal is moved left. In this case the decimal is moved 6 places, as you are converting from μCi to Ci, which are 6 decimal places apart.

  4 2 3 0 0 0 μCi = 0.423 Ci

D. Convert 3.43×10^6 μCi to mCi.

  3.43×10^3

  Because there are three units difference between μCi and mCi, the exponent can be changed by 3 units. Since you are converting from small units to larger ones, you need fewer of them. The exponent must therefore become smaller.

Problems:

1. Convert 7.5×10^5 µCi to mCi
2. Convert 8.4×10^7 mCi to µCi
3. Convert 2.5×10^4 kBq to MBq
4. Convert 12.1×10^6 µCi to Ci
5. Convert 5.2×10^4 GBq to MBq
6. Convert 5.0×10^5 kBq to MBq
7. Convert 7.5×10^2 mCi to µCi
8. Convert 2.1×10^6 µCi to mCi
9. Convert 6.7×10^2 MBq to GBq
10. Convert 10.5×10^6 mCi to µCi
11. Convert 2 mCi to µCi
12. Convert 0.2 mCi to µCi
13. Convert 75 µCi to mCi
14. Convert 1.1 MBq to kBq
15. Convert 6 MBq to kBq and GBq
16. Convert 0.65 mCi to µCi
17. Convert 1076 µCi to mCi and Ci
18. Convert 1.3 Ci to µCi
19. Convert 2.1 GBq to MBq
20. Convert 0.670 GBq to MBq

References:

Christian & Waterstram-Rich (6th Ed.), p. 2–3.
Harbert & da Rocha, p. 479
Iturralde, p. 492–493.

9. Converting between curie and becquerel

Principles:

According to the International System (SI) of units that were accepted as standard measurements by the International Commission on Radiological Units (ICRU) in 1975, the becquerel (Bq) is the preferred unit of measurement for radioactivity. It is equivalent to one disintegration per second (dps).

Although the Bq is the accepted unit, many texts and practitioners continue to use the curie (Ci) out of habit, tradition, or preference.

The conventional curie units are usually converted to becquerels as follows.

curies (Ci) to gigabecquerels (GBq)
millicuries (mCi) to megabecquerels (MBq)
microcuries (μCi) to kilobecquerels (kBq)

---

* Note: Because 1 Ci equals 3.70×10^{10} dps or Bq, you will always have a larger number of Bq than Ci when converting between the commonly used units as listed above. Always check your answer to be sure it complies with this rule.

I-20 How to convert curies to becquerels:

Multiply the number of curies by the equivalent number of becquerels.

    1 Ci = 37 GBq
    1 mCi = 37 MBq
    1 μCi = 37 kBq

i.e., MBq = (mCi)(37 MBq/mCi).

I-21 How to convert becquerels to curies:

Multiply the number of becquerels by the equivalent number of curies.

    1 Bq = 2.7×10^{-11} Ci
    1 GBq = 0.027 Ci or 27 mCi
    1 MBq = 0.027 mCi or 27 μCi
    1 kBq = 0.027 μCi

i.e., mCi = (MBq)(0.027 mCi/MBq) or μCi = (MBq)(27 μCi/MBq).

Examples:

A. Convert 100 μCi to kBq.

   If 1 μCi = 37 kBq, then (100 μCi)(37 kBq/μCi) = 3,700 kBq or 3.70×10^3 kBq

B. Convert 50 mCi to MBq.

   (50 mCi)(37 MBq/mCi) = 1,850 or 1.85×10^3 MBq

---

* Note: In actuality you are using a direct proportion. (See Basic Math Skills, Section 7.)

$$\frac{37\,\text{MBq}}{1\,\text{mCi}} = \frac{X\,\text{MBq}}{50\,\text{mCi}} \qquad X = \frac{(37\,\text{MBq})(50\,\text{mCi})}{1\,\text{mCi}} = 1,850\,\text{MBq or } 1.85 \times 10^3$$

This is NOT an inverse proportion as was used to change WITHIN the metric system. (See Basic Math Skills Section 8.) You are not changing to a different size of units, but to a different system.

C. Convert 560 MBq to mCi.

   If 1 MBq equals 0.027 mCi, then (560 MBq)(0.027 mCi/MBq) = 15 mCi.

   You can also use the "1 mCi equals 37 MBq" conversion to obtain the same results. Again, a direct proportion is used:

$$\frac{37\,\text{MBq}}{1\,\text{mCi}} = \frac{560\,\text{MBq}}{X\,\text{mCi}} \qquad (37\,\text{MBq})(X\,\text{mCi}) = (560\,\text{MBq})(1\,\text{mCi})$$

$$X = \frac{(560\,\text{MBq})(1\,\text{mCi})}{37\,\text{MBq}} = 15\,\text{mCi}$$

Problems:

Convert the following to becquerel units as indicated.

1. Convert 15 μCi to kBq
2. Convert 0.50 μCi to kBq
3. Convert 0.50 mCi to MBq
4. Convert 25 mCi to MBq
5. Convert 1.1 mCi to GBq
6. Convert 1575 μCi to kBq
7. Convert 752 mCi to GBq
8. Convert 808 Ci to MBq
9. Convert 268 mCi to GBq
10. Convert 75 Ci to kBq

Convert the following to curie units as indicated.

11. Convert 185 MBq to μCi
12. Convert 9.25 MBq to mCi
13. Convert 7.79 GBq to mCi
14. Convert 581 MBq to mCi
15. Convert 4.1 MBq to μCi
16. Convert 24,790 kBq to μCi
17. Convert 5.21 kBq to Ci
18. Convert 1,687 kBq to mCi
19. Convert 3.1 MBq to μCi
20. Convert 9,100 GBq to Ci

References:

Christian & Waterstram-Rich (6th Ed.), p. 5–7.
Early & Sodee (2nd Ed), p. 36–37.
Iturralde, p. 485–486.

10. Converting between rad and gray

Principles:

The traditional unit for absorbed dose is the rad (**r**adiation **a**bsorbed **d**ose). The International System (SI) unit is the gray (Gy).

These units are used to measure the amount of energy deposited in tissue by ionizing radiation.

I-22 How to convert rad to grays:

Multiply the number of rad by the equivalent number of Gy.

> 1 rad = 0.01 Gy
> 1 mrad = 0.01 mGy

i.e., Gy = (rad)(0.01 Gy/rad)

I-23 How to convert grays to rad:

Multiply the number of Gy by the equivalent number of rad.

> 1 Gy = 100 rad
> 1 mGy = 100 mrad

i.e., mrad = (mGy)(100 mrad/mGy)

---

* Note: Because 1 rad equals 1/100th of a Gy, you will always have fewer Gy than rad when converting between equivalent tradition units and SI units. Always check your answer to be sure it complies with the rule.

Example:

A.   Convert 5 rad to grays.

  (5 rad)(0.01 Gy/rad) = 0.05 Gy or 50 mGy

> *** Note:** When converting between the traditional and the SI system, you are using a direct proportion. (See Basic Math Skills Section 7.)
>
> $$\frac{0.01\,\text{Gy}}{1\,\text{rad}} = \frac{X\,\text{Gy}}{5\,\text{rad}} \qquad X = \frac{(0.01\,\text{Gy})(5\,\text{rad})}{1\,\text{rad}} \qquad X = 0.05\,\text{Gy}$$
>
> This is NOT an inverse proportion as was used to change WITHIN the metric system. (See Basic Math Skills, Section 8.) You are not changing to a different size of units, but to a different system.

B.   Convert 0.2 mGy to mrad.

(0.2 mGy)(100 mrad/mGy) = 20 mrad

Problems:

1.   Convert 66 mrad to mGy and μGy.
2.   Convert 1.8 rad to Gy and mGy.
3.   Convert 700 mrad to mGy.
4.   Convert 3.9 mrad to mGy and μGy.
5.   Convert 1.5 mGy to mrad.
6.   Convert 60 mGy to mrad and rad.
7.   Convert 0.75 mGy to mrad.
8   Convert 3 μGy to μrad and mrad.

References:

Christian & Waterstram-Rich (6th Ed.), p. 5–7.
Early & Sodee (2nd Ed), p. 65.
Iturralde, p. 480–482, 487.

11. Converting between rem and sievert

Principles:

The traditional unit for dose equivalent is the rem (**r**oentgen **e**quivalent **m**an). The International System (SI) unit is the sievert (Sv).

These units are used to measure the potential effects of an absorbed dose (rad) based on the type of radiation involved (quality factor, Q).

I-24 How to convert rem to sieverts:

Multiply the number of rem by the equivalent number of Sv.

    1 rem = 0.01 Sv
    1 mrem = 0.01 mSv

i.e., Sv = (rem)(0.01 Sv/rem)

I-25 How to convert sieverts to rem:

Multiply the number of Sv by the equivalent number of rem.

    1 Sv = 100 rem
    1 mSv = 100 mrem

i.e., mrem = (mSv)(100 mrem/mSv)

---

* Note: The relationship between rem and Sv is the same as that between rad and Gy, so learning one is learning the other.

---

* Note: Because 1 rem equals 1/100th of a Sv, you will always have fewer Sv than rem when converting between equivalent tradition units and SI units. Always check your answer to be sure it complies with the rule.

Examples:

A.   Convert 5 rem to sieverts.

    (5 rem)(0.01 Sv/rem) = 0.05 Sv or 50 mSv

> * **Note:** When converting between the traditional and the SI system, you are using a direct proportion. (See Basic Math Skills Section 7.)
>
> $$\frac{0.01\,\text{Sv}}{1\,\text{rem}} = \frac{X\,\text{Sv}}{5\,\text{rem}} \qquad X = \frac{(0.01\,\text{Sv})(5\,\text{rem})}{1\,\text{rem}} \qquad X = 0.05\,\text{Sv}$$
>
> This is NOT an inverse proportion as was used to change WITHIN the metric system. (See Basic Math Skills Section 8.) You are not changing to a different size of units, but to a different system.

B.   Convert 35 mrem to mSv.

   (35 mrem)(0.01 mSv/mrem) = 0.35 Sv

C.   Convert 0.3 Sv to rem.

   (0.3 Sv)(100 rem/Sv) = 30 rem

Problems:

1.   Convert 0.1 rem to Sv and mSv.
2.   Convert 0.5 rem to Sv and mSv.
3.   Convert 50 rem to Sv and mSv.
4.   Convert 5000 mrem to mSv.
5.   Convert 7.2 mSv to mrem and rem.
6.   Convert 0.08 mSv to mrem.
7.   Convert 0.03 Sv to rem.
8.   Convert 0.005 Sv to rem and mrem.

References:

Christian & Waterstram-Rich (6th Ed.), p. 5–7.
Early & Sodee (2nd Ed), p. 65–66.
Iturralde, p. 480–482, 487.

12. Converting between pound and kilogram

Principles:

The traditional U.S. unit for human weight is the pound (lb), while the International System (SI) unit is the kilogram (kg).

1 lb = 0.45 kg or 1 lb = 454 g
1 kg = 2.2 lb

As with the curie-to-becquerel conversions, you are using a direct proportion. (See Basic Math Skills, Sections 7 and 9.) However, by utilizing the two equivalents shown above, a simplified equation can be used.

I-26 How to convert from pounds to kilograms:

kg = (lb)(0.45 kg/lb)

* **Note:** You can also convert pounds to kilograms by dividing weight in lb by 2.2 lb/kg. The answer will be minimally different. The method shown above is used in this book.

I-27 How to convert from kilograms to pounds:

lb = (kg)(2.2 lb/kg)

---

* **Note:** Because 1 lb equals about 1/2 kg, you will always have about twice as many lb as kg when converting between equivalent traditional units and SI units. Always check your answer to be sure it complies with the rule.

Examples:

A.   Convert 155 lb to kg.

(155 lb)(0.45 kg/lb) = 70 kg

* **Note:** This is the weight of the "reference man" which is used to set standard adult doses.

B.   If a child weighs 12 kg, how much does he or she weigh in pounds?

(12 kg)(2.2 lb/kg) = 26 lb

Problems:

Convert the following weights in pounds to kilograms.

1.   15.4 lb
2.   17 lb
3.   136 lb
4.   34 lb
5.   102 lb
6.   44 lb
7.   83 lb
8.   179 lb
9.   205 lb
10.   236 lb

Convert the following weights in kilograms to pounds.

11.   22 kg
12.   96 kg
13.   15 kg
14.   73 kg
15.   9 kg
16.   3 kg
17.   70 kg
18.   43 kg
19.   29 kg
20.   12 kg

References:

Iturralde, p. 501.
Venes (21st Ed.), p. 2474.

13. Logs, natural logs, and antilogs

Principles:

The graphing of data such as radioactive decay versus time produces a curve rather than a straight line. Because a straight line provides a more accurate graph, logarithms and semi-logarithmic graph paper may be employed to produce a straight line when a curve would be produced on linear graph paper. (See Basic Math Skills Section 15.)

The logarithm (log) of a number is the power to which a base must be raised to produce that number. In base 10, the number 10 is raised to a given power to produce the desired number. For example, $10^3 = 1,000$, therefore the logarithm to base 10 (written $\log_{10}$) equals 3. In other words, $\log_{10} 1,000 = 3$.

If $b^x = N$, then $x = \log_b N$.

Because base 10 is so commonly used, the abbreviation $\log_{10}$ is usually shortened to log. When any other base is being used, it will be written as a subscript following log, such as $\log_3$ or $\log_e$.

In nuclear medicine, base e is used in several situations. Radioactive decay (half-lives) and attenuation of photons (half-value layers) both require the use of base e for problem solving.

Base e or Euler's number is an irrational number (an infinite number, or one having no end). It is equal to 2.718..., with the dots indicating its infinite status. Logarithms to the base e are referred to as natural logarithms (natural log or ln).

An antilogarithm (antilog) or natural antilogarithm is the inverse of the log or ln, respectively. The antilog in base 10 is expressed as 10^x. If the log of 1,000 = 3, then the antilog of 3 = 1,000 or 10^3. The natural antilog is expressed as e^x. If the ln of 2 is 0.693, then the natural antilog of 0.693 is 2 or $e^{0.693} = 2$.

Before the advent of handheld scientific calculators, cumbersome logarithm charts were needed. Scientific calculators will have a LOG key and an LN key. The antilogs will have their own keys or may be found as alternate functions for the LOG and LN keys.

I-28 How to calculate logs, natural logs, antilogs, and natural antilogs:

Refer to the instruction booklet that came with your scientific calculator to determine how to utilize the log (LOG), natural log (LN), antilog (10^x), and natural antilog (e^x) functions on your instrument.

---

* Note: Logs are traditionally recorded to the hundredth or thousandths place (i.e., to the third or fourth decimal place).

Examples:

A. Find the log of 10,000.

     Answer: log 10,000 = 4. Note that 10,000 is written in exponential form as 10^4.

B. Find the ln of 25.

     Answer: ln 25 = 3.219

C. Find the antilog of 4 (10^4) using the 10^x function key.

     Answer: $10^4 = 10,000$

D. Find the natural antilog of 3.219 ($e^{3.219}$) using the e^x function.

     Answer: $e^{3.219} = 25$

Problems:

Using a scientific calculator, find the log of the following numbers.

1. 28
2. 196
3. 5,760
4. 0.391

Using a scientific calculator, find the antilog of the following numbers.

5. 2.625
6. 0.477
7. 3.226
8. 1.749
9. −0.908
10. −2.274
11. 1.532
12. 3.878

Using a scientific calculator, find the natural log (ln) of the following numbers.

13. 34
14. 2,800
15. 0.360
16. 4.69
17. 4,860
18. 45
19. 564
20. 4,264

Using a scientific calculator, find the natural antilog of the following numbers.

21. 0.693
22. −0.693
23. 1.556
24. −3.11
25. 4.304
26. 0.466
27. 8.77
28. −1.483
29. −2.631
30. −0.806

References:

Christian & Waterstram-Rich (6th Ed.), p. 7–9.

14. Solving equations with an unknown in the exponent

Principles:

There are occasions when the unknown in an equation appears as an exponent or part of an exponent. The use of logs and natural logs will allow the unknown to be removed from the exponent.

As shown in Basic Math Skills, Section 13, the inverse of an exponent is its log.

If $b^x = N$, then $\log_b N = x$. For example, if $10^2 = 100$, then $\log_{10} 100 = 2$.

The same is true of natural logs and natural antilogs.

If $e^x = Y$, then $\ln Y = x$. For example, if $e^{0.693} = 2$, then $\ln 2 = 0.693$.

I-29 How to move an unknown out of the exponent:

1. Isolate the component containing the exponent with the unknown (x).
2. Simplify the side of the equation not containing x.
3. Take the log (for base 10) or ln (for base e) of both sides of the equation. The exponent now becomes a whole number or a decimal.
4. Isolate and solve for x.

Examples:

A. Solve for x: $(4)(10^{4x}) = 100$.

    1. Isolate the component containing x: $10^{4x} = \dfrac{100}{4}$.

    2. Simplify the side of the equation not containing x: $10^{4x} = 25$.

    3. Take the log of each side of the equation: $\log 10^{4x} = \log 25 \quad 4x = 1.398$.

    4. Isolate and solve for x: $x = \dfrac{1.398}{4} = 0.35$.

B. Solve for x: $50 = (30)(e^{0.693x})$.

    1. Isolate the component containing x: $\dfrac{50}{30} = e^{0.693x}$.

    2. Simplify the side of the equation not containing x: $1.667 = e^{0.693x}$.

    3. Take the ln of each side of the equation: $\ln 1.667 = \ln e^{0.693x} \quad 0.511 = 0.693x$.

    4. Isolate and solve for x: $x = \dfrac{0.511}{0.693} = 0.74$.

C. Solve for x: $18 = (15) \left(e^{(0.693)\left(\frac{2.9}{x}\right)} \right)$.

1. Isolate the component containing x: $\dfrac{18}{15} = e^{(0.693)\left(\frac{2.9}{x}\right)}$.

2. Simplify the side of the equation not containing x: $1.2 = e^{(0.693)\left(\frac{2.9}{x}\right)}$.

3. Take the ln of each side of the equation:

$\ln 1.2 = \ln e^{(0.693)\left(\frac{2.9}{x}\right)}$ $0.182 = \dfrac{(0.693)(2.9)}{x}$.

4. Isolate and solve for x: $x = \dfrac{(0.693)(2.9)}{0.182} = 11$.

Problems:

Solve for x in each of the following equations.

1. $74 = 10^{2.37x}$

2. $48 = (22)\left(10^{8.46x}\right)$

3. $173 = (0.6)\left(10^{(0.551)\left(\frac{x}{4.1}\right)}\right)$

4. $1.7 = e^{0.931x}$

5. $10.5 = (8.6)\left(e^{1.35x}\right)$

6. $110 = (12)\left(e^{(0.443)\left(\frac{x}{0.5}\right)}\right)$

7. $0.12 = (120)\left(e^{-(0.693)\left(\frac{x}{0.03}\right)}\right)$

8. $3.1 = 57e^{-(0.693)\left(\frac{x}{0.11}\right)}$

9. $7.5 = 120e^{-(0.693)\left(\frac{0.24}{x}\right)}$

10. $8.6 = 25e^{-(0.693)\left(\frac{20}{x}\right)}$

11. $2.4 = 3.2e^{-(0.693)\left(\frac{28}{x}\right)}$

12. $281 = 473e^{-(0.693)\left(\frac{4.5}{x}\right)}$

References:

Christian & Waterstram-Rich (6th Ed.), p. 7–9, 11–17.
Saha (4th Ed), p. 62.

15. Graphing on linear and semi-log papers

You will need linear and semi-log graph paper to complete this section.

Principles:

The horizontal axis of a graph is called the abscissa and is designated the x-axis. The x-axis represents the independent variable. The vertical axis is called the ordinate, and is designated the y-axis. The y-axis represents the dependent variable. In Chart 1 below, the percent activity remaining (y-axis) is dependent upon the elapsed time (x-axis).

When drawn on linear paper, a graph showing elapsed time (x) versus the percent of radioactivity remaining (y) will produce a curve rather than a straight line. This is because radioactive decay is not a linear process. If it were, the same **amount of radioactivity** would be lost in each half-life. For example, if you started with 100 mCi, 50 mCi would be lost during the first half-life and 50 mCi more would be lost in the second. If radioactive decay followed a linear progression, all of a radioactive substance would be decayed within two half-lives. This, of course, is not true.

In reality, the same **percentage of radioactivity** decays within each half-life (i.e., 50% of the amount present at the beginning of each half-life). Therefore, if you started with 100 mCi, there would be 50 mCi at the end of one half-life, 25 mCi at the end of two half-lives, 12.5 mCi at the end of three, and so forth. On linear graph paper, such a geometric progression will produce a curved line (see Chart 1).

Decay of Tc99m

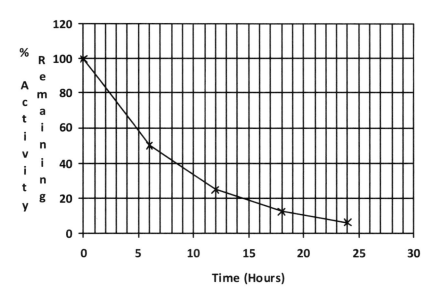

Chart 1.

For convenience a straight line is preferred, so data can be extrapolated between the discrete points (known data) used to create the line. Extrapolated data from a straight line will be more accurate than from a curve.

To convert the curve to a straight line, the logs of the y values are used and the data is graphed on semi-log paper (see Chart 2). (See Basic Math Skills Section 13.)

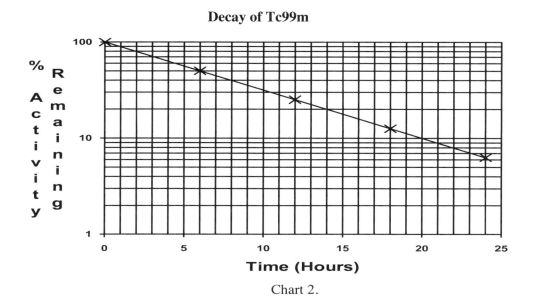

Chart 2.

* **Note:** On a semilog graph, as shown above, the y-axis is divided into 1-unit segments for the first 10 segments; the second 10 are in 10-unit segments; the third, if they were used, would be in 100-unit segments. The x-axis remains constant in its divisions.

I-30 How to determine values between the discrete data points on a graph:

1. Read from the point of interest on one axis, such as the 20-hour mark on Chart 2, to the graphed line.
2. Now read directly across to the opposing axis to obtain the corresponding data, in this case 10% of activity remaining. The graph shows that at 20 hours, 10% of activity remains.

Although you have used only a limited number of discrete points, the graph allows calculation of data anywhere between the points.

* **Note:** The more discrete data points used to create a graph, the more accurate the extrapolated data. Compare Chart 3 to Chart 4 (next page), which demonstrate the same data. On Chart 3, only 3 points are plotted. On Chart 4, an additional 4 points are plotted to more accurately determine the true shape of the curve.

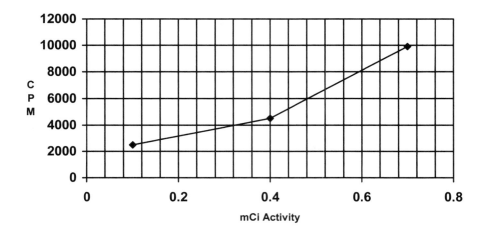

Chart 3.

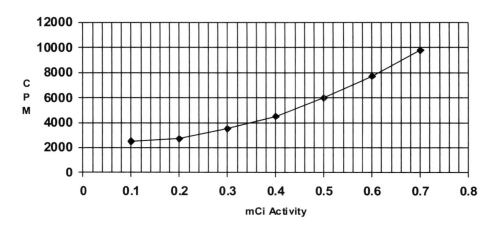

Chart 4.

Examples:

A. Using Chart 3, calculate the activity present when 3,000 cpm are acquired.

    Read from the y-axis to intercept of graphed line, then read down to the x-axis.

    Answer: At 3,000 cpm, 0.180 mCi should be present.

B. Using Chart 4, calculate the activity present when 3,000 cpm are acquired.

    Answer: At 3,000 cpm, 0.240 mCi are actually present.

    The use of only 3 points to create Chart 3 resulted in a 25% error in this extrapolated data. (See Statistics Section 1.)

Problems:

1. Use Chart 1 to determine the percent activity of Tc99m remaining at 3 hours.
2. Use Chart 2 to determine the percent activity of Tc99m remaining at 3 hours.
3. In actuality, 70.7% of the Tc99m activity will remain at 3 hours. Which method of graphing, linear or semilog, gave the most accurate result?
4. Use Chart 1 to determine the percent activity of Tc99m remaining at 21 hours.
5. Use Chart 2 to determine the percent activity of Tc99m remaining at 21 hours.
6. In actuality, 8.8% of the Tc99m activity will remain at 21 hours. Which method of graphing, linear or semilog, gave the most accurate result?
7. According to Chart 3, how many mCi are present when 7,000 cpm are acquired?
8. According to Chart 4, how many mCi are present when 7,000 cpm are acquired?
9. Using to Chart 4, calculate how many cpm should be acquired when 0.640 mCi are placed in the counter.
10. Using to Chart 4, calculate how many cpm should be acquired when 0.350 mCi are placed in the counter.
11. Graph the following data on semilog paper with "time" on the x-axis and "percent activity remaining" on the y-axis. Determine the half-life of the radionuclide, the point at which 50% of the activity remains.

Time in Hours	% Activity Remaining
20	83
40	69
60	57
80	47
100	39
120	32

12. Graph the following data on semilog paper with "time" on the x-axis and "percent activity remaining" on the y-axis. Determine the half-life of the radionuclide, the point at which 50% of the activity remains.

Time in Hours	% Activity Remaining
4	81
8	66
12	53
16	43
20	35

13. Extend the graph in Problem 11 to determine the approximate time at which 10% of the activity remains.
14. Using linear paper, graph the data in Problem 12. Extend the graph to estimate the time at which 10% of the activity remains.

References:

Chandra (6th Ed.), p. 22–23.
Cherry, Sorenson & Phelps (3rd Ed.), p. 35–36.
Christian & Waterstram-Rich (6th Ed.), p. 16–18.

1. Percent error or percent difference

Principles:

When one value is expected and a different one obtained, the percent difference or percent error involved in the measurement can be calculated. The difference between the expected value and the one actually obtained is divided by the expected value to give the error in the form of a fraction. This is also referred to as the relative error. More commonly the fraction is multiplied by 100% to give a percent error or percent difference.

II-1 How to calculate the percent error or percent difference:

$$\text{percent error or percent difference} = \left| \frac{\text{expected} - \text{actual}}{\text{expected}} \right| \times 100\% .$$

The symbol $|\ |$ denotes the absolute value. If a negative number is obtained, the minus sign is simply dropped and the number becomes positive. For example, a -6 is converted to 6. The percent error is expressed as a positive number.

* Note: The above equation is most often written without the absolute symbol. You can assume that it is implied.

Examples:

A. A long-lived calibration standard is known to contain 80 μCi of activity at this time. The dose calibrator gives a reading of 72 μCi. What is the percent error in the measurement?

$$\frac{80\mu Ci - 72\mu 2\mu}{80\mu 0\mu} \times 100\% = 10\%$$

B. The above source gives a reading of 83 μCi in the dose calibrator. What is the percent error of the measurement?

$$\frac{80\mu Ci - 83\mu 3\mu}{80\mu 0\mu} \times 100\% = 3.8\%$$

Note that the absolute value of the numerator was used, so the percent error is expressed as a positive number.

Problems:

1. If a source is calculated to be 25 mCi, but measures 21 mCi, what is the percent error?

2. A dose calibrator gives a reading of 3.42 mCi for a radioactive source that has been calibrated to contain 3.10 mCi. What is the percent difference?

3. One technologist processed an ejection fraction and obtains a value of 59.7%. A second technologist processed the data and obtained a value of 62.2%. What is the percent difference between the two values?

4. A Cs137 stick source is counted in a well counter each morning to determine the precision of the instrument. On Monday a count of 1,356 cpm is obtained. On Tuesday the counting rate is 1,193 cpm. What is the percent difference?

5. A long-lived standard typically produces a counting rate of 703 cpm. What is the percent difference, if it is now producing 647 cpm?

6. A unit dose is calibrated to contain 22.4 mCi. What is the percent error if the dose calibrator measures the dose at 23.7 mCi?

7. An automatic pipettor is calibrated to deliver 1.0 ml. It is determined that 0.92 ml are delivered instead. What is the percent error?

8. A radiopharmacy technologist has prepared 438 doses. Seven did not meet the required dose range standards. What is the technologist's percent of error?

9. A nuclear medicine department schedules 172 patients during 1 week. If 22 fail to show up for their tests, what is the percent cancellation?

10. Duplicate samples are prepared and counted during a blood volume test. One sample produces 2,640 cpm and the other produces 3,346 cpm. What is the percent difference between the two samples?

References:

Christian & Waterstram-Rich (6th Ed.), p. 3.

2. Counting rate determination

Principles:

The counting rate is defined as the number of events detected per unit time. Camera and well counter counting rates are measured in counts per second (cps) or counts per minute (cpm).

II-2 How to calculate a counting rate:

$$\text{counting rate} = \frac{\text{counts}}{\text{time}}$$

Examples:

A. A total of 933,000 counts were acquired in 3.0 minutes. What is the counting rate?

$$\frac{933,000 \text{ counts}}{3 \text{ minutes}} = 311,000 \text{ cpm}$$

B. 150,000 counts were obtained in 0.5 minutes. What is the counting rate?

$$\frac{150,000 \text{ counts}}{0.5 \text{ minutes}} = 300,000 \text{ cpm}$$

Problems:

Determine the counting rate in **cpm** for each of the following. Round to the appropriate number of significant figures. (See Basic Math Skills Section 1.)

1. 74,035 counts in 2.0 minutes
2. 13,952 counts in 12.0 minutes
3. 12,361 counts in 5.0 minutes
4. 571,200 counts in 3.0 minutes
5. 3,291,500 counts in 2.0 hours

Determine the counting rate in **cps** for each of the following. Round to the appropriate number of significant figures. (See Basic Math Skills Section 1.)

6. 9,026 counts in 20 seconds
7. 60,472 counts in 0.5 minutes
8. 3,318 counts in 2.0 minutes
9. 7,376 counts in 15 seconds
10. 34,573 counts in 60 seconds

Additional Applications:

11. At a counting rate of 850 cpm, how long will it take to acquire 10,000 counts?

12. How much time is needed to acquire a 30,000,000 count flood, if the flood source produces 244,000 cpm?

13. How long will it take to collect 2 million counts, if the flood source provides 718,500 counts in 5.0 minutes?

References:

Harbert & da Rocha, Vol. 1, p. 73.

3. Effects of background on counts and counting rates

Principles:

Background radiation is always present due to solar radiation, natural radiation from sources within the earth, and from man-made sources. Whenever a radioactive source is counted with a detector (camera, G-M counter, well counter, uptake probe, or dose calibrator), you must account for background radiation.

When counting samples in a well counter or uptake probe, a background count is acquired first, and subtracted from each sample count in order to eliminate mathematical error due to background radiation. (The effects of background when using other radiation detectors are discussed in other sections.)

Some important definitions:

gross counts—The total number of counts acquired with the radiation source present. Gross counts are also referred to as total counts.

background counts—The counts acquired when no radiation source is present.

net counts—The actual counts produced by the radiation source.

II-3 How to determine the net counts:

    net counts = gross counts − background counts

Example:

A. A red blood cell mass blood sample gives the following data when counted in a well counter. Determine the net counts of the sample.

    sample   8,750 cpm
    background   350 cpm

    8,750 cpm − 350 cpm = 8,400 cpm

II-4 How to determine the net counting rate:

$$\text{net counting rate} = \frac{\text{gross counts - background counts}}{\text{time}}$$

Examples:

A. If a Cs137 stick source gives the following data when counted in a well counter, what is the net counting rate in cpm?

Cs137 source   3,550,000 counts in 3.00 minutes
background   822 counts in 3.00 minutes

$$\frac{(3,550,000 \text{ counts}) - (822 \text{ counts})}{3.00 \text{ min}} = 1,183,059 \text{ cpm}$$

Round the answer to significant figures (see Basic Math Skills, Section 1):

The counting rate is 1,180,000 cpm.

B. The following counts are acquired for a patient having a thyroid uptake study. Calculate the net counts per minute for the patient's thyroid.

thyroid   4,218 counts in 3.00 minutes
body background   1,333 counts in 3.00 minutes

$$\frac{(4,218 \text{ counts}) - (1,333 \text{ counts})}{3.00 \text{ min}} = 962 \text{ cpm}$$

---

* Note: It is important to note that background has a much greater effect on small numbers than on large numbers. Failing to subtract background in example A would not affect the results of an equation in which the counting rate of the Cs137 stick source was used. The counting rate, in significant figures, without background subtraction is still 1,180,000 cpm. However, failure to subtract background for the thyroid uptake value in Example B will substantially change the results of the calculation, and, therefore, the results of the patient's test. Without background subtraction, the patient's counting rate is 1,406 cpm, which is 30% greater than the true counting rate.

---

* Note: There are some situations, such as a red cell mass study, in which various samples are counted for different time periods. The patient sample may be counted for 10 minutes because it has a very low activity, while the standard may be counted for 3 minutes because it has a relatively high activity. If the patient sample is counted for only 3 minutes, the accuracy of the measurement could be compromised. When different counting times are involved, a background count should be acquired for each counting time and subtracted from the gross counts, so in this case, a 10-minute background count is subtracted from the patient sample counts, and a 3-minute background count is subtracted from the standard counts. The net counts are then calculated for each sample, so each datum is entered into the equation as cpm.

Problems:

Calculate the net counts, then round to the appropriate number of significant figures.

1. sample   82,977 counts
    background   509 counts

2. sample   35,457 counts
    background   1,233 counts

3. sample   96,027 cpm
    background   590 counts

4. sample   7,664 cpm
    background   754 counts

Calculate the net counting rate in cpm, then round to the appropriate number of significant figures.

5. sample   73,815 counts acquired in 3.0 minutes
    background   947 counts acquired in 3.0 minutes

6. sample   6996 counts acquired in 5.0 minutes
    background   319 counts acquired in 5.0 minutes

7. sample   9,736 counts acquired in 2.0 minutes
    background   868 counts acquired in 2.0 minutes

8. sample   8,153 counts acquired in 10.0 minutes
    background   1,309 counts acquired in 10.0 minutes

9. sample   26,623 counts acquired in 15.0 minutes
    background   977 counts acquired in 15.0 minutes

10. sample   9,241 counts acquired in 20.0 minutes
    background   597 counts acquired in 20.0 minutes

Additional Applications:

11. A sample is counted for 0.5 minutes to give 1,624 counts with a background count of 107 counts in 0.5 minutes. The same sample is counted for 3.0 minutes, giving 10,750 counts with a background of 590 counts in 3.0 minutes. What is the net counting rate for each acquisition? What is the percent difference in the 0.5-minute count as compared to the 3-minute count? (See Statistics Section 1.)

References:

Cherry, Sorenson & Phelps (3rd Ed.), p. 137.
Christian & Waterstram-Rich (6th Ed.), p. 24–25.
Saha (4th Ed.) p. 27–28.

4. Mean, median, and mode

Principles:

The term "average" is commonly used to describe the arithmetic mean. It is the sum of a series of values, divided by the number of values in the series. The median is the middle number of a series of values that have been arranged in numerical order. The mode is the value that occurs most frequently in a data series.

---

* **Note:** Actually mean, median, and mode are all terms denoting an average. An average is a measure of central tendency. It is typical of a series of values.

II-5 How to calculate the mean:

$$\text{mean} = \frac{\text{sum of all values}}{\text{number of values}} \quad \text{or} \quad \bar{n} = \frac{\sum n}{N}$$

Where: $\sum$ is the summation symbol, which indicates that the values immediately following the symbol are to be summed.

$\bar{n}$ = mean of values
n = individual values
N = total number of values

II-6 How to determine the median:

1. Arrange the series of values in numerical order, referred to as a ranked series.
2. If the series contains an odd number of values, then the middle value is the median.
3. If the series contains an even number of values, then the number that falls halfway between the two middle values is the median. To find this number, add the two middle values and divide by two.

$$\frac{\text{mid value}_1 + \text{mid value}_2}{2}$$

II-7 How to determine the mode:

1. Arrange the series of values in numerical order.
2. Determine which value occurs most frequently.
3. If two different values occur with maximum frequency, then the series is bimodal. If three different values occur with maximum frequency, then the series is trimodal.
4. If no value occurs more than once, then no mode exists for the series.

Examples:

A.   A Co57 source was counted repeatedly in a dose calibrator providing the following results. Determine the median, mode, and mean of the data series.

    52.8   52.3   52.3   52.7   52.3   52.4   52.5

Rearrange the series into ranked order.

    52.8   52.7   52.5   52.4   52.3   52.3   52.3

The median is the middle value in the series: 52.4
The mode is the value that occurs most frequently: 52.3

Calculate the mean: $\dfrac{52.8 + 52.7 + 52.5 + 52.4 + 52.3 + 52.3 + 52.3}{7} = 52.5$

> *** Note:** In this example, the median, mode, and mean are each a different number. The mean is actually greater than both the most frequently occurring value (mode) and the middle value in the ranked series (median).

B.   Four hours after administration of radioactive iodine, a patient's thyroid is counted. The following values are obtained. Determine the median, mode, and mean of the series of counts.

    6,372
    6,388
    6,423

The median or middle number in the ranked series is 6,388. No mode exists in this case, as no number is repeated.

Calculate the mean: $\dfrac{6423 + 6388 + 6372}{3} = 6394$

C.   Determine the median for the following series of values:

    250   276   280   293

Because there is an even number of values, the median will fall halfway between to two middle values.

$\dfrac{276 + 280}{2} = 278$

Problems:

For problems 1–4, determine the mode, median, and mean for the series of numbers.

1. 173, 137, 192, 135, 187, 174, 174

2. 27, 41, 14, 86, 60, 62, 93, 60, 54, 75, 60

3. 6,809, 6,886, 6,855, 6,893, 6,808

4. 57,161, 60,805, 57,449, 57,527, 60,493

5. Calculate the median and mean: 910, 756, 903, 516.

6. A radioactive sample has been counted 4 times. Calculate the median and mean for the values obtained.

    10,836, 11,439, 10,486, 10,357.

7. A series of samples is pipetted from a standard solution. Calculate the mean.

    76,062   75,935   76,433   76,080   75,901

References:

Cherry, Sorenson & Phelps (3rd Ed.), p. 132.
Christian & Waterstram-Rich (6th Ed.), p. 21–22.
Itturalde, p. 190–191, 195.

5. Standard deviation of a series of values

Principles:

If a long-lived radioactive source was counted in a well counter repeatedly and the results were plotted on a graph, the graph would produce a bell-shaped curve. This curve would be very similar to the normal curve or Gaussian curve produced whenever a large population is analyzed. For example, a normal curve is produced if the certification exam scores of all nuclear medicine technologists sitting for the test in 1995 are plotted on a graph.

The curve produced by the radioactive source will take the shape of a Poisson distribution. This is a slightly different distribution as compared to a Gaussian distribution. The peak of the curve is shifted slightly to the left of the peak of the Gaussian curve. The shift in the peak results from the randomness of radioactive decay.

When large numbers, such as high counts, are used, a Gaussian or normal bell curve can be used to estimate values. You can therefore use the processes applied to the normal or Gaussian distribution to perform statistical calculations in most nuclear medicine procedures. Some texts use the terms Poisson and Gaussian interchangeably.

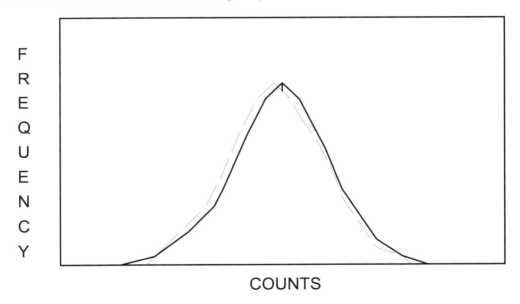

solid line = Gaussian or normal distribution
broken line = Poisson distribution

The standard deviation (SD or σ) describes the dispersion or distribution of values around the mean value. It describes the variance within the data series.

The standard deviation is an indicator of the precision of a series of values. The smaller the standard deviation, the more similar the values are to one another.

* Note: The term "precision" is used to define the reproducibility of results. For example, if a radiopharmaceutical dose is repeatedly measured in a dose calibrator and very similar activities are obtained each time, then the results are precise.

Precision must not be confused with accuracy. The term "accuracy" describes how close to the true value a number actually is. If the above-mentioned dose is measured while the dose calibrator well is contaminated with radioactive material, then the results may be reproducible (precise) for a period of time, but they are not accurate. They do not represent the true activity of the dose.

precision = reproducibility
accuracy = true value

The smaller the standard deviation, the more closely the values are related to the mean. A larger standard deviation shows they are distributed further from the mean.

The standard deviation is often expressed as the mean value $\pm\ \sigma$, for example $10,355 \pm 310$.

II-8 How to calculate the standard deviation for a population or series of values:

$$SD = \sqrt{\frac{\sum\left(n-\overline{n}\right)^2}{N-1}}$$

where: $\sum$ is the summation symbol, which indicates that the values immediately following the symbol are to be summed.

$\overline{n}$ =   mean of values
n =   individual values
N =   total number of values

OR

Utilize the standard deviation function on your scientific calculator. Check the instrument's instruction booklet for the proper key sequence.

* Note: In order for calculator results to match the SD calculations in this book, the σxn-1 function must be used as opposed to the σxn function.

* **Note:** In the above equation N-1 denotes the degrees of freedom. The number of degrees of freedom is defined as the number of values in the sample, minus the number of parameters that are estimated from the sample. For example, the standard deviation is to be determined for a series of 10 counts that were obtained from a long-lived radioactive source. The sample consists of 10 values. Each value is, in reality, an estimate of the true counting rate of the source. It is an estimate because of the randomness of radioactive decay; the variability in the response of the counting instrument; and the instrument's deadtime and efficiency. The counting rate parameter is, therefore, estimated and N-1 should be used in the calculation of the standard deviation.

Many texts utilize a slightly different equation for the standard deviation:

$$SD = \sqrt{\frac{\sum(n - \overline{n})^2}{N}}$$

This does not account for the estimation of a parameter. In nuclear medicine, the equation shown in Shadowbox II-8 is usually more appropriate.

Examples:

A. Calculate the standard deviation for the following series of numbers: 175, 180, 178, 169, 184.

Calculate the mean $(\overline{n})$: $\overline{n} = \dfrac{175 + 180 + 178 + 169 + 184}{5} = 177.2$.

Calculate $(n - \overline{n})^2$ for each value:

$(175 - 177.2)^2 = -2.2^2 = 4.84$

$(180 - 177.2)^2 = 2.8^2 = 7.84$

$(178 - 177.2)^2 = 0.8^2 = 0.64$

$(169 - 177.2)^2 = -8.2^2 = 67.24$

$(184 - 177.2)^2 = 6.8^2 = 46.24$

Calculate the $\sum(n - \overline{n})^2$: $4.84 + 7.84 + 0.64 + 67.24 + 46.24 = 126.8$.

Calculate the SD: $SD = \sqrt{\dfrac{126.8}{5-1}} = \sqrt{31.7} = 5.6$.

B. Calculate the standard deviation for a series of counts acquired over a patient's thyroid 24 hours after administration of radioiodine.

33,890   34,230   33,770

Calculate $\overline{n}$: $\overline{n} = \dfrac{33,890 + 34,230 + 33,770}{3} = \dfrac{101,890}{3} = 33,963$

Calculate $\left(N - \overline{N}\right)^2$ for each value:
$$(33,890 - 33,963)^2 = -73^2 = 5,329$$
$$(34,230 - 33,963)^2 = 267^2 = 71,289$$
$$(33,770 - 33,963)^2 = -193^2 = 37,249$$

Calculate the $\sum \left(n - \overline{n}\right)^2$: $5,329 + 71,289 + 37,249 = 113,867$.

Calculate the SD: $SD = \sqrt{\dfrac{113,867}{3-1}} = \sqrt{56,934} = 239$.

Problems:

1. A radioactive source is measured five times to obtain the following values. Calculate the standard deviation.

    27.2 μCi   27.6 μCi   27.9 μCi   26.8 μCi   27.4 μCi

2. Three samples are withdrawn from a standard solution using a semi-automatic pipetting device. What is the standard deviation if the samples provide the following counts?

    13,967 cpm   14,472 cpm   14,229 cpm

3. Background counts are repeatedly acquired on a well counter. What is the standard deviation of the values obtained?

    127 cpm   112 cpm   143 cpm   133 cpm   147 cpm   159 cpm

4. Four technologists calculated an ejection fraction from a particular patient's images. If they obtained the following values, what is the standard deviation?

    44.5%   41.5%   43.2%   43.7%

5. A single sample was measured in a dose calibrator 5 different times. What is the standard deviation if the following activities were obtained?

    10.2 mCi   10.8 mCi   11.4 mCi   9.7 mCi   9.6 mCi

6. Five aliquots of a radioactive solution are measured in a well counter. Calculate the standard deviation.

    18,426   18,691   17,766   18,443   18,059

References:

Cherry, Sorenson & Phelps (3rd Ed.), p. 134.
Christian & Waterstram-Rich (6th Ed.), p. 21–27.
Early & Sodee (2nd Ed.), p. 185–187.
Harbert & da Rocha, Vol. 1, p. 70–72.

6. Confidence intervals and the standard deviation of a single value

Principles:

In a normal distribution, a given percentage of values will always fall within a specified number of standard deviations (SD or σ) above and below the mean, as shown in the following diagram.

The diagram demonstrates a normal distribution with the standard deviations and confidence intervals marked.

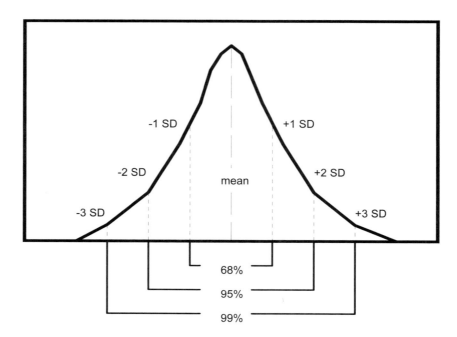

Number of Standard Deviations	Confidence Interval or Percentage of Values Within This Range
1	68%
2	95%
3	99%

The number of standard deviations used can also be referred to as the confidence interval (CI) or level of confidence. For example, you would be confident that 68% of count values fall within ±1 SD from the mean. You would be confident that 95% of count values fall within ±2 SD from the mean and the 99% of count values fall within ±3 SD from the mean.

The 95% level of confidence is most commonly used in nuclear medicine procedures. If a value falls within this range, it is accepted. It is assumed that the variation of the value from the mean results from the randomness of decay, and the inherent error produced by slight variations in performance of electronic equipment and measuring devices, such as well counters, semi-automatic pipettes, and automatic pipettes.

A predetermined number (often the mean counts from a standard or control sample) and the standard deviation are used to determine if a value is acceptable or if it may indicate a procedural error or equipment malfunction. Values falling within two standard deviations are usually considered acceptable in nuclear medicine. If they fall outside of this range, their variation from the mean is considered too extreme and therefore probably indicates malfunction of equipment or an error in procedure.

In many situations, you would be calculating the standard deviation for an individual value rather than a series.

---

* Note: In reality a single value cannot deviate from itself. You are actually estimating the SD of an underlying distribution using the single value. This is possible because the value occurs within a Poisson distribution. (See Statistics Section 5.)

Because a Poisson distribution is created by the randomness of radioactive decay, it has a characteristic that a Gaussian or normal curve (see Statistics Section 5) does not have. The standard deviation of a single value is approximately equal to the square root of the value: $SD \approx \sqrt{n}$.

II-9 How to calculate the standard deviation from a single value at a desired confidence interval:

This number represents the range of acceptable values at that level of confidence.

CI = confidence interval

For the 68% confidence interval (±1 SD): $CI_{68\%} = n \pm \sqrt{n}$ or $CI_{68\%} = n \pm 1\ SD$,

where n = the single value

For the 95% confidence interval (±2 SD): $CI_{95\%} = n \pm 2\sqrt{n}$ or $CI_{95\%} = n \pm 2\ SD$.
For the 99% confidence interval (±3 SD): $CI_{99\%} = n \pm 3\sqrt{n}$ or $CI_{99\%} = n \pm 3\ SD$.

Examples:

A. Calculate the standard deviation of 1,000 counts.

$$SD = \sqrt{1,000\ ct} = 32\ counts$$

B.   What range of values is included in 1SD of 1,000 counts? 2SD? 3SD?

$$1\text{SD or } CI_{68\%}: 1,000 \text{ ct} \pm \sqrt{1,000} = 1,000 \text{ ct} \pm 32 \text{ or } 968 \text{ to } 1,032 \text{ counts}$$

$$2\text{SD or } CI_{95\%}: 1,000 \text{ ct} \pm 2\sqrt{1,000} = 1,000 \text{ ct} \pm 63 \text{ or } 937 \text{ to } 1,063 \text{ counts}$$

$$3\text{SD or } CI_{99\%}: 1,000 \text{ ct} \pm 3\sqrt{1,000} = 1,000 \text{ ct} \pm 95 \text{ or } 905 \text{ to } 1,095 \text{ counts}$$

C.   At the 95% level of confidence, what range of values would be accepted if a radioactive standard produced 56,100 cpm?

$$CI_{95\%} = 56,100 \text{ cpm} \pm 2\sqrt{56,100} = 56,100 \text{ cpm} \pm 474$$

Therefore the range of values at $CI_{95\%}$ would be 55,626 to 56,574 cpm.

At the 95% confidence level, values falling between 55,626 cpm and 56,574 cpm will be accepted. Values that fall below or above this range will be investigated.

D.   A long-lived radioactive calibration standard should produce a reading of 120 μCi in a dose calibrator. At the 95% confidence level, what range of values will be accepted?

$$CI_{95\%} = 120 \ \mu Ci \pm 2\sqrt{120} = 120 \ \mu Ci \pm 22 \text{ or } 98 \text{ to } 142 \ \mu Ci$$

Problems:

Calculate the standard deviation at the 68% level of confidence:

1.   10,763
2.   24,298
3.   644

Calculate the standard deviation at the 95% level of confidence:

4.   9,768
5.   14,820
6.   1,864,000

Calculate the standard deviation at the 99% level of confidence:

7.   847
8.   112,500
9.   64,100

For each of the following calculate the range of values covered by 1SD or the 68% confidence interval.

10. 100,000 counts
11. 28,000 counts
12.   4,000 counts

For each of the following calculate the range of values covered by 2SD or the 95% confidence interval.

13. 11,000 counts
14. 2,600 counts
15. 48,700 counts

For each of the following calculate the range of values covered by 3SD or the 99% confidence interval.

16. 854,000 counts
17. 12,000 counts

18. What range of values would be included at the 68% confidence interval if a sample averaged 7,882 counts?

19. Determine the acceptable range of counts at the 99% level of confidence for a source that gives 49,691 cpm.

20. A Cs137 stick source gives an average count of 60,629 cpm. At the 95% confidence interval, what range of counts would be acceptable if the source is to be used for daily well counter tests?

21. If a source produces a counting rate of 3,733 cpm, what is the acceptable range of values at the 95% level of confidence?

22. Calculate the acceptable range at the 99% confidence level for a calibration source that produces 92,537 cpm.

23. If a standard solution produces a counting rate of 134 cpm, what is the acceptable count range at the 95% confidence interval?

References:

Chandra (6th Ed.), p. 27–28.
Cherry, Sorenson & Phelps (3rd Ed.), p. 134–135.
Christian & Waterstram-Rich (6th Ed.), p. 23–25.
Early & Sodee (2nd Ed.), p. 185–187.
Harbert & da Rocha, Vol. 1, p. 70–76.
Saha (4th Ed.), p. 27–28.

7. Percent error or coefficient of variation for a series of values

Principles:

The percent error or coefficient of variation (CV) for a series of values is a measure of precision. The smaller the CV, the less variation there is between values in a series of measurements and the greater the precision. The CV is frequently used to demonstrate pipette precision, intra-assay precision, and inter-assay precision.

II-10 How to calculate the coefficient of variation or percent error for a series of values:

The CV or percent error at 1SD or the 68% confidence interval (see Statistics Section 6):

$$CV = \frac{\text{standard deviation}}{\text{mean}} \times 100\% \quad \text{or} \quad CV = \frac{\sigma}{n} \times 100\% \quad \text{or} \quad CV = \frac{SD}{n} \times 100\%$$

* Note: The above equations are simply three different ways of expressing the same mathematical operation. They will all produce the same answer.

* Note: The CV for the 68% confidence interval could also be represented by the symbol $CV_{68\%}$. If no subscript appears after the CV, you can assume the 68% confidence interval or one standard deviation is being utilized.

---

* Note: The CV or percent error for 2 or 3 standard deviations can also be determined.

CV at 2SD or the 95% confidence interval: $CV_{95\%} = \frac{2SD}{n} \times 100\%$

CV at 3SD or the 99% confidence interval: $CV_{99\%} = \frac{3SD}{n} \times 100\%$

Examples:

A. Calculate the CV for a series of samples with a standard deviation of 0.14 and a mean of 4.12 µg/dl.

$$\frac{0.14}{4.12} \times 100\% = 3.4\%$$

B. A series of measurements is made with an automatic pipettor. What is the CV if the SD is 0.36 and the mean is 11.73?

$$\frac{0.36}{11.73} \times 100\% = 3.1\%$$

Problems:

1. What is the coefficient of variation for a series of measurements with a mean of 8,945 and a standard deviation of 260?

2. Calculate the % error for a series of values for which the mean is 2.89 and SD is 0.49.

3. If the standard deviation is 199 and the mean is 6,443, what is the CV?

4. Calculate the coefficient of variation at the 68% confidence interval for a series of control samples with a mean value of 1.73 µg/dl and a standard deviation of 0.12.

5. If the mean value is 651 cps and the standard deviation is 23, what is the CV?

6. A semi-automatic pipettor is used to prepare a series of samples that have a mean count of 10,521 cpm and a standard deviation of 236. What is the CV_{68}?

7. Ten samples of a standard solution are pipetted with a semi-automatic pipettor. The samples are then counted in a well counter to determine the precision of the pipettor. The mean of the 10 values is 1.41 and the standard deviation is 0.21. What is the CV_{68}?

Additional Applications:

8. A Cs137 stick source is counted in a well counter each morning for quality control testing. The CV_{68} is determined on a weekly basis and must be less than 10% to be acceptable. For a particular week the mean value is 22,952 cpm and the standard deviation is 1,123. Does the CV fall within the acceptable limit?

9. A Cs137 source is counted in an uptake probe each day. The CV is determined on a weekly basis. The mean value for this week is 25,284 cpm and the standard deviation is 1,015. Calculate the CV_{68}, CV_{95}, and CV_{99} for the week.

---

* Note: As you widen the confidence interval from 68% to 99%, you increase the possibility that subsequent values will fall within it, but you are also increasing the percent error inherent in the value. In other words, an individual value is less and less likely to be close to the true value.

As you widen the confidence interval, you are also accepting a decrease in precision, i.e., an increase in variability from one value to another.

References:

Christian & Waterstram-Rich (6th Ed.), p. 24–25.
Early & Sodee (2nd Ed.), p. 780, 786.

8.   Error inherent in a single value

Principles:

The percent standard deviation (%SD) can be used to determine the degree of error inherent in any single value in a Poisson distribution. (See Statistics Section 5.) The percent standard deviation is also referred to as the percent relative standard deviation (%RSD), percent uncertainty, or the percent error.

II-11 How to calculate the percent standard deviation (%SD) or percent error of a single value:

1 standard deviation or the 68% confidence interval: $\%SD = \dfrac{100\%}{\sqrt{N}}$

2 standard deviations or the 95% confidence interval: $\%SD = \dfrac{(2)(100\%)}{\sqrt{N}}$

3 standard deviations or the 99% confidence interval: $\%SD = \dfrac{(3)(100\%)}{\sqrt{N}}$

For the derivation of these simplified equations see Chandra, Saha, or Harbert & da Rocha (Vol I).

Examples:

A.   What is the % SD at the 68% confidence interval if 1,000 counts are obtained?

$$\%SD = \frac{100\%}{\sqrt{1,000}} = \frac{100}{31.6} = 3.2\%$$

B: What is the %SD at the 68% confidence level if 10,000 counts are obtained?

$$\%SD = \frac{100\%}{\sqrt{10,000}} = \frac{100\%}{100} = 1.0\%$$

C.   What is the % SD at the 95% level of confidence if 20,000 counts are obtained?

$$\%SD = \frac{(2)(100\%)}{\sqrt{20,000}} = \frac{200}{141} = 1.4\%$$

D.   What is the % SD at the 95% confidence interval if 50,000 counts are obtained?

$$\%SD = \frac{(2)(100\%)}{\sqrt{50,000}} = \frac{200}{224} = 0.9\%$$

> *** Note:** Remember that the %SD is also called the percent error or percent uncertainty. Compare the results of Examples A and B, as well as C and D. The more counts acquired for a specific confidence level, the more likely the number is to be close to the true value, i.e., the smaller the error or uncertainty. The fewer counts acquired, the greater the uncertainty that the number obtained is close to the true value.

Problems:

For each of the following calculate the %SD (% error or % uncertainty) at the 68% confidence interval.

1.   8,000 counts
2.   46,500 counts
3.   121,500 counts
4.   1,400 counts

For each of the following calculate the %SD (% error or % uncertainty) at the 95% confidence interval.

5.   21,750 counts
6.   6,210 counts
7.   58,920 counts
8.   225,000 counts

For each of the following calculate the %SD (% error or % uncertainty) at the 99% level of confidence.

9.   5,600 counts
10. 821 counts
11. 10,800 counts
12. 23,860 counts

References:

Chandra (6th Ed.), p. 27–28.
Cherry, Sorenson & Phelps (3rd Ed.), p. 134–135.
Early & Sodee (2nd Ed.). p. 185–187.
Harbert & da Rocha, Vol. 1, p. 72–73.
Saha (4th Ed.), p. 26–28.

9. Determination of counts required for statistical significance

Principles:

The percent standard deviation equation can be used to determine the minimum number of counts needed to assure a specified percent error is not exceeded at a desired level of confidence.

II-12 How to determine the minimum number of counts required for a desired statistical significance:

1. Utilize the appropriate percent error (%SD) equation based on the desired confidence level. The level most commonly used in nuclear medicine is 95%.

$$1 \text{ standard deviation or the } 68\% \text{ confidence interval: } \% \text{ error} = \frac{100\%}{\sqrt{N}}$$

$$2 \text{ standard deviations or the } 95\% \text{ confidence interval: } \% \text{ error} = \frac{(2)(100\%)}{\sqrt{N}}$$

$$3 \text{ standard deviations or the } 99\% \text{ confidence interval: } \% \text{ error} = \frac{(3)(100\%)}{\sqrt{N}}$$

2. Since the desired percent error will be a given, you are solving for N in each case.
3. Isolate N.
4. Solve for N. To remove the square root sign from the N, square both sides of the equation.

Examples:

A. Determine the minimum counts that need to be acquired in order to obtain less than a 1% error at the 95% confidence interval (2 standard deviations), when counting an assay sample.

$$1\% = \frac{(2)(100\%)}{\sqrt{N}} \qquad \sqrt{N} = \frac{200}{1} \qquad \left(\sqrt{N}\right)^2 = \left(\frac{200}{1}\right)^2 \qquad N = 40,000$$

---

* Note: This is one case in which a percent is NOT converted to its decimal form for use in an equation. The equation defines it as a percent. If you change it to a decimal, the answer will be drastically changed, as shown below.

$$0.01 = \frac{(2)(100\%)}{\sqrt{N}} \qquad N = 4,000,000,000$$

B. The protocol for the red cell mass study is being prepared. Calculate the minimum number of counts that must be acquired in order to assure a 2% error at the 95% confidence interval.

$$2\% = \frac{(2)(100)}{\sqrt{N}} \qquad \sqrt{N} = \frac{200}{2} \qquad \left(\sqrt{N}\right)^2 = \left(\frac{200}{2}\right)^2 \qquad N = 10,000$$

> *** Note:** Compare the results of Examples A and B. Note that fewer counts are required when a larger % standard deviation or % error is allowed, because less precision is being required.

Problems:

1. How many counts are required to obtain a 2% error (% SD) at the 68% confidence interval?

2. How many counts are required to obtain a 5% error at the 68% confidence interval?

3. How many counts must be obtained to assure an error of 0.5% at the 68% confidence interval?

4. If an error of 5% is acceptable, how many counts should be acquired for the 95% level of confidence?

5. How many counts must be acquired to assure a 0.3% error at the 95% confidence interval?

6. How many counts must be acquired in order to obtain a % standard deviation no greater than 0.7% at the 95% confidence level?

7. How many counts must be obtained for a 2% error at the 99% confidence interval?

8. What is the minimum number of counts that must be acquired in order to assure a 1% error at the 99% confidence interval?

9. How many counts must be obtained if a 0.5% error is desired at the 99% confidence interval?

References:

Christian & Waterstram-Rich (6th Ed.), p. 24–25.
Early & Sodee (2nd Ed.), p. 185–187.

10. Standard deviation of a counting rate

Principles:

The standard deviation (SD) of a counting rate is calculated differently than the SD of an individual count. The length of time over which the sample is counted affects the standard deviation of the counting rate. The longer the counting period, the smaller the SD. Acquisition for a longer time period decreases the effects of inherent variations in counting instrument performance and the randomness of radioactive decay. The reliability of the acquired value therefore increases.

The standard deviation for a single value designates the inherent error in measurement.

II-13 How to calculate the standard deviation of a counting rate:

At the 68% confidence interval or 1SD: $\sigma_c = \sqrt{\dfrac{c}{t}}$

where: c = counting rate
         t = time over which counts were acquired

* Note: You must first calculate the counting rate, then the SD_c or σ_c. In reality, the count has been divided by the time twice during standard deviation calculation.

At the 95% confidence interval or 2SD: $2\sigma_c = 2\sqrt{\dfrac{c}{t}}$

At the 99% confidence interval or 3SD: $3\sigma_c = 3\sqrt{\dfrac{c}{t}}$

Examples:

A. What is the standard deviation at the 68% confidence interval for a sample producing 5,240 counts in 2 minutes?

$$c = \frac{5,240 \text{ counts}}{2 \text{ min}} = 2,620 \text{ cpm} \qquad \sigma_c = \sqrt{\frac{2,620 \text{ cpm}}{2 \text{min}}} \qquad \sigma_c = \sqrt{1,310} = 36$$

Therefore the measured counting rate is 2,620 cpm ± 36.

* Note: On the basis of this calculation, there is a 68% certainty that the true counting rate is between 2,584 and 2,656 cpm.

B.   What is the standard deviation at the 68% confidence interval for 26,200 counts acquired in 10 minutes?

$$c = \frac{26{,}200 \text{ counts}}{10 \text{ min}} = 2{,}620 \text{ cpm} \qquad \sigma c = \sqrt{\frac{2{,}620 \text{ cpm}}{10 \text{ min}}} \qquad \sigma c = \sqrt{262} = 16$$

Therefore the counting rate is 2,620 cpm± 16.

---

* Note: According to the calculation, there is a 68% probability that the true counting rate is between 2,604 and 2,636 cpm.

The counting rates in Examples A and B are the same, but the standard deviation decreases as the counting time increases. In other words, counting longer increases the potential accuracy of the measurement.

C.   What is the standard deviation for a sample producing 1,625,200 counts in 3 minutes? What range of values is included in 1 standard deviation?

$$c = \frac{1{,}625{,}200 \text{ counts}}{3 \text{ min}} = 541{,}733 \text{ cpm} \qquad \sigma_c = \sqrt{\frac{541{,}733 \text{ cpm}}{3 \text{ min}}}$$

$$\sigma_c = \sqrt{180{,}578} = 425$$

Therefore the counting rate is 541,733 cpm ± 425. The range of values covered by 1 SD is 541,308 to 542,158 cpm.

Problems:

Calculate the range of values in cpm covered by 1 standard deviation for the following counting rates.

1.   65,340 counts in 5 minutes
2.   8,610 counts in 10 minutes
3.   110,000 counts in 3 minutes
4.   5,752 counts in 12 minutes

Calculate the range of values in cpm covered by 2 standard deviations for the following counting rates.

5.   35,030 counts in 2 minutes
6.   175,377 counts in 15 minutes
7.   908,900 counts in 20 minutes
8.   12,410 counts in 3 minutes

Calculate the range of values in cpm covered by 3 standard deviations for the following counting rates.

9. 4,078 in 2 minutes
10. 395,400 in 12 minutes
11. 11,050 in 6 minutes
12. 5,260 in 1 minute

Additional Applications:

13. Calculate the range of values covered by 2 standard deviations for the following counting rates.

    a) 8,526 in 1 minute
    b) 17,052 counts in 2 minutes
    c) 25,578 counts in 3 minutes
    d) 42,630 counts in 5 minutes
    e) 85,260 counts in 10 minutes

---

* Note: All of the counts in Problem 13 result in a counting rate of 8,426 cpm, but as the counting time increases, the SD decreases. In other words, the obtained counting rate is more and more likely to reflect the true counting rate the longer counts are acquired. The acceptable range of values, therefore, becomes narrower.

References:

Chandra (6th Ed.), p. 27–28.
Cherry, Sorenson & Phelps (3rd Ed.), p. 134–135.
Christian & Waterstram-Rich (6th Ed.), p. 24–25.
Early & Sodee (2nd Ed.), p. 185–187.
Saha (4th Ed.), p. 26–28.

11. Propagation of errors

Principles:

Every measurement contains a degree of error. When more than one measurement is used in an equation, the errors in measurements combine to increase the standard deviation (σ or SD) or the propagated error. The magnitude of their effect depends upon the calculations performed.

II-14 How to determine the standard deviation of a sum or a difference:

$$\sigma = \sqrt{N_x + N_y}$$

where: N_x = one value

N_y = a value that is added to or subtracted from the first value

---

When calculations involve division or multiplication of values, the combined standard deviation equations become more complex. However, we will not deal with them here.

Examples:

A.   Calculate the standard deviation of the net counts for a sample providing 8,600 cpm from which a background count of 320 cpm is subtracted (i.e., 8,600 − 320 = 8,280 cpm).

$$\sigma = \sqrt{8,600 \text{ cpm} + 320 \text{ cpm}} \qquad \sigma = \sqrt{8,920 \text{ cpm}} \qquad \sigma = 94 \text{ cpm}$$

The net counts for the sample equal 8,280 cpm ± 94.

---

* Note: Even though 320 is subtracted from 8,600 to obtain the net counts, the values are added in the standard deviation equation. This is because error increases with each value that is added to an equation involving detection of radioactive events. The error increases because each value has an inherent error in its measurement due to detector performance and the randomness of radioactive decay.

B.   Calculate the standard deviation for a sample providing 1,420 cpm and a background count of 210 cpm.

$$\sigma = \sqrt{1,420 \text{ cpm} + 210 \text{ cpm}} \qquad \sigma = \sqrt{1,630 \text{ cpm}} \qquad \sigma = 40 \text{ cpm}$$

The net counts for the sample equal 1,210 cpm ± 40.

Problems:

Calculate the propagated error or combined standard deviation in each of the following cases.

1.   Patient K.B. has a thyroid count of 850,200 cpm and a thigh count (body background) of 2,570 cpm. What is the standard deviation of the net count?

2.   What is the standard deviation of the net count if a sample provides 12,500 cpm and background is 480 cpm?

3.   A red blood cell mass study sample gives 98,891 cpm with a background count of 815 cpm. What is the standard deviation of the net count?

4.   If a background check results in 825 cpm and a sample produces 8,384 cpm, what is the propagated error?

5.   Calculate the propagated error for a thyroid uptake having the following values:

     thyroid   58,377 counts
     thigh   1,704 counts

6.   A sample produces 11,324 cpm. A background count gives 1,792 cpm. What is the standard deviation of the net count?

7.   If a background acquisition provides 620 cpm and a sample produces 32,967 cpm, what is the standard deviation of the net count?

References:

Chandra (6th Ed.), p. 27–29.
Cherry, Sorenson & Phelps (3rd Ed.), p. 135–136.
Christian & Waterstram-Rich (6th Ed.), p. 24–25.
Harbert & da Rocha, Vol. 1, p. 73–75.
Saha (4th Ed.), p. 28.

Chapter III. Radiation Protection

1. Conversion of counts per minute to disintegrations per minute using well counter efficiency

Principles:

The counts per minute (cpm) obtained from a sample counted in a well counter demonstrate the number of events (photons) detected by the instrument. However, cpm do NOT indicate the actual amount of radioactivity in the sample, because not every photon interacts with the crystal or is registered by the electronics (due to dead time).

In order to determine the actual activity of a sample, the well counter's efficiency for the energy being measured must be taken into account. Efficiency mathematically describes the percentage of a known activity that is actually detected by the scintillation counter or imaging device.

➤ **Regulations:** According to DOT 49CFR173.443, package wipe tests must be recorded in disintegrations per unit time rather than counts per minute.

Disintegrations per minute (dpm) is the most convenient unit, as most wipes are counted for 1 minute each.

Disintegrations per minute better represent the actual amount of radioactivity present on a survey swab than do counts per minute (cpm). To convert cpm to dpm, divide the cpm by the well counter efficiency.

---

* **Note:** Because detector efficiency is less than 100% or unity (1), dpm will always be greater than the cpm.

III-1 How to convert counts per minute to disintegrations per minute using the well counter efficiency:

$$dpm = \frac{\text{gross cpm} - \text{background cpm}}{\text{efficiency expressed as decimal}}$$

Examples:

A. A wipe test swab produces a gross count of 1,225 cpm in a well counter with a 56% efficiency. The background is 395 cpm. Calculate the dpm produced by the swab.

$$\frac{1,225 \text{ cpm} - 395 \text{ cpm}}{0.56} = 1,482 \text{ dpm}$$

B.   A wipe test swab produces 2,439 cpm in a well counter with an efficiency of 32%. The background count is 280 cpm. How many dpm are being produced by the swab?

$$\frac{2,439 \text{ cpm} - 280 \text{ cpm}}{0.32} = 6,747 \text{ dpm}$$

Problems:

1.   A wipe test swab produces a gross count of 662 cpm in a well counter with a 38% efficiency. The background count is 312 cpm. Calculate the dpm.

2.   How many dpm are being produced by a swab with a counting rate of 346 cpm in a well counter with a 54% efficiency? The background is 209 cpm.

3.   If a wipe gives 1,084 cpm, the background is 159 cpm, and the well counter has a 47% efficiency, how many dpm are being produced by the wipe?

4.   A weekly wipe test sample is found to produce 1,270 cpm. The well counter gives a background count of 150 cpm and has a 35% efficiency. How many dpm are being produced by the sample?

5.   Calculate the radioactivity present on a wipe test swab in dpm given the following data:

     gross counts for swab   736 cpm
     background   428 cpm
     well counter efficiency   0.43

6.   The gross counts obtained for a wipe test swab are 3,470 cpm in a well counter with an efficiency of 29%. If the background was 197 cpm, how much radioactivity (in dpm) is present on the swab?

7.   A well counter has an efficiency of 42%. A swab gives a gross count of 1,095 cpm and a background count of 334 cpm. How many dpm are being produced by the swab?

---

* Note: Note the significant increase in the dpm as the cpm rise and/or the efficiency falls. Using cpm as a standard for determining contamination would be deceptive as to the true level of contamination present.

Additional Applications:

---

* Note: The standard of practice requires a facility to establish a trigger level for wipe tests and area surveys. This is the level at which the radiation safety officer must be notified of contamination, so that he or she can investigate the cause of the contamination and institute practices to prevent repeat occurrences. A common trigger level is 22,000 dpm, but a lower trigger can be set.

---

8. The following are the results of a weekly hot lab wipe test using a well counter with a efficiency of 48%. The background is 183 cpm. Do any of the wipes exceed a trigger level of 2,000 dpm?

Area	CPM
a. L-block	2,640
b. dose calibrator key pad	467
c. handle of lead-lined waste can	3,210
d. sink	1,340
e. counter	321
f. vial storage area	429

➤ **Regulations:** NRC 10CFR20 requires the NRC and the carrier be notified immediately if a radioactive shipping package demonstrates removable contamination that exceeds 22,000 dpm per 100 cm^2 of package surface.

9. Following are the cpm obtained for package wipe tests. According to NRC regulations, is any notification action required? Well counter efficiency is 0.38 and background is 252 cpm.

Package	CPM
A	1,954
B	426
C	12,137

10. The following package wipe test results were obtained in a well counter with an efficiency of 51% and background count of 314 cpm. Must the NRC and carrier be notified concerning any of these packages?

Package	CPM
A	856
B	957
C	9,523

References:

Christian & Waterstram-Rich (6th Ed.), p. 206.
Early & Sodee (2nd Ed.), p. 325, 329, 331.
Steves & Wells (3rd Ed.), p. 6.
US DOT 49CFR173.443
US NRC 10CFR20.1906

2. Exposure rate constants

Principles:

The exposure rate produced by a quantity of a radionuclide can be estimated using the exposure rate constant (Γ), which is also called the gamma constant. The constant has been calculated based on the energies involved and applies only to gamma and x-ray photons. Constants are expressed either as $\dfrac{R \cdot cm^2}{mCi \cdot h}$ at 1 cm (also written as $R \cdot cm^2/mCi \cdot h$ at 1 cm) or as $\dfrac{\mu Gy \cdot m^2}{GBq \cdot h}$ at 1 m (also written as $\mu Gy \cdot m^2/GBq \cdot h$).

In order to estimate the exposure rate, you must know the exposure rate constant, the activity, and the distance from the source to the area of concern.

The exposure rate is expressed in units such as R/h, mR/h, μGy/h.

III-2 How to calculate the exposure rate based on the gamma constant:

$$X = \frac{n\Gamma}{d^2}$$

where: X = exposure rate in units of R/h or μGy/h
          n = activity
          Γ = exposure rate constant (also called gamma constant)
          d = distance

* Note: The units of activity and distance must match those of the gamma constant.

Examples:

A. What is the exposure rate at 1 cm from an unshielded 20 mCi dose of Tc99m. The exposure constant is 0.59 $R \cdot cm^2/mCi \cdot h$ at 1 cm.

$$X \text{ R/h} = \frac{(20 \text{ mCi})}{(1 \text{ cm})^2} \times 0.59 \frac{R \cdot cm^2}{mCi \cdot h} = 11.8 \text{ R/h or } 11{,}800 \text{ mR/h at 1 cm}$$

Notice how the units of the terms cancel out.

---

* Note: A common Tc99m dose is about 20 mCi. Observe the exposure rate of 11,800 mR/h or 200 mR/min when the dose is unshielded. (See Radiation Protection Section 5, for a demonstration of the effectiveness of shielding radioactive materials.)

B. A 6-mCi dose of Ga67 is left unshielded. If the exposure rate constant is 0.76 R · cm²/mCi · h at 1 cm, what is the exposure rate at 10 cm?

$$X \text{ R/h} = \frac{(6 \text{ mCi})}{(10 \text{ cm})^2} \times 0.76 \frac{\text{R} \cdot \text{cm}^2}{\text{mCi} \cdot \text{h}} = 0.046 \text{ R/h or } 46 \text{ mR/h at } 10 \text{ cm}$$

C. What is the exposure rate from a 0.11-GBq dose of Tl201 at 1 m if the exposure constant is 12.16 μGy · m²/GBq · h?

$$X \text{ μGy/h} = \frac{(0.11 \text{ GBq})}{(1 \text{ m})^2} \times 12.16 \frac{\text{μGy} \cdot \text{m}^2}{\text{GBq} \cdot \text{h}} = 1.3 \text{ μGy/h at } 1 \text{ m}$$

Problems:

1. What is the exposure rate at 1 cm from an unshielded dose containing 15 mCi Tc99m if the exposure constant is 0.59 R·cm²/mCi · h at 1 cm?

2. What is the exposure rate for the dose in Problem 1 at 10 cm? At 1 m?

✻ Note: Note the significant decrease in the exposure rate as the distance from the Tc99m source increases.

---

3. The exposure rate constant for Tl201 is 0.45 R·cm²/mCi · h at 1 cm. What is the exposure rate at 4 cm for an unshielded 3-mCi dose?

4. What is the exposure rate at 15 cm (about 6 in) for a 2-mCi capsule of I123? The exposure constant is 1.55 R · cm²/mCi · h at 1 cm.

5. What is the exposure rate for the same capsule if it was I131 instead, which has an exposure constant of 2.17 R · cm²/mCi · h at 1 cm?

6. A vial of In111 contains 8 mCi. If Γ = 2.05 R·cm²/mCi · h at 1 cm, what is the exposure rate at 3 cm?

7. A Co57 check source with an activity of 0.05 μCi is permanently attached to a Geiger counter. If Γ = 0.56 R · cm²/mCi · h at 1 cm, what is the exposure rate to a technologist who sits 30 cm (about 1 ft) from the unshielded source?

8. While preparing a dose, you drip Tc99m behind the L-block. The spill contains 0.3 mCi. What is your exposure rate at 15 cm above the spot? Γ = 0.59 R · cm²/mCi · h at 1 cm.

References:

Chandra (6ᵗʰ Ed.), p. 169.
Cherry, Sorenson & Phelps (3ʳᵈ Ed.), p. 434.
Harbert & da Rocha, Vol. 2, p. 31–33.
Saha (4ᵗʰ Ed.), p. 211–212.

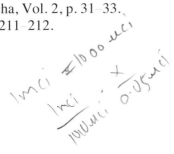

3. Radiation dose versus time

Principles:

There is a direct linear relationship between radiation dose and time. The radiation dose increases in a linear fashion as the time of exposure increases. The dose resulting from exposure is expressed as the total effective dose-equivalent (TEDE) and is measured in rem, mrem, mSv, or μSv.

---

* Note: When dealing with x-rays and gamma rays that have energies greater than 30 keV, R, rad, and rem are essentially equivalent for whole-body exposures. Therefore a survey meter reading of 20 mR/h can be assumed to produce an exposure rate of 20 mrad/h and an effective dose-equivalent of 20 mrem/h. You are usually concerned with measuring exposure (R) for the purpose of determining the radiation dose to workers or patients (effective dose-equivalent, rem, or Sv). Therefore, in this book, rem rather than R will be used, unless the sole focus of the question is a Geiger counter reading, at which time R will be used.

For a detailed explanation and comparison of R, rad, and rem, see the references listed at the end of this section.

III-3 How to calculate the total radiation dose based on the time of exposure:

total dose = (dose rate)(time).

* Note: The dose rate and the time must be expressed in the same units of time. If necessary, convert one to match the other.

Examples:

A. If a technologist is exposed to a source with a dose rate of 3.0 mrem/h for a period of 2 hours, what is the total radiation dose?

(3.0 mrem/h)(2 h) = 6.0 mrem.

B. If the technologist is exposed to the source for 20 minutes, what is total radiation dose?

Convert 3.0 mrem/h to 3.0 mrem/60 min.

$$\left(\frac{3.0 \text{ mrem}}{60 \text{ min}}\right)(20 \text{ min}) = 1.0 \text{ mrem}$$

C. You are next to a source with a dose rate of 15 μSv/h. What will be your total radiation dose if you are exposed for 4 hours?

(15 μSv/h)(4 h) = 60 μSv

Problems:

1. If you are exposed for 50 minutes to a source that has an exposure rate of 3.0 mrem/h, what will your the total radiation dose be?

2. If a source has an exposure rate of 0.35 mrem/h, what is the total radiation dose to a technologist who is exposed for 4 hours?

3. (a) What is the total radiation dose for a technologist who is exposed for 11 minutes to a source with a dose rate of 5.8 mrem/h? (b) What is the total radiation dose if the technologist cuts the exposure time to 6 minutes?

4. An area of undetected contamination has an exposure rate of 3.2 mrem/h. What will be the total radiation dose to a technologist who works over the contamination for 90 minutes?

5. A poorly shielded vial of I131 produces a radiation dose of 35 mrem/h. What is the total radiation dose to a technologist who works beside the source for (a) 10 minutes? (b) 25 minutes?

6. If exposure to a source results in a radiation dose of 16 μSv/h, what is the total radiation dose for a technologist who works next to the source for 2.5 hours?

7. A technologist has worked for 6 minutes with a source that has a dose rate of 85 μSv/h. What is the technologist's total radiation dose for this exposure?

Additional Applications:

➢ **Regulations:** NRC 10CFR20 sets the total effective dose-equivalent (TEDE) for occupationally exposed individuals and members of the general public. Occupationally exposed workers can receive up to 5 rem/y (0.05 Sv or 50 mSv). Members of the general public can receive up to 0.1 rem/y (1.0 mSv). The fetus of an occupationally exposed female is not to receive more than 0.5 rem (5 mSv) during gestation after written declaration of the pregnancy.

8. The department's secretary sits at a desk that is placed next to the wall of the hot lab. The Mo99/Tc99m generator that is stored on the opposite side of the wall from the desk is not sufficiently shielded. The secretary is being exposed to a radiation dose of 1.5 mrem/h. What is her total radiation dose for:

   (a) an 8-hour work day?
   (b) a 40-hour work week?
   (c) 4 weeks at 40 hours per week?

9. As an occupationally exposed worker, the aforementioned secretary is monitored for exposure. (a) On the basis of the above monthly exposure, will she exceed the yearly TEDE limit? (b) If she declares a pregnancy, when will she have to stop working because the TEDE limit for her fetus has been reached?

References:

Chandra (6th Ed.), p. 181.
Cherry, Sorenson & Phelps (3rd Ed.), p. 405–406.
Christian & Waterstram-Rich (6th Ed.), p. 201, 216–219.
Early & Sodee (2nd Ed.), p. 65–67, 323–324.
Iturralde p. 487.
Saha (4th Ed.), p. 189–190, 337–339.
Steves & Wells (3rd Ed.), p. 5.
US NRC 10CFR20.1201, 20.1207, 20.1208, 20.1301

4.   Radiation dose versus distance from source

Principles:

There is an inverse geometric relationship between the radiation dose and the distance from a source of radiation. Radiation is emitted symmetrically from a source, with photons traveling in all directions. The paths of the emissions diverge from one another to a greater degree the farther from the source you move.

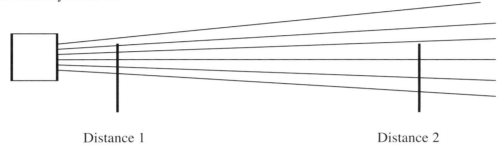

Distance 1   Distance 2

Close to the source, you interact with many emissions. As you move further from the source, the number of interactions drops off rapidly, by the square of the distance. This is referred to as the Inverse Square Law.

This relationship can be expressed by two equations. Any element in the equation can be the unknown (*X*).

1. $\dfrac{I_1}{I_2} = \dfrac{\left(D_2\right)^2}{\left(D_1\right)^2}$ To solve, cross-multiply, then isolate and solve for *X*.

2. $\left(I_1\right)\left(D_1\right)^2 = \left(I_2\right)\left(D_2\right)^2$ This equation is produced when you cross-multiply to solve equation 1. To solve, isolate and solve for *X*.

Both equations will produce the same answer. This author prefers the second equation and will use it here, because experience has shown there is less likelihood of arranging the elements incorrectly.

III-4 How to calculate the radiation dose based on the distance (Inverse Square Law):

$$\left(I_1\right)\left(D_1\right)^2 = \left(I_2\right)\left(D_2\right)^2$$

Where: I_1 = intensity at original distance (D_1)

I_2 = intensity at new distance (D_2)

* **Note:** This is an inverse proportion. (See Basic Math Skills Section 7.)

Examples:

A. You are standing 1 foot from a radioactive source and receiving a radiation exposure dose of 20 mrem/h. If you move to a position 2 feet from the source, what will be your rate of exposure?

$$(20 \text{ mrem/h})(1 \text{ ft})^2 = (2 \text{ ft})^2 (x)$$

Isolate and solve for x: $X = \dfrac{(20 \text{ mrem/h})(1 \text{ ft})^2}{(2 \text{ ft})^2} = \dfrac{20}{4} = 5 \text{ mrem/h}$

---

* **Note:** By doubling the distance you have decreased the exposure rate to one quarter of the original dose rate.

B. If you move to a point 3 feet from the source in Example A, what will be your rate of exposure?

$$(20 \text{ mrem/h})(1 \text{ ft})^2 = (3 \text{ ft})^2 (x)$$

$$x = \dfrac{(20 \text{ mrem/h})(1 \text{ ft})}{9 \text{ ft}} = \dfrac{20}{9} = 2.2 \text{ mrem/h}$$

C. A technologist is standing 6 inches from a radioactive source, which results in an exposure rate of 10 mrem/h. To what distance must the technologist move to decrease the exposure to a background level of 0.05 mrem/h?

$$(6 \text{ in})^2 (10 \text{ mrem/h}) = (x)^2 (0.05 \text{ mrem/h})$$

$$x^2 = \dfrac{(6 \text{ in})^2 (10 \text{ mrem/h})}{0.05 \text{ mrem/h}} = \dfrac{360}{0.05} = 7{,}200$$

$$x^2 = 7{,}200$$

To eliminate the exponent take the square root of each side of the equation.

$$\sqrt{x^2} = \sqrt{7{,}200} \qquad x = 85 \text{ in or} \approx 7 \text{ ft}$$

Problems:

1. When a radioactive source produces 160 mrem/h at 1 meter, what is the exposure rate at 3 meters?

2. If a source produces an exposure rate of 350 mrem/h at 3 inches from the surface, what is the exposure rate at 36 inches?

3. What is the exposure rate from the source in Problem 2 at 6 feet from the surface?

4. If a technologist is exposed to a dose rate of 80 mrem/h when standing 2 feet from a radioactive source, what will be the dose rate at 3 feet from the source?

5. A radioactive source produces 20 mrem/h at 1 foot. How far away must a technologist stand to decrease the exposure rate to 2 mrem/h?

6. If a source produces an exposure rate of 50 mrem/h at 3 inches from the source, how far away must you stand to reduce the exposure rate to 0.5 mrem/h?

7. How far away must you stand from the source in Problem 6 to decrease the exposure rate to 0.05 mrem/h?

Additional Applications:

➤ **Regulations:** NRC 10CFR20 sets the total effective dose-equivalent (TEDE) for workers over the age of 18 at 5 rem/y or 5,000 mrem/y (0.05 Sv/y or 50 mSv/y). For members of the general public, the TEDE is 0.1 rem/y or 100 mrem/y (1.0 mSv/y).

➤ **Regulations:** NRC 10CFR20 requires employees to participate in an **ALARA** program, which strives to minimize radiation exposure to a level **A**s **L**ow **A**s **R**easonably **A**chievable. The suggested level is 10% of the TEDE. Ideally, then, an occupationally exposed worker would receive a whole-body dose of no more than 0.5 rem/y or 500 mrem/y (0.05 Sv/y or 50 mSv/y).

It is important to note that the NRC does not regulate the actual ALARA level, but it does require that one be established by a facility and that a reasonable effort be made to remain below it.

8. a). If you work 1,960 h/y (49 wk × 40 h/wk) and intend to accumulate no more than 10% of the TEDE, what is the maximum average exposure rate in mrem/h to which you should be exposed? (See Radiation Protection, Section 2.)
   b) If you are standing 2 feet from a radiation source that is producing an exposure rate of 1.5 mrem/h, how far must you move from the source to achieve the maximum average exposure that will allow you to maintain ALARA exposure levels?

➤ **Regulations:** NRC 10CFR20 gives the limit for exposure to the extremities as 50 rem/y (0.50 Sv/y or 500 mSv/y).

9. A radiopharmacist has an average exposure rate of 35 mrem/h when not using long-handled tongs for placing doses and vials in a dose calibrator. The source of radioactivity is 1 inch from the hand when tongs are not used. What will the exposure rate be if 12-inch tongs are used?

➤ **Regulations:** According to NRC 10CFR20, members of the public must not receive an exposure from external sources that exceeds 2 mrem (0.02 mSv) in any hour when in an unrestricted area. The NRC expressly states 2 mrem **in any hour** not 2 mrem **per hour**. If 2 mrem per hour was the acceptable limit, then exposure rates could be averaged. The NRC is striving to minimize the public's exposure and therefore requires that exposure in unrestricted areas never exceed 2 mrem (0.02 mSv) in any hour.

10. A sealed generator is placed 12 inches from a wall bordering a public hallway. If readings in the hallway show a person would receive an exposure rate of 3.5 mrem/h, determine how far back the generator must be moved in order to comply with NRC regulations.

11. Weekend deliveries of a generator are made to a hot lab that opens onto a public hallway. If the package produces a dose rate of 100 mrem/h at 2 inches from the package surface, how far from the door must the package be placed when delivered?

References:

Chandra (6th Ed.), p. 169.
Cherry, Sorenson & Phelps (3rd Ed.) , p. 405–406.
Christian & Waterstram-Rich (6th Ed.), p. 68, 71.
Early & Sodee (2nd Ed.), p. 67–71, 323–326, 332.
Saha (4th Ed.), p. 210–211.
Steves & Wells (3rd Ed.), p. 2.
US NRC 10CFR20.1101, 20.1201, 20.1301.
US NRC NUREG-1556.

5. Radiation dose versus shielding

Principles:

Shielding decreases exposure rates according to the thickness and density of the shielding material used, and the type and energy of radiation involved.

The denser the material, the higher the probability that a photon or particle will collide with an atom of the shielding material. By increasing the thickness of shielding, you increase the probability of an interaction because the photon must pass though more atoms before exiting the shield.

A low-energy radionuclide is more likely to lose all its energy to interactions within the shield than high-energy radionuclide. Because of its mass, a beta particle is more likely to interact with shielding material than is a photon. The thickness and density of materials needed to shield betas of a given energy are significantly less than that needed for the same energy photons. Alpha particles will require even less.

The effectiveness of a shielding material is measured in half-value layers (HVL). For example, the HVL of lead is 0.27 mm for the 140 keV photon of Tc99m and 3.0 mm for the 364 keV photon of I131.

Each HVL will decrease the exposure rate to one half its original intensity.

> *** Note:** This is identical to the decrease in activity that occurs with each half-life of a radionuclide.

Number of HVLs	Percent of Original Exposure Rate	Fraction of Original Exposure Rate
0 (in air)	100%	1.0
1	50%	0.50
2	25%	0.25
3	12.5%	0.125
4	6.3%	0.063
5	3.1%	0.031
6	1.6%	0.016
7	0.8%	0.008
8	0.4%	0.004
9	0.2%	0.002
10	0.1%	0.001

> *** Note:** You do not need to memorize this chart, as you can quickly produce it yourself. Each fraction is simply one half of the preceding fraction.

III-5 How to calculate the change in exposure rate due to shielding:

The change in intensity, and therefore exposure rate, can be calculated using the above chart.

1.   Calculate the number of half value layers that have been added.
2.   Use the chart to find the fraction of the original exposure rate.
3.   Multiply the original exposure rate by the fraction.

The following equation is used when fractions of half-value layers are involved.

$$I = I_o e^{-(0.693)(x/\mathrm{HVL})}$$

Where: I   =   exposure rate (intensity) being calculated

   I_O =   original exposure rate (intensity)

   e   =   2.718...
             A constant known as Euler's number. On a scientific calculator, this may be
             represented as either an e^x key or INV ln x. (See Basic Math Skills, Section
             13.) e^x and ln x are the inverse of one another.
             0.693 is the natural log of 2. It represents the halving of values with the
             addition of each HVL. See Cherry Sorenson & Phelps, (3rd Ed.), p. 33 for the
             derivation.

   x =   thickness of shielding material

   HVL   =   half value layer for given shielding material

* Note: Note the similarity of this equation to the radioactive decay equation in Radiopharmacy, Section 1.

Examples:

A.   The half-value layer of lead for Ga67 is 0.10 cm. A vial of Ga67 is stored in a lead shield
     that is 0.7 cm thick. If the exposure rate for the unshielded vial is 730 mR/h, what will it be
     when the vial is placed in the shield?

     Calculate the number of HVLs that have been added: $\dfrac{0.7 \text{ cm}}{0.1 \text{ cm} / \text{HVL}} = 7 \text{ HVL}$.

     Refer to the chart above for the fraction of original exposure rate: 0.008
     Calculate the exposure rate after the vial has been shielded:

     (730 mR/h)(0.008) = 5.8 mR/h

* Note: The same results will be obtained by using the equation $I = I_o e^{-(0.693)(x/\mathrm{HVL})}$. When HVLs are added in whole numbers, the HVL chart is quick and simple. If fractions of HVLs are added, the chart provides an estimate of the exposure rate, but the equation is needed for an accurate determination.

B. The half-value layer of lead for Tc99m is 0.3 mm. If a radiopharmaceutical dose is producing 11 R/h, what will be the exposure rate if the dose is placed in a lead syringe shield that has a thickness of 2.5 mm?

$$I = 11\,\text{R/h}\,e^{-(0.693)\left(\frac{2.5\,\text{mm}}{0.3\,\text{mm}}\right)} = 11e^{-5.775} = (11)(0.0031) = 0.034\,\text{R/h or 34 mR/h}$$

To check this answer, refer to the HVL chart above. The 2.5 mm used for the shield is equivalent to 8 1/3 HVLs. According to the chart, 8 HVLs will decrease the exposure rate to 0.4% of its original intensity.

(0.004)(11 R/h) = 0.044 R/h

Since the actual thickness of lead used is an additional 1/3 HVL thicker, the answer of 0.034 R/h looks reasonable.

C. If a shielded source of I131 gives an exposure rate of 60 mR/h, how many HVLs must be placed in front of it to reduce the rate to 2 mR/h? The half-value layer of lead is 0.30 cm for I131.

$$2\,\text{mR/h} = 60\,\text{mR/h} \times e^{-(0.693)\left(\frac{x\,\text{cm}}{0.3\,\text{cm}}\right)}$$

Isolate the component containing x: $\dfrac{2\,\text{mR/h}}{60\,\text{mR/h}} = e^{-(0.693)\left(\frac{x\,\text{cm}}{0.3\,\text{cm}}\right)}$

To move x out of the exponent take the natural log (ln) of each side of the equation. (Remember the inverse of e^x is the ln of e. See Basic Math Skills Section 14.)

$$0.033 = e^{-(0.693)\left(\frac{x\,\text{cm}}{0.3\,\text{cm}}\right)} \qquad \ln 0.033 = \ln e^{-(0.693)\left(\frac{x\,\text{cm}}{0.3\,\text{cm}}\right)} \qquad -3.4 = -(0.693)\left(\frac{x}{.03}\right)$$

Isolate and solve for x: $x = \dfrac{(-3.4)(0.3)}{-0.693} = 1.5\,\text{cm lead}$

To double check the answer, obtain an estimate using the HVL chart. 2 mR/h is about 3% of 60 mR/h. According to the chart, about 5 HVLs would be needed.

(5 HVL)(0.30 cm/HVL) = 1.5 cm

Problems:

For each of the following problems, assume that the exposure rate is measured at the same distance before and after shielding.

1. A radioactive source produces an exposure rate of 15 mR/h outside a 1-HVL shield. If an additional 2 half-value layers are added, what will the resultant exposure rate be?

2. An unshielded Tc99m vial is generating an exposure rate of 8850 mR/h. What will the exposure rate when the vial is placed in a shield with the thickness of 10 HVLs?

3.   A point source that gives an exposure rate of 0.05 mR/h is stored in a lead container that is 6 HVLs thick. What will be the exposure rate outside the shield?

4.   The half-value layer of lead is 0.27 mm for Tc99m. A dose generates 5,300 mR/h before being shielded. What will be the exposure rate after the dose is placed in a shield made with 0.90 mm of lead?

5.   A thicker shield is to be used for the above dose. The shield is made of 3.8 mm lead. What will be the exposure rate after shielding?

∗ Note: A 3.8-mm shield is only 1/8th inch thick. Observe the dramatic decrease in the exposure rate when the dose is placed in the shield. You should be acutely aware of the impact of shielding.

➤ **Regulations:** NRC 10CFR20 states, "The licensee shall use, to the extent practical, procedures and engineering controls based upon sound radiation protection principles to achieve occupational doses and doses to members of the public that are as low as is reasonably achievable (ALARA)." Therefore, syringe shields must be used whenever doses are being drawn up and injected.

6.   A shielded dose of Tl201 registers as 25 mR/h on an ionization survey meter held 4 inches from the surface. If the HVL for lead is 0.2 mm, what will be the reading at 4 inches after the shielded dose is placed in a lead pig constructed of 1.35-mm-thick lead?

7.   A Mo99 generator produces 90 mR/h at 1/2 meter away from the spot where technologists stand to prepare doses. If lead bricks 9 cm thick are placed in front of the generator, what will be the new exposure rate at 1/2 meter? The HVL of lead for Mo99 is 0.7 cm.

8.   A shielded vial of I131 gives a reading of 30 mR/h at 1 meter. If the vial is placed in a drawer lined with 5 mm of lead, what will the 1-meter exposure rate be? The HVL of lead for I131 is 0.21 mm.

Additional Applications:

9.   A sealed Co57 dose calibrator source produces 0.15 mR/h unshielded at 1 foot from the vial. How many 0.2-mm HVLs must be placed in front of the source in order to decrease the exposure rate to the background level of 0.01 mR/h?

➤ **Regulations:** NRC 10CFR20 requires unrestricted areas of public access to have exposure rates that do not exceed 2 mrem (0.02 mSv) in any hour. This exposure rate from a photon-producing source would be indicated by an ionization survey meter reading of 2 mR/h.

10. A Mo99 generator is located next to a wall shared by a public hallway. The reading in the hallway is 6.4 mR/h. How much shielding must be added to decrease the exposure rate to 2 mR/h? The HVL for Mo99 is 0.7 cm of lead.

11. A survey meter reading taken outside the shield surrounding a radionuclide storage area gives a reading of 12.8 mR/h. Only Tc99m is being stored. The HVL for lead is 0.27 mm.

How much lead must be added to bring the reading down to a background reading of 0.02 mR/h?

References:

Chandra (6th Ed.), p. 5960, 169–170.
Christian & Waterstram-Rich (6th Ed.), p. 14–16.
Early & Sodee (2nd Ed.), p. 79 80.
Saha (4th Ed.), p. 212.
Steves & Wells (3rd Ed.), p. 2–3.
US NRC 10CFR20.1101, 1301.

6. Effective half-life calculations from biological and physical half-lives

Principles:

The effective half-life (T_e) is used to estimate the patient's radiation dose after administration of a radiopharmaceutical. The effective half-life takes into account both the physical and biological half-lives.

The physical half-life (T_p) is immutable. It will be the same regardless of where the radionuclide is, what it is attached to, or the environmental conditions to which it is subjected. The biological half-life (T_b), however, will vary depending upon which pharmaceutical is used. The physical half-life of Tc99m is always 6 hours. However, the biological half-life of a Tc99m-labeled pharmaceutical will be dependent upon the pharmaceutical's behavior within the patient's body.

The biological half-life varies from patient to patient, because it is affected by metabolism, pathological conditions, radiochemical impurities, age, function of the excretory system, etc. The biological half-life, therefore, is an estimate. Because the biological half-life is an estimate, the effective half-life is also an estimate.

The effective half-life combines the physical and biological half-lives in a way that allows a reasonable estimation of the length of time a person is irradiated by a particular radiopharmaceutical.

III-6 How to calculate the effective half-life:

$$T_e = \frac{T_p \times T_b}{T_p + T_b}$$

where: T_e = effective half-life
         T_p = physical half-life
         T_b = biological half-life

Examples:

A. If the physical half-life of a radionuclide is 12 hours and the biological half-life of the pharmaceutical is 4 hours, what is the effective half-life?

$$T_e = \frac{12\,h \times 4\,h}{12\,h + 4\,h} = \frac{48}{16} = 3\,h$$

B. Calculate the effective half-life for radiopharmaceutical *X*.

$$T_p = 75 \text{ hours}$$

$$T_b = 98 \text{ hours}$$

$$T_e = \frac{75\,h \times 98\,h}{75\,h + 98\,h} = \frac{7{,}350}{173} = 42\,h$$

Problems:

1. Calculate the effective half-life for Tc99m albumin colloid using the following data:

$$T_p = 6 \text{ hours}$$

$$T_b = 11 \text{ hours}$$

2. When red blood cells are tagged *in vitro* with Tc99m, the majority have a biological half-life of 29 hours. What is the effective half-life? Tc99m T_p = 6 hours.

3. With a physical half-life of 73 hours and a biological half-life of about 10 days, what is the effective half-life of Tl201 thallous chloride?

4. About 17% of injected Ga67 gallium citrate is excreted from the body with a biological half-life of 30 hours. The remaining 83% has a biological half-life of 25 days. What are the effective half-lives for these two fractions if T_p = 78 hours?

5. Xe133 has a biological half-life of 0.37 minutes in the lungs, where 68% of the administered dose concentrates. What is the T_e if T_p = 5.3 days?

---

* Note: Observe what happens to the effective half-life when the T_p and the T_b are drastically different from one another. When the biological half-life is very short as compared to the physical half-life, then $T_e = T_b$.

The reverse is also true. If the biological half-live is very long compared to the physical half-life, then $T_e = T_p$. For example, Tc99m sulfur colloid is released from the liver cells only when they die. The biological half-life is, therefore, in terms of years, while the physical half-life is 6 hours. The effective half-life would, therefore, be 6 hours.

---

6. When injected, P32 sodium phosphate has a biological half-life of 49 days. With a physical half-life of about 14 days, what is the effective half-life?

7. Orally administered P32 sodium phosphate is excreted more rapidly than the IV preparation. It has a biological half-life averaging 5 days. What is the effective half-life for the orally administered radiopharmaceutical?

References:

Chandra (6th Ed.), p. 24–26.
Christian & Waterstram-Rich (6th Ed.), p. 14.
Early & Sodee (2nd Ed.), p. 41.
Kowalsky & Fallon p. 81, 239–240.

Chapter IV. Instrumentation

1. Calculation of acceptable ranges for dose calibrator accuracy and constancy

Principles:

The dose calibrator accuracy test determines how close a measurement is to the true value. Constancy or precision testing assures the reproducibility of results. If a radiopharmaceutical dose is repeatedly measured in a dose calibrator and very similar activities are obtained each time, then the results are precise. However, the results may or may not be accurate. If a dose is measured while the dose calibrator well is contaminated with radioactive material, then the results may be reproducible (precise) for a period of time, but they are not accurate. They do not represent the true activity of the dose.

> *** Note:**   precision = reproducibility
> accuracy = true value

➤ **Regulations:** NRC 10CFR35 requires calibration of a dose calibrator in accordance with the nationally recognized standard of practice or the manufacturer's instructions.

The standard of practice requires an accuracy test be performed upon installation and annually thereafter. A minimum of two sources should be used and at least one source must produce gamma emissions between 100 keV and 500 keV. The sources must have an activity of not less than 50 μCi and must be certified by the manufacturer as being within 5% of the stated activity. The most commonly used sources are Co57 (122 keV) and Cs137 (662 keV).

The standard of practice also requires constancy testing to be performed at the beginning of each work day. The test must be performed on a frequently used setting and must use a sealed source having an activity of not less than 50 μCi. If a wide range of radionuclides is administered to patients, two or more long-lived sources must be used.

If a facility has a dose calibrator with pre-set channel buttons, such as buttons marked Tc99m, Tl201, Mo99, etc., then each channel should be checked for precision on a daily basis using a long-lived source.

> *** Note:** The daily pre-set channel check does not provide a measurement of accuracy. However, once an initial reading is established for each channel, subsequent readings that fall within plus or minus 10% of the initial reading demonstrate that the setting remains constant.

It is convenient to use the same sources to test for both precision and accuracy. If accuracy is established once a year, then daily constancy measurements of the same sources assure not only precision, but accuracy.

According to the standard of practice a dose calibrator must be replaced or repaired if errors in accuracy or precision exceed ±10%. Some licensees adopt a stricter error limitation of 5%, to assure corrective action will be undertaken before the readings fall outside acceptable levels. If the ±-5% limit is written into the facility's license, then that limit cannot be exceeded even though the percent error is still below standard of practice levels.

IV-1 How to calculate the acceptable range of dose calibrator readings for a given source:

1. Examine the source's label to determine the calibration date and the activity at the time of calibration as certified by the manufacturer.
2. Determine the elapsed time from the calibration date to the specified day.
3. Use a decay calculation to determine the "expected activity" on the specified day. (See Radiopharmacy Sections 1 and 2.)
4. Calculate 10% of the expected activity. X = (expected activity)(0.10)
   If your institution's license specifies a 5% range, then multiply by 0.05, instead of 0.10.
5. To determine the acceptable range, add and subtract 10% or 5% (depending upon your institution's license) from the expected activity.

Examples:

A. Calculate the 10% acceptable range for a 140 µCi source.

   (140 µCi)(0.10) = 14.0 µCi
   140 ± 14.0 = 126–154 µCi

   If the actual dose calibrator accuracy or constancy reading falls within this range, it is acceptable. If it falls below or above these readings the instrument cannot be used until it is repaired.

B. Calculate the 5% acceptable range for a source with an expected activity of 208 µCi.

   (208 µCi)(0.05) = 10.4 µCi
   208 ± 10.4 = 198–218 µCi

Problems:

Calculate the 10% acceptable range for each of the following.

1. 1.34 mCi
2. 195 µCi
3. 62.6 µCi
4. 81.3 µCi

Calculate the 5% acceptable range for each of the following.

5.   260 µCi
6.   148 µCi
7.   90.4 µCi
8.   76.2 µCi

Additional Applications:

9.   If a source contained 153 µCi of Ba133 (T_p = 10.66 y) on June 1, 2005, what would be the 10% acceptable activity range if the source is used for a dose calibrator accuracy test on June 1, 2007? (See Radiopharmacy Sections 1, 2, and 3.)

10. A Co57 (T_p = 270 d) source contained 76.0 µCi on May 1. What is the 5% acceptable range when the source is used for a dose calibrator precision test on May 31?

11. On March 1, 1998, a Cs137 (T_p = 30.0 y) source was calibrated to contain 63.8 µCi. What is the 10% acceptable activity range when the source is used for dose calibrator accuracy testing on March 1, 2006?

12. A Co57 (T_p = 270 d) source is being used for dose calibrator accuracy. It is 90 days since it was certified to contain 122 µCi. Will a reading of 90.2 µCi fall within the 10% acceptable range?

13. A Ba133 (T_p = 10.66 y) source had a certified activity of 96.2 µCi 8 years ago. Will an accuracy test reading of 49.9 µCi fall within the standard acceptable range?

References:

Christian & Waterstram-Rich (6th Ed.), p. 86–88.
Early & Sodee (2nd Ed.), p. 213–214.
Steves & Wells (3rd Ed.), p. 39–40.
US NRC 10CFR35.60.

2. Percent error for dose calibrator accuracy and constancy

Principles:

See Instrumentation Section 1 for an explanation of accuracy and constancy (also called precision) and a description of the NRC regulations and standards of practice that apply to these tests.

IV-2 How to determine the accuracy or constancy of a given dose calibrator reading:

A simple percentage calculation is utilized. (See Statistics Section 1.)

$$\text{percent error or percent difference} = \frac{|\text{expected reading} - \text{actual reading}|}{\text{expected reading}} \times 100\%$$

* Note: Observe that the absolute value of the difference between expected and actual readings is used. If a negative number is obtained in the numerator, the negative sign is simply ignored. Because the absolute value is used, reversing the elements of the numerator will still yield the same % error or % difference.

Examples:

A. What is the percent error in accuracy if the expected dose calibrator reading is 1.35 mCi and the actual reading is 1.26 mCi?

$$\frac{|1.35 \text{ mCi} - 1.26 \text{ mCi}|}{1.35 \text{ mCi}} \times 100\% = 6.67\% \quad \frac{25 \text{ s}}{60 \text{ s/min}} = 0.42 \text{ min}$$

This percent error is within the standard of practice limits, so the dose calibrator can be used.

B. What is the percent error in constancy if the expected activity of a source is 78.5 µCi and the actual activity reading is 70.1 µCi?

$$\frac{|78.5 \text{ } \mu\text{Ci} - 70.1 \text{ } \mu\text{Ci}|}{78.5 \text{ } \mu\text{Ci}} \times 100\% = 10.7\%$$

This percent error exceeds the standard of practice limits, so the dose calibrator cannot be used. It must be repaired or replaced.

---

* Note: When limits are exceeded, you should check the instrument setting, review the calculations, and repeat the test. Human error is a common cause of poor test results. If test results are acceptable, but near the limits, this should be reported to the person responsible for overseeing instrument quality control and maintenance, so early intervention can prevent an emergency situation at a later date.

C. Community Medical Center has written a 5% error limitation into its NRC license. Can a dose calibrator be used if the expected activity of a calibration source is 233 µCi and the actual activity reading is 238 µCi?

$$\frac{|233\,\mu Ci - 238\,\mu Ci|}{233\,\mu Ci} \times 100\% = 2.14\%$$

The percent error falls within the acceptable 5% limitation, so the instrument can be used.

Problems:

Unless otherwise stated, the standard of practice is 10%.

1. The expected value of a dose calibrator accuracy source is 198 µCi and the actual reading is 187 µCi. Does the actual value fall within the 10% acceptable range?

2. If a source reads 1.03 mCi in a dose calibrator when the expected activity is 0.96 mCi, can the instrument be used according to the standard of practice?

3. A dose calibrator source is expected to contain 52.3 µCi. The actual reading is 47.1 µCi when the precision test is performed. Is this acceptable according the standard of practice?

4. A facility's license sets a maximum error of 5% for dose calibrator precision. If the expected activity is 77.3 µCi and the actual reading is 79.6 µCi, is the precision acceptable?

5. Do the results of a dose calibrator accuracy test conform to the standard of practice if the actual reading for a 1.36 mCi source is 1.21 mCi?

6. If 5% precision is required, would a dose calibrator meet the requirement with the following results?

expected reading	97.9 µCi
actual reading	92.1 µCi

Additional Applications:

7. A Cs137 (T_p = 30.0 y) source was calibrated to contain 126 µCi on June 3, 2006. Is a dose calibrator operating with acceptable precision if the activity reading for the source is 116.3 µCi on June 5, 2010?

8. Determine if a dose calibrator precision test conforms to the standard of practice using the following data. A Ba133 source is being used. The half-life of Ba133 is 10.66 years.

calibration date	9-10-80
activity at calibration	154 µCi
current date	9-6-95
current reading	54.8 µCi

9. A dose calibrator was tested for accuracy on June 1, 2009. A Co60 (T_p = 5.26 y) source was used. It was calibrated on March 5, 2007 to contain 80.2 μCi. Did the instrument conform to the standard of practice if the current reading was 53.2 μCi?

10. Memorial Hospital uses a Cs137 (T_p = 30.0 y) source to evaluate dose calibrator accuracy. The source contained 85.2 μCi on April 15, 1992, and gave a reading of 58.2 μCi on August 14, 2010. Did the dose calibrator's performance conform to the standard of practice?

References:

Early & Sodee (2nd Ed.), p. 213–214.
O'Connor, p. 48–49.
Steves & Wells (3rd Ed.), p. 39–40.

3. Dose calibrator geometry and percent error for syringes

Principles:

➢ **Regulations:** 10CFR35 requires calibration of a dose calibrator in accordance with the nationally recognized standard of practice or the manufacturer's instructions.

The standard of practice requires a dose calibrator be tested for geometry dependence when it is installed and after repairs. Because geometric dependence is very stable, more frequent testing is not necessary.

Testing must cover the range of volumes and volume configurations for which it will be used. Volume ranges refer to the various volumes used in radiopharmaceutical vials (see Instrumentation Section 4), while volume configurations refer to the different sizes of syringes used to administer patient doses.

The percent error of an expected reading is determined.

According to the standard of practice, a correction factor must be calculated if the error exceeds plus or minus 10%. The correction factor must be applied each time that size syringe or volume is used. (See Instrumentation Section 6.) Some licensees adopt a stricter error limitation of 5%. If this limit is written into the facility's license, then a correction factor must be utilized when the ±5% limit is exceeded.

IV-3 How to determine dose calibrator geometry dependence for a particular size syringe:

1. Place 2 to 20 mCi of Tc99m sodium pertechnetate in a vial.
2. Determine the actual activity using the dose calibrator.
3. Using the syringe to be tested, withdraw a commonly used activity in a commonly used volume.
4. Measure the activity in the syringe and the activity remaining in the vial.
5. Calculate the expected reading for the dose in the syringe:
    expected activity of dose = vial activity before dose – vial activity after dose
6. Calculate the percent error. (See Statistics Section 1.)

$$\% \text{ error} = \frac{|\text{expected reading} - \text{actual reading}|}{\text{expected reading}} \times 100\%$$

7. Some protocols require the measuring of several volumes for each syringe size.

---

* Note: Various volumes for a particular size syringe can also be tested using the same method used to check geometry dependence for vials. (See Instrumentation Section 4.) However, care must be taken not to lose any of the radioactive material as the incremental volumes are added to the syringe, as this would invalidate the test.

Examples:

A. During geometry testing the following results are obtained for a 3-ml syringe. What is the percent error for this size syringe?

    original activity in vial   46.8 mCi
    remaining activity in vial after withdrawal of dose   25.9 mCi
    actual syringe activity   20.2 mCi

    Calculate the expected reading: 46.8 mCi – 25.9 mCi = 20.9 mCi

    Apply data to percent error equation: $\dfrac{|20.9 \text{ mCi} - 20.2 \text{ mCi}|}{20.9 \text{ mCi}} \times 100\% = 3.3\%$

    This percent error is acceptable according to the standard of practice 10% tolerance.

B. A 5-ml syringe is typically used to draw up Tc99m HMPAO tagged white blood cells for reinjection. Given the following data, determine the percent error attributable to syringe geometry.

    original activity in vial   31.6 mCi
    remaining activity in vial after withdrawal of dose   17.2 mCi
    actual syringe activity   12.8 mCi

    Calculate the expected reading: 31.6 mCi – 17.2 mCi = 14.4 mCi

    Apply data to percent error equation: $\dfrac{|14.4 \text{ mCi} - 12.8 \text{ mCi}|}{14.4 \text{ mCi}} \times 100\% = 11\%$

    The percent error exceeds the standard of practice limitation of 10%, so a correction factor must be calculated and applied whenever a 5-ml syringe is used to administer a patient dose. (See Instrumentation Section 6.)

Problems:

Unless otherwise stated, the standard of practice is 10%.

1. Calculate the percent error due to geometry for a 3-ml syringe.

    original vial activity   94.5 mCi
    vial activity after dose   71.7 mCi
    syringe activity   21.6 mCi

2. Would a correction factor be needed for a 5-ml syringe if the following data were obtained during geometry testing?

    vial before dose   52.3 mCi
    vial after dose   41.9 mCi
    syringe activity   9.7 mCi

3. Determine if a correction factor is needed for a 3-ml syringe based on the results of a geometry test.

vial before dose	67.1 mCi
vial after dose	44.9 mCi
syringe activity	19.3 mCi

4. Use the following geometry test data to determine if a correction factor is needed.

vial before dose	33.8 mCi
vial after dose	24.3 mCi
syringe activity	10.6 mCi

5. A dose calibrator is being tested for dependence on geometry. Would a correction factor be needed if a syringe measured 5.5 mCi, and the vial measured 57.6 mCi before the dose was withdrawn and measured 52.3 mCi afterward?

6. Determine if a correction factor is needed for a 5-ml syringe based on the results of a geometry test.

vial before dose	112.3 mCi
vial after dose	66.7 mCi
syringe activity	44.9 mCi

References:

Christian & Waterstram-Rich (6th Ed.), p. 87.
Early & Sodee (2nd Ed.), p. 213–214.
NRC 10CFR35.60.
O'Connor, p. 53.
Steves & Wells (3rd Ed.), p. 40–41.

4. Dose calibrator geometry and percent error for vials

Principles:

See Instrumentation Section 3 for an explanation of geometry and a description of the NRC regulations and the standards of practice that apply.

IV-4 How to calculate the percent error in dose calibrator readings for various volumes within a vial:

1. Place 2 to 10 mCi of Tc99m in a very small volume (1–2 drops) in a 30-ml vial.
2. Assay the activity in the dose calibrator.
3. Add 2 ml saline, agitate to mix, and assay.
4. Continue to add saline in 2-ml increments, until a volume of 20 ml or more is reached. Agitate and assay after each addition.
5. Calculate the percent error for each volume using the following equation. Typically the 4- or 8-ml volume reading is used as the reference (expected value) to which all other volumes are compared.

$$\% \text{ error} = \frac{\left|\text{expected reading} - \text{actual reading}\right|}{\text{expected reading}} \times 100\%$$

(See Statistics Section 1.)

Examples:

A. Using the following data, determine if volume affects geometry for a volume of 10 ml. The 8-ml reading is used as the reference value (expected reading).

    8 ml   2.04 mCi
    10 ml   1.98 mCi

$$\frac{\left|2.04 \text{ mCi} - 1.98 \text{ mCi}\right|}{2.04 \text{ mCi}} \times 100\% = 2.9\%$$

According to the standard of practice (±10%), the percent error is acceptable.

B. A 2-ml volume gives a reading of 2.26 mCi. If the 4-ml volume, which is being used as the reference point of a geometry test, gives a reading of 2.10 mCi, what is the percent error for the 2-ml volume?

$$\frac{\left|2.10 \text{ mCi} - 2.26 \text{ mCi}\right|}{2.10 \text{ mCi}} \times 100\% = 7.6\%$$

The percent error is within the standard of practice tolerance (±10%).

Problems:

Unless otherwise stated, the standard of practice is 10%.

1. The 4-ml volume is being used as the reference (expected value) for a dose calibrator geometry test. If the 20-ml volume gives a reading of 2.34 and the 4-ml volume gives a reading of 2.63 mCi, is a correction factor needed when a 20-ml volume is used?

2. During a dose calibrator geometry test, the 8-ml reference produced a reading of 1.94 mCi and the 6-ml volume produced a reading of 1.89 mCi. What is the percent error? Is a correction factor needed?

3. If the 8-ml reference is read as 2.71 mCi and the 16-ml volume is read as 2.60 mCi, will a correction factor be needed when a 16-ml solution is measured in the dose calibrator?

4. Determine if a 20-ml volume is affected by geometry when measured in the dose calibrator.

10-ml reference	2.06 mCi
20-ml solution	1.84 mCi

5. What is the percent error produced when a 2-ml sample is measured in a dose calibrator? The 8-ml volume is used as the geometry test standard.

8-ml reference	2.43 mCi
2-ml solution	2.26 mCi

6. A 16-ml volume produces a reading of 1.69 mCi during a dose calibrator geometry test. If the reference solution gives a reading of 1.73 mCi, will a correction factor be needed when a 16-ml volume is used?

7. What is the percent error caused by geometry when an 18-ml volume is measured in a dose calibrator? The 18-ml volume provides a reading of 2.17 mCi and the 4-ml reference gives a reading of 2.38 mCi. Is this an acceptable level according to the standard of practice?

8. The following data were acquired during a dose calibrator geometry test. Is a correction factor needed when a 4-ml solution is calibrated?

8-ml reference	2.17 mCi
4-ml solution	2.30 mCi

References:

Christian & Waterstram-Rich, (6th Ed.), p. 87.
Early & Sodee, (2nd Ed.), p. 213–214.
O'Connor, p. 53.
Steves & Wells (3rd Ed.), p. 40–41.
US NRC 10CFR35.60.

5. Dose calibrator linearity of response and percent error

Principles:

Dose calibrator linearity of response refers to the accuracy of readings over a wide range of activities.

➤ **Regulations:** 10CFR35 requires calibration of a dose calibrator in accordance with the nationally recognized standard of practice or the manufacturer's instructions.

The standard of practice specifies the range as the highest activity to be measured in the dose calibrator down to 30 μCi or less.

> *** Note:** In a department that uses a generator, the highest amount of Tc99m activity is likely to be the first generator eluate. In a department that uses bulk Tc99m, the highest activity is likely to be the bulk vial upon its arrival. In a department that uses only unit doses, the highest activity will be the highest patient dosage administered. If large I131 therapeutic dosages are used, this activity will need to be considered when determining the highest activity.

According to the standard of practice, linearity is to be tested upon installation, after repair, and at least quarterly. If an error greater than 10% is found, then a correction factor must be applied each time a dose of that level is measured. (See Instrumentation, Section 6.) Some licensees adopt a stricter error limitation of 5%, to assure corrective action will be undertaken before the readings fall outside acceptable levels. If the 5% limit is written into the facility's license, then that limit cannot be exceeded even though the percent error is still below standard of practice level.

There are two methods for testing linearity of response: the decay method and the shielding or attenuation method (lineator).

For the decay method, an activity of Tc99m is measured at various time intervals with pre-calibration and decay factors applied to determine expected values. Intervals such as 6, 12, 24, 30, 48, and 72 hours are chosen to provide a wide range of activities. The test must be continued until the activity being measured is equal to or less than 30 μCi. The percent error of each reading is calculated, as shown in Shadowbox IV-5.

Usually the 30-hour activity is used as the reference, so pre-calibration and decay factors for each time interval are applied to the 30-hour activity to determine the expected value as shown on the chart below.

Time interval from initial measurement	Time interval from 30-hour activity	Pre-calibration (PCF) or decay factor (DF) applied to 30-hour activity to determine expected activity
Initial activity	−30	PCF = 32
6 hours	−24	PCF = 16
12 hours	−18	PCF = 8
24 hours	−6	PCF = 2
30 hours	0	N/A
48 hours	+18	DF = 0.125
52 hours	+24	DF = 0.0625
72 hours	+42	DF = 0.0078

* **Note:** The exact timing of the intervals is not important, so long as the correct pre-calibration or decay factor is used. For example, your protocol specifies a 48-hour interval, but you are not able to make the measurement until 48.5 hours have passed. You can still perform the test, but the 18.5-hour decay factor must be used. (Refer to the table above to see that 48 h is 18 h after the 30-h reference measurement, so the decay factor is figured from the time of that measurement.) Using the 18-hour decay factor instead of 18.5 hours will produce erroneous results.

The activity from each interval can also be plotted on a semilogrithmic graph. The x-axis is time and the y-axis is activity. A best fit line is generated. Using the point furthest from the best fit line, the percent error is determined. If the error is within the acceptable limit, the instrument passes.

For the shielding method, a source containing Tc99m is placed in the dose calibrator. Shields of various thicknesses and in specified combinations are placed around the source and readings obtained. The shields are engineered to attenuate the activity to a specific degree providing activities over a wide range. Factors are applied to the readings depending upon which shields are used. The percent error for each reading is calculated.

The shielding method allows for more rapid evaluation of linearity. It must, however, be performed rapidly, so the decay of the radionuclide does not affect the results.

On first use of the shields, the decay method must be performed at the same time to prove accurate correlation between the two methods. Thereafter, the shielding method alone is acceptable, unless damage to the shields is suspected.

The calculations needed for the shield test vary according to manufacturer, so they will not be discussed here. Complete instructions should accompany the shields.

IV-5 How to determine linearity of response for a dose calibrator using the Tc99m decay method:

1. An activity similar to the highest patient dose administered is placed in a vial and assayed in the dose calibrator at time zero.
2. The vial is assayed repeatedly at specific intervals until the activity reaches 30 μCi or less.
3. Usually the 30-hour activity is used as the reference. Pre-calibration and decay factors for each time interval are applied to the 30-hour activity to determine the expected value. (See Radiopharmacy Sections 1 and 2, and the table above.)
4. Calculate the percent error for each activity level (i.e. time interval):

$$\% \text{ error} = \frac{|\text{expected reading} - \text{actual reading}|}{\text{expected reading}} \times 100\%$$

(See Statistics Section 1.)

Examples:

A.   The expected activity for a 48-hour linearity test reading is 158 μCi. The actual reading is
     175 μCi. What is the percent error at this level of activity?

$$\frac{|158\,\mu Ci - 175\,\mu Ci|}{158\,\mu Ci} \times 100\% = 10.8\%$$

The percent error exceeds the standard of practice of 10%, so a correction factor must be
used each time a dose of this level is measured. (See Instrumentation Section 6.)

B.   At the 6-hour interval, the dose calibrator reading was 76.3 mCi. The 30-hour interval
     reading was 4.84 mCi. What is the expected activity for the 6-hour interval? What is the
     percent error at this level of activity?

The 6-hour interval is 24 hours prior to the 30-hour interval, so the 24-hour pre-calibration
factor is applied to the 30-hour interval activity. PFC = 16 (see table above).

Expected activity at 6-hour interval: (4.84 mCi)(16) = 77.4 mCi

Percent error: $\dfrac{|77.4\,\text{mCi} - 76.3\,\text{mCi}|}{77.4\,\text{mCi}} \times 100\% = 1.4\%$

According to the standard of practice this percent error is acceptable.

Problems:

Use the table above to find the appropriate pre-calibration or decay factors when needed.
Unless otherwise stated, the standard of practice is 10%.

1.   A decayed source is expected to produce an activity of 37.2 mCi during a dose calibrator
     linearity test. The actual reading is 37.6 mCi. What is the percent error?

2.   A linearity source is expected to produce a reading of 45.3 mCi, but reads 40.1 mCi instead.
     What is the percent error? Will a correction factor be needed?

3.   If the expected activity of a linearity source is 8.6 mCi and the actual reading is 8.0, what is
     the percent error? Will a correction factor be needed?

4.   Will a correction factor be needed if a linearity source reads 26.1 μCi as opposed to the
     expected value of 29.2 μCi?

5.   A linearity source should give a reading of 95.4 μCi. The actual reading is 96.8 μCi. Is a
     correction factor needed?

6.   If the 30-hour interval reading is 3.28 mCi and the 8-hour-interval reading is 375 μCi, what
     is the percent error at the 48-hour interval?

7.   The 30-hour interval activity of a linearity source is 2.85 mCi. What is the percent error if a
     reading of 5.45 mCi is obtained at the 24-hour interval?

8.   A linearity source read 154.2 mCi at 8:00 am on Monday and the reading at 2:00 pm Tuesday (the 30-h reference) was 4.72 mCi. What is the percent error for the linearity reading from Monday?

9.   The 30-hour reading of a linearity source was 1.74 mCi on Wednesday at 1:00 pm. If the dose calibrator readout for the source was 28.8 mCi at 1:00 pm on Tuesday, is a correction factor needed?

References:

Christian & Waterstram-Rich (6th Ed.), p. 87.
Early & Sodee (2nd Ed.), p. 211 212.
O'Connor, p. 49–52.
Steves & Wells (3rd Ed.), p. 40.
US NRC 10CFR35.60.

6. Calculation and use of correction factors for dose calibrator geometry and linearity

Principles:

When dose calibrator linearity or geometry tests exceed the standard of practice tolerance of 10%, a correction factor must be applied to any subsequent doses of that activity or particular geometry. Some licensees adopt a stricter error limitation of 5%, to assure corrective action will be undertaken before the readings fall outside acceptable levels. If the 5% limit is written into the facility's license, then that limit cannot be exceeded even though the percent error is still below standard of practice level.

IV-6 How to calculate a correction factor:

$$\text{correction factor} = \frac{\text{expected activity}}{\text{actual activity}}$$

* Note: If you have trouble remembering this equation, you can easily figure it out. If the actual value is less than the expected value, then the correction factor must be greater than 1. In other words, the actual value must be made larger, and this can only be done by multiplying it by a number greater than 1.

If the actual value is greater than the expected value, then the correction factor must be less than 1. The actual value must be made smaller to achieve accuracy. Multiplying it by a number less than 1 will cause the actual value to decrease.

IV-7 How to apply a correction factor:

When a dose is calibrated, it is then multiplied by the appropriate correction factor to obtain the accurate activity reading.

true activity = (actual activity reading)(correction factor)

Examples:

A. The expected reading for a geometry test on a 5-ml syringe was 2.95 mCi. The actual reading was 2.63 mCi. Calculate the correction factor.

$$\frac{2.95 \text{ mCi}}{2.63 \text{ mCi}} = 1.12$$

* Note: As with decay factors, correction factors have no units.

B. If a correction factor of 1.18 is required for a 5-ml syringe, what will be the true activity of a dose with a reading of 12.6 mCi?

(12.6 mCi)(1.18) = 14.9 mCi

Problems:

1. Calculate the correction factor for the 10-µCi dose level if the expected value is 8.04 µCi and the actual value is 9.83 µCi.

2. A 1-ml syringe gives a reading of 0.35 µCi when the expected activity is 0.39 µCi. Determine the correction factor.

3. The lineated activity of a source is expected to be 847 µCi. The actual reading is 937 µCi. What correction factor should be used?

4. A volume of 20 ml is expected to have an activity of 5.63 mCi. What correction factor should be used if the actual reading is 4.99 mCi?

5. What would be the true activity of a 522-µCi dose if a correction factor of 0.89 is required at this level of activity?

6. If a correction factor of 1.16 is required, what is the true activity of a 76.8-µCi dose?

7. A correction factor of 0.84 is used for a 1-ml syringe. What is the true activity of a dose measuring 45.2 µCi?

8. A 2-ml volume requires the use of a correction factor of 1.17. If the actual reading is 8.23 mCi, what is the true activity?

Additional Applications:

9. For doses greater than 100 mCi, a correction factor of 1.19 is used. A therapeutic I131 dose of 120 mCi is needed. If the dose measures 120.8 mCi prior to correction, how much activity is being administered?

10. A minimum activity of 200 µCi is needed for a pediatric study. If the dose calibrator reading is 206 µCi and a correction factor of 0.87 is required, what is the true dose? Does this dose fall below the recommended minimum?

References:

Christian & Waterstram-Rich (6th Ed.), p. 87.
Early & Sodee (2nd Ed.), p. 212–213.
Steves & Wells (3rd Ed.), p. 40–41.

7. Energy resolution (full width at half-maximum)

Principles:

The energy resolution test evaluates the sharpness of a photopeak produced when a scintillation instrument is exposed to a monoenergetic radionuclide. A relatively sharp, bell-shaped peak indicates proper functioning of the equipment. Widening of the bell indicates a malfunction of some system component, such as inconsistent multiplication of electrons in the photomultiplier (PM) tubes; a breakdown of the crystal-to-PM tube seal; or deterioration of the crystal.

In order to evaluate energy resolution, a long-lived, monoenergetic source such as Cs137 is used. Its gamma photopeak (E_γ) occurs at 662 keV.

The source is measured over a wide range of energies and the data are graphed. The width of the resulting peak is measured at half the peak's height. The percent energy resolution is calculated as shown below. According to the standard of practice, the percent energy resolution should fall between 8% and 12% for Cs137.

---

* Note: A peak that is too narrow is unacceptable, as is a peak that is too wide. Even under normal circumstances, there is a certain amount of incomplete energy absorption by the crystal; small discrepancies in the number of electrons produced by the dynodes; instances of coincidental photon events; and other inherent electronic inconsistencies that result in a widening of the peak from its theoretical spike. If the photopeak is too sharp, it suggests that normal events are not being detected and/or reproduced properly.

IV-8 How to determine energy resolution:

1. Measure a Cs137 source starting at about 100 units below the 662-keV photopeak and ending about 100 units above it, using a 20-unit window.
2. Graph the data with the energy on the x-axis and the number of counts on the y-axis.
3. Determine the half-maximum or half the height of the peak:

$$half - maximum = \frac{maximum\ counts}{2}$$

4. Find the half-maximum count on the y-axis of the chart and draw a line from the half-maximum point on the y-axis through both sides of the bell curve.
5. Drop lines to the x-axis from the points where the half-maximum line and the bell curve intersect on both the upward and downward slopes of the bell curve. The x-axis values mark the limits of the full width at half-maximum (FWHM).
6. To calculate the spread at FWHM: upper limit − lower limit = FWHM in keV
7. Apply the FWHM to the percent energy resolution equation:

$$\%\ energy\ resolution = \frac{FWHM\ in\ keV}{energy\ of\ radionuclide\ in\ keV} \times 100\%$$

Examples:

A. Calculate the percent energy resolution for the following peak that was produced with a Cs137 source. $E_\gamma = 662$ keV.

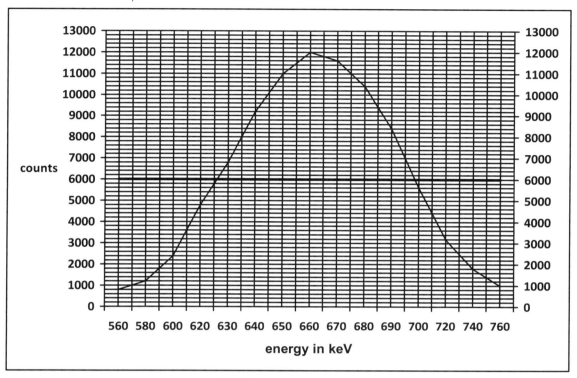

Determine the half-maximum: $\dfrac{12,000 \text{ counts}}{2} = 6,000$ counts

Determine the energies at half-maximum and calculate FWHM: $698 - 626 = 72$ keV

Calculate the percent energy resolution: $\dfrac{72 \text{ keV}}{662 \text{ keV}} \times 100\% = 10.9\%$

This value is within the acceptable range.

Problems:

1. The energy range at half-maximum for a Cs137 source is from 635 keV to 689 keV. What is the percent energy resolution, and is it acceptable?

2. Determine the percent energy resolution for Cs137 when the energy spread at half-maximum is 611 keV to 713 keV. Is the instrument performing within standard limits?

3. If the energy spread for Cs137 is 630 keV to 694 keV at half-maximum, does the instrument have an acceptable percent energy resolution?

4. Determine if the percent energy efficiency for Cs137 is acceptable using the following graph.

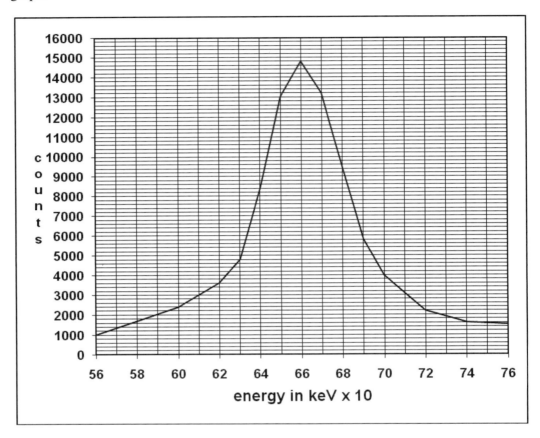

5. A Cs137 source produced the following energy resolution curve. Is it within acceptable standards?

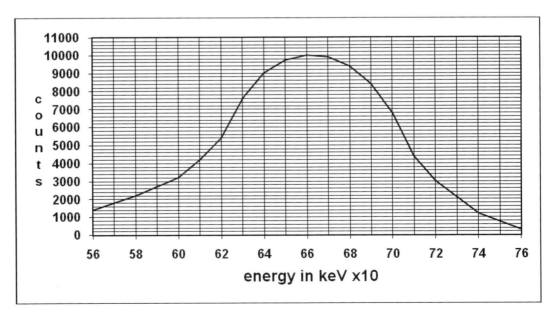

6. Using the Cs137 energy resolution graph below, determine if the instrument meets the standard limits for the test.

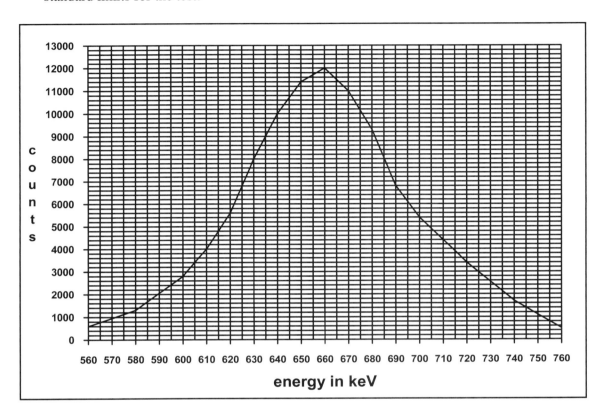

References:

Chandra (6th Ed.), p. 79, 89–90.
Cherry, Sorenson & Phelps (3rd Ed.), p. 230–231.
Christian & Waterstram-Rich (6th Ed.), p. 64, 71, 87.
Early & Sodee (2nd Ed.), p. 165–167, 179.
Steves & Wells (3rd Ed.), p. 41–42.

8.   Well counter or uptake probe constancy (precision) using chi square

Principles:

A series of data obtained by counting a single radioactive sample repeatedly will always demonstrate variation. To determine if the variation is due to the natural randomness of radioactive decay or is due to inconsistency in instrument performance, a chi-square test is performed.

The chi-square test allows you to determine how close a series of counts would come to a true Poisson distribution. (See Statistics Section 5.) It provides a measure of the precision or the constancy of an instrument's performance.

Since it is time consuming and inconvenient to count every patient test sample multiple times, you would want to be certain that an instrument was supplying a reliable value for a single or duplicate sample count. If the instrument passes the chi-square test, then individual values can be used with confidence.

After calculating the chi-square (χ^2), its P value is obtained using a chi-square table. The P value indicates the acceptability of the data variation based on a Poisson distribution.

Chi-Square Table
(See Appendix B for an expanded Chi-Square Table.)

Degrees of Freedom	$P = 0.95$	$P = 0.90$	$P = 0.50$	$P = 0.10$	$P = 0.05$
4	0.711	1.064	3.357	7.779	9.488
9	3.325	4.168	8.343	14.684	16.919
14	6.571	7.790	13.339	21.064	23.685
19	10.117	11.651	18.338	27.204	30.144

* Note: Some chi-square charts are based on the number of determinations used instead of the degrees of freedom. In that case you would refer to the line using 10 determinations to find the acceptable P value range rather than 10-1. (See the note concerning degrees of freedom that follows Shadowbox II-8.)

For the purpose of testing a well counter or an uptake probe, the χ^2 is acceptable if it falls between P values of 0.9 and 0.1.

A P value of 0.5 shows the variation in data are exactly as expected according to the Poisson distribution.

A P value that falls below 0.1 indicates that it is unlikely the variation produced by the instrument would match a Poisson distribution. The variation appears to be too great. Instrument malfunction must be considered.

A P value that exceeds 0.9 is probably too good to account for randomness. Electrical background noise could contribute to lack of variation.

If the chi-square value falls between a *P* value of 0.9 and 0.1 it is acceptable to use a single or small number of values when counting a radioactive sample. It can be assumed that a single value has an acceptably high probability of falling within the normal Poisson distribution that would be produced by obtaining a large number of counts from the sample.

IV-9 How to determine precision using the chi-square value:

1. Obtain at least 10 counts of at least 10,000 counts each.

* **Note:** Sample count values for a chi-square test should be 10,000 or greater to assure statistical reliability. (See Statistics Sections 8 and 9.) A sample count is obtained at 10,000 counts, then the instrument is set to stop at that preset time.

2. Calculate chi-square (χ^2) using either equation:

$$\chi = \frac{\sum \left(n - \bar{n}\right)^2}{\bar{n}} \quad \text{or} \quad \chi = (N-1)\frac{(SD)^2}{\bar{n}} \quad \text{(See Christian or Cherry for derivation.)}$$

Where: Σ is the summation symbol, which indicates that the values immediately following the symbol are to be summed

   n = individual values

   $\bar{\eta}$ = mean value

   N   = number of values used

   SD   = standard deviation (See Statistics, Section 5.)

* **Note:** The second equation is particularly easy if a scientific calculator is used that has statistical functions. In order for the two equations to produce identical results, the standard deviation key using n-1 weighting must be used. If the SD key using n weighting is used, the results will be lower than with the traditional n-1 weighting method. (See Statistics Section 5.)

3. The value of χ^2 is applied to the chi-square table according to the degrees of freedom used.

   Degrees of Freedom = N-1, where N = the number of values used.

Although many nuclear medicine departments now have computer programs that will calculate the chi-square, manual calculation with a pocket calculator is simple if you use the step-by-step method demonstrated in Examples A and B.

First calculate the mean ($\bar{n}$), then calculate $n - \bar{n}$ for each value, and square the number $\left(n - \bar{n}\right)^2$. Calculate the sum of the $\left(n - \bar{n}\right)^2$ values, then solve chi-square equation.

Calculators with standard deviation function keys allow use of the even simpler equation shown in the shadowbox and demonstrated in both examples.

Examples:

A. Calculate the χ^2 for the following data that was obtained from a sample counted in a well counter. Determine if the variation in counts is acceptable.

	n	$n - \bar{n}$	$\left(n - \bar{n}\right)^2$
1	14,231	45	2,025
2	14,103	−83	6,889
3	14,267	81	6,561
4	14,391	205	42,025
5	14,088	−98	9,604
6	14,219	33	1,089
7	14,112	−74	5,476
8	14,097	−89	7,921
9	14,183	−3	9
10	14,166	−20	400

$$\Sigma\, n = 141,857 \qquad\qquad \Sigma\left(n - \bar{n}\right)^2 = 81,999$$

$$\bar{n} = \frac{14,1857}{10} = 14,186 \qquad\qquad \chi = \frac{\Sigma\left(n - \bar{n}\right)^2}{\bar{n}} = \frac{81,999}{14,186} = 5.780$$

OR

Use the standard deviation function keys on your calculator and apply the results to the simplified equation:

$$(9)\frac{(95.451)^2}{14,186} = (9)\frac{9,110.9}{14,186} = 5.780$$

Degrees of Freedom = N–1   10–1 = 9

Refer to the chi-square table on page 122. At 9 degrees of freedom, 5.780 falls between the *P* values 0.9 and 0.1, which are 4.168 to 14.684, respectively. It is therefore acceptable.

B. Calculate the chi-square value for counts acquired with a thyroid uptake probe. Is instrument precision acceptable?

	n	$n - \bar{n}$	$(n - \bar{n})^2$
1	12,512	247	61,009
2	12,535	270	72,900
3	12,257	−8	64
4	12,126	−139	19,321
5	12,223	−42	1,764
6	12,167	−98	9,604
7	12,196	−69	4,761
8	12,265	0	0
9	12,142	−123	15,129
10	12,228	−37	1,369

$\Sigma\, n = 122{,}651$ $\qquad\qquad$ $\Sigma\left(n - \bar{n}\right)^2 = 185{,}921$

$$\bar{n} = \frac{12{,}2651}{10} = 12{,}265 \qquad \chi = \frac{\sum\left(n - \bar{n}\right)^2}{\bar{n}} = \frac{18{,}5921}{12{,}265} = 15.159$$

$$\text{OR}$$

Use the standard deviation function keys on your calculator and apply the results to the simplified equation:

$$(9)\frac{(143.728)^2}{12{,}265} = (9)\frac{20{,}657.9}{12{,}265} = 15.159$$

Degrees of Freedom = N–1   10–1 = 9

Refer to the chi-square table (Appendix B). At 9 degrees of freedom 15.159 falls above the *P* value for 0.1, which is 14.684. It is therefore unacceptable.

Problems:

1. A well counter gave the following results for a Cs137 stick source. Calculate the chi-square and determine its acceptability.

13,777	13,715
13,765	13,529
13,575	13,557
13,511	13,783
13,615	13,678

2. The following data were obtained when a vial of Co57 standard was counted in a well counter. Is the chi-square value acceptable?

11,553	11,610
11,721	11,412
11,773	11,569
11,628	11,395
11,580	11,672

3. Do the values obtained from an uptake probe meet standard chi-square limits?

13,824	13,829
13,787	13,754
13,815	13,793
13,776	13,793
13,762	13,792

4. The following counts were obtained from a well counter using a Cs137 stick source. Is the chi-square value acceptable?

10,867	10,112
9,817	10,456
10,621	9,954
10,328	10,473
9,992	10,373

5. What is the chi-square value for a well counter that produced the following values for a long-lived sealed source? Is instrument precision acceptable?

11,148	11,126
11,126	11,255
11,356	11,254
11,141	11,139
11,211	11,116

References:

Cherry, Sorenson & Phelps (3rd Ed.), p. 140–142.
Christian & Waterstram-Rich (6th Ed.), p. 25–27.
Early & Sodee (2nd Ed.), p. 189–193.
Steves & Wells (3rd Ed.), p. 42, Appendix B.

9. Well counter efficiency

Principles:

   A calculation of well counter efficiency determines the percentage of emissions produced by a radioactive source that are actually detected by the instrument.

➢ **Regulations:** DOT 49CFR173.443 requires the results of wipe tests to be reported in disintegrations per minute (dpm). In order to convert counts per minute (cpm) to dpm, you must know the efficiency of the well counter.

---

* Note: It is not necessary to know the efficiency when performing tests that compare patient samples to a standard. If samples and standards are counted with the same geometry and compared to one another in a single equation, values in the form of dpm are not needed. The instrument's efficiency, therefore, need not be known.

   Calculation of the efficiency requires a source of known activity. Sealed sources with activities calibrated and guaranteed by the manufacturer are commonly used.

   The proportion of emissions occurring at the selected energy must also be known (mean number per disintegration).

IV-10 How to calculate well counter efficiency:

$$\%\text{efficiency} = \frac{\text{counts per unit time}}{(\text{disintegrations per unit time})(\text{mean number per disintegration})} \times 100\%$$

Where: counts per unit time   =   cpm or cps produced by source during preset time
          disintegrations per unit time   =   dpm or dps produced by the activity (μCi) used
                                                                     for the test
          mean number per disintegration =   abundance of emissions at selected energy setting
                                                                     in decimal form

To determine the disintegrations per unit time, multiply the μCi of activity used by the dpm or dps for 1 μCi.

* Note: The units of time in the numerator and denominator must match. If you use cpm in the numerator, then dpm must be used in the denominator. 1 μCi $= 3.7 \times 10^4$ dps . To convert dps to dpm: (3.7×10^4 dps)(60 s) $= 2.22 \times 10^6$ dpm or 2,220,000 dpm/μCi.

Examples:

A. The current activity of Cs137 stick source is 0.2 μCi. Cs137 has an 85% abundance at 662 keV. A 1-minute acquisition produces 1,750,000 counts. What is the well counter efficiency?

Convert 85% to its decimal form: 0.85.

$$\frac{175,000 \text{ cpm}}{(0.2 \ \mu\text{Ci})(2,220,000 \text{ dpm/}\mu\text{Ci})(0.85)} \times 100\% = 46\%$$

---

* Note: The activity of the source, 0.2 μCi, is converted to disintegration per minute by multiplying it by the number of dpm in 1 μCi. (0.2 μCi)(2,220,000 dpm/μCi)

B. An I131 source is known to contain 1.2 μCi. I131 has an 83.8% abundance at 364 keV. What is the well counter efficiency, if the source has a counting rate of 999,000 cpm?

$$\frac{999,000 \text{ cpm}}{(1.2 \ \mu\text{Ci})(2,220,000 \text{ dpm/}\mu\text{Ci})(0.838)} \times 100\% = 45\%$$

Problems:

1. A 0.3-μCi source of Cs137 gives a counting rate of 294,000 cpm in a well counter. What is the counter efficiency? Cs137 has an 85% abundance at 662 keV.

2. What is the well counter efficiency for Cs137 if a 1.6-μCi source produces 664,000 cpm?

3. A Cs137 source containing 0.41 μCi activity provides 240,000 cpm. What is the well counter efficiency?

4. A Co57 source with a known activity of 0.22 μCi produces a counting rate of 335,700 cpm. If Co57 has an abundance of 87% for a 122 keV gamma ray, what is the efficiency of the instrument?

5. What would be the instrument efficiency if the above source produced a counting rate of 256,800 cpm?

6. If an I131 source with an activity of 0.95 μCi produced a counting rate of 830,000 cpm, what would the well counter efficiency be? I131 has an 83.8% abundance at 364 keV.

7. A 1.8 μCi I131 source gives 1,335,000 cpm. What is the well counter efficiency?

References:

Cherry, Sorenson & Phelps (3rd Ed.), p. 186–188.
Early & Sodee (2nd Ed.), p. 180.
US DOT 49CFR173.443.

10. Window calculations: Centerline plus percent window

Principles:

The pulse height analyzer window for gamma cameras is usually set as a percent window around a centerline. The centerline is the energy of the photon being imaged and the percent window is a percent of that energy. The window is usually centered symmetrically around the centerline, so a 20% window is 10% below the centerline and 10% above it.

It should be noted that many of the newer generation of cameras are now using asymmetrical windows. In these cases the window is not centered around the centerline, but is shifted to the right to eliminate most of the Compton scatter coming from the patient.

IV-11 How to determine the energies that will be accepted in a symmetrical pulse height analyzer window with a centerline and percent window setting:

$$\text{energies within window} = \text{centerline energy} \pm \frac{\text{energy in keV} \times \text{percent window as decimal}}{2}$$

Examples:

A. If a pulse height analyzer is set for a 20% window for Tc99m, what energies will be accepted? Tc99m has an energy of 140 keV.

$$140\,\text{keV} \pm \frac{140\,\text{keV} \times 0.20}{2} = 140\,\text{keV} \pm 14\,\text{keV or } 126\,\text{keV to } 154\,\text{keV}$$

B. What energies are included in a 15% pulse height analyzer window set around the 69-keV Hg201 peak used during thallium imaging?

$$69\,\text{keV} \pm \frac{69\,\text{keV} \times 0.15}{2} = 69\,\text{keV} \pm 5\,\text{keV or } 64\,\text{keV to } 74\,\text{keV}$$

Problems:

1. What energies will be accepted by a 15% window set around the 140-keV Tc99m peak?

2. If a 20% window is set around the 296-keV peak of Ga67, what energies will be accepted by the pulse height analyzer?

3. What energies are included if a 20% window is used for the 93-keV peak of Ga67? The 185-keV window?

4. When a 30% window is used for the 364-keV gamma photopeak of I131, which energies are imaged? A 20% window? A 10% window?

5. If a 20% window is used for both the 171-keV and 245-keV photopeaks of In111, will the windows overlap?

Additional Applications:

6. A Tc99m study is to be performed immediately following completion of a Tl201 study. If a 25% Tc99m window is used, will the 68- to 80-keV x-rays produced by Tl201 be detected?

7. A patient who recently had a gallium scan is to have an In111 oxine tagged white blood cell study. Will the 184 keV gallium peak fall within a 20% window with a centerline of 171 keV?

References:

Early & Sodee, (2nd Ed.), p. 167–169.
Mettler & Guiberteau, (5th Ed.), p. 21.
Palmer, et al., p. 33–34.

11. Window Calculations: Upper and Lower Level Discriminators

Principles:

The spectrometers used with well counters and uptake probes may utilize an upper level discriminator (ULD) and a lower level discriminator (LLD) to determine the energies to be accepted by the pulse height analyzer (PHA). Each discriminator is set at a specific energy (keV) or voltage (V).

The LLD is set at a specific energy (keV). The ULD may be either independent or dependent. An independent ULD is set at an energy in the same way as the LLD. A dependent ULD defines the number of units the window extends above the LLD or threshold.

For example, if a window is to include 145 to 175 keV, then the LLD or threshold would be set at 145 keV. An independent ULD would be set at 175 keV. A dependent ULD, however, would be set at 30, so as to include 30 keV above the 145-keV threshold. This is frequently referred to as the window.

Discriminator settings can be determined in two ways.

1. A percentage of the energy can be used to determine window width settings, as was done with the centerline method in the previous section. (See Instrumentation, Section 10.)

2. The second method utilizes a window that includes the 75% of the photopeak surrounding the highest counting rate. This eliminates the tails of the bell curve where the majority of the inappropriate events occur.

IV-12 How to determine the energy setting for an upper and lower level discriminator on a spectrometer pulse height analyzer using a centerline and percent window.

1. Determine the energies to be included in the window:

$$\text{energies within window} = \text{centerline energy} \pm \frac{\text{energy in keV} \times \text{percent window as decimal}}{2}$$

2. Use the minimum energy as the LLD or threshold.
3. Use the maximum energy as the independent ULD or determine the window width for a dependent ULD as follows:

$$\text{maximum keV} - \text{minimum keV} = \text{window width in keV.}$$

IV-13 How to determine the energy setting for an upper and lower level discriminator on a spectrometer pulse height analyzer using 75% of the photopeak:

Identify 75% of the peak width as follows:

1. Obtain a spectrum of the primary photopeak by counting at 10-keV increments, beginning about 100 keV below the photopeak energy to about 100 keV above it, using a 20-unit window. Graph the data with counts on the y-axis versus energy on the x-axis.
2. Identify the 75% of the peak which is acceptable, by finding the full width at 25% maximum.

   To determine the 25% maximum: (maximum counts)(0.25)

3. Find the 25% maximum cpm on the y-axis of the chart and draw a line from it through both sides of the bell curve.
4. Drop a line from the intercept point on both sides of the bell curve down to the x-axis. These are the energy settings to be used for the LLD and the ULD.
5. To determine the dependent ULD setting:

   maximum keV – minimum keV = window width in keV

6. To calculate the percent window which has actually been selected:

$$\% \text{ window} = \frac{\text{ULD setting} - \text{LLD setting}}{\text{photopeak energy}} \times 100\%$$

Examples:

A. If a 20% window centered around the 159-keV I123 peak is desired, what would be the LLD and independent ULD settings?

$$159 \text{ keV} \pm \frac{159 \text{ keV} \times 0.20}{2} = 159 \text{ keV} \pm 16 \text{ keV}$$

The LLD will be set at 143 keV and the ULD will be set at 175 keV.

B.   Determine the LLD and ULD settings for a Cs137 spectrum so you utilize the highest 75% of the peak. Determine the percent window that is actually covered by these settings. $E_\gamma = 662$ keV.

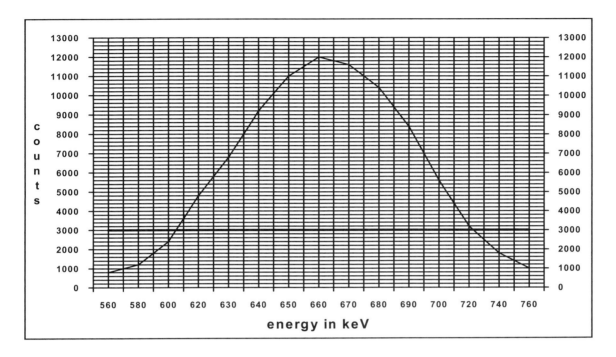

To determine 25% maximum: (12,000 counts)(0.25) = 3,000 counts

Draw a line from the 25% point on the y-axis through the bell curve. Drop lines to the x-axis from the points where the 25% line and the bell curve intersect. The x-axis values are the LLD and ULD settings.

LLD = 605   ULD = 722.

Determine actual percent window: $\dfrac{722-605}{662\,\text{keV}} \times 100\% = 18\%$

---

* Note: Although you have used 75% of the photopeak, a 75% window has NOT been created. As seen above, the window width is a function of the sharpness or spread of the bell curve.

Problems:

1.   What will the LLD and independent ULD settings be for a 10% window around the 159-keV I123 peak?

2.   Determine the LLD and independent ULD settings required for a 3% Cs137 window. The primary photopeak is 662 keV.

3.   If a 10% window is wanted for counting Co57 samples, what LLD and ULD must be used? The primary photopeak is 122 keV.

4. If a 10% window for Cs137 is desired, what threshold and window would be selected (LLD and dependent ULD)? The primary photopeak is 662 keV.

5. A spectrum of an I123 source was acquired. The central 75% of the peak fell between 146 and 172. At what settings should the threshold and window be set to cover this range?

6. Determine the threshold and window settings that will provide a 10% window for Co57. The primary photopeak is 122 keV.

7. If a 20% window is needed for the 364-keV peak of I131, what threshold and window settings must be used?

8. What threshold and window settings will be needed to provide for 75% of the photopeak if the spectrum for Cs137 gives the following values at 25% maximum? What percent window is being used?

    lower limit = 618
    upper limit = 708
    $E_\gamma = 662$ keV

9. What percent window is utilized when a Co57 ($E_\gamma = 122$ keV) source is counted with an LLD of 110 keV and ULD of 130 keV?

10. Determine the LLD and ULD settings for a Cr51 spectrum so the highest 75% of the peak is used. ($E_\gamma = 320$ keV.) What percent window is actually covered by these settings?

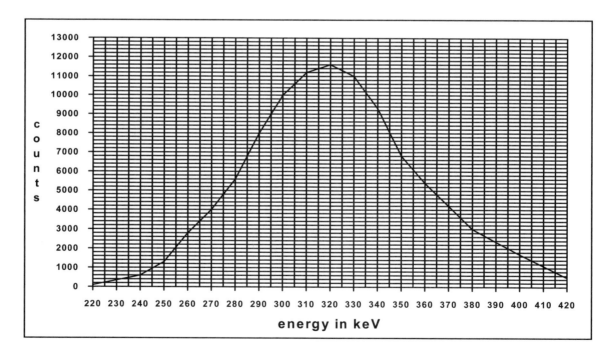

11. Use the central 75% of the photopeak to determine the LLD and ULD settings for Co58. ($E_\gamma = 810$ keV.) What percent window is actually being used?

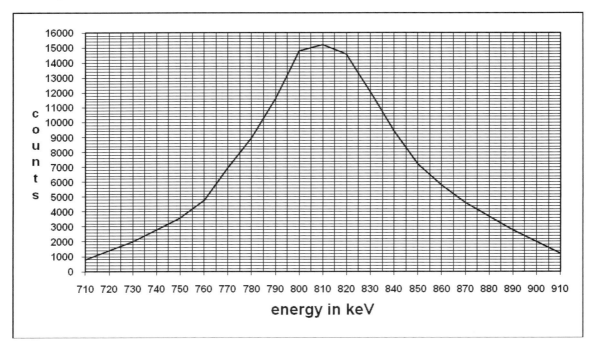

12. Determine the threshold and window settings needed for inclusion of 75% of the for Cr51 photopeak. ($E_\gamma = 320$ keV.) What percent window is actually being used?

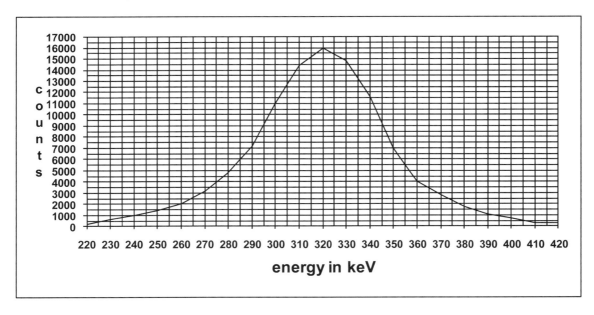

References:

Early & Sodee (2nd Ed.), p. 141–147, 158–162, 167–169.
Cherry, Sorenson & Phelps (3rd Ed.), p. 217–218.
Steves & Wells (3rd Ed.), p. 30 32.

12. Camera sensitivity

Principles:

Tracking camera sensitivity is a useful method for detecting subtle changes in instrument performance. Day-to-day or week-to-week comparisons allow early detection of potential problems. This allows for planned preventative maintenance as opposed to emergency repairs when a problem becomes significant enough to visualize on floods.

A known activity of radionuclide is required. Counting geometry must be identical each time the test is performed on an instrument.

Sensitivity is expressed as counts per minute per microcurie.

---

* Note: There are no established acceptable ranges for gamma camera sensitivity, because sensitivity is dependent upon many factors, including collimator, crystal thickness, and number of PM tubes. Different collimators used on the same camera will produce different sensitivities. The value of the sensitivity measure is in its comparison to previous values obtained from the same instrument over a period of time.

IV-14 How to calculate gamma camera sensitivity:

$$\text{sensitivity as cpm/}\mu\text{pm} = \frac{\text{source cpm} - \text{background cpm}}{\text{source activity in } \mu\text{Ci}}$$

Examples:

A. Calculate the sensitivity of a camera that produces 26,657 cpm with a 152-µCi source. Background was 340 cpm.

$$\frac{26{,}657\,\text{cpm} - 340\,\text{cpm}}{152\,\mu\text{Ci}} = 173\,\text{cpm/}\mu\text{Ci}$$

B. What is the sensitivity of a camera if a 110-µCi source gives 48,286 cpm and the background is 1,252 cpm?

$$\frac{48{,}286\,\text{cpm} - 1{,}252\,\text{cpm}}{110\,\mu\text{Ci}} = 428\,\text{cpm/}\mu\text{Ci}$$

Problems:

1. If a 185-µCi source produces 57,508 cpm, what is the camera's sensitivity? The background was 850 cpm.

2. Calculate the sensitivity of a camera that gives a counting rate of 32,131 cpm with a 134-μCi source and a background reading of 988 cpm.

3. When a 108-μCi source is used, 44,645 cpm are obtained for a given camera. What is the instrument's sensitivity if the background reading is 1,122 cpm?

4. What is the sensitivity of a camera that produces 59,876 cpm when exposed to a 173-μCi source? Background is 755 cpm.

5. Calculate the sensitivity for a camera that produces 51,819 cpm in response to a 127-μCi source. A background count of 547 cpm was obtained.

Additional Applications:

6. According to the protocol for Hospital X, preventative maintenance is scheduled whenever a camera shows a 10% decrease in sensitivity over time. According to the data below, when should the call for service have been made? Use the May 1 value as the reference standard to which other values are compared. Assume background has already been subtracted from each value. (See Statistics, Section 1.)

Date	Activity in μCi	CPM
May 1	153	44,210
May 2	157	44,109
May 3	144	40,659
May 4	150	41,203
May 5	149	38,112
May 8	160	40,276
May 9	141	32,998

7. Camera sensitivity is to be adopted as a quality control indicator for your nuclear medicine department. Weekly values have been acquired for two months. They are to be averaged and used as the standard for comparison. Calculate the standard value −10%. Assume background has already been subtracted from each value.

Week	Activity in μCi	CPM
1	122	48,329
2	138	56,856
3	119	46,172
4	145	59,305
5	136	53,176
6	130	53,820
7	147	56,301
8	139	54,905

References:

Early & Sodee (2nd Ed.), p. 272–273.
Steves & Wells (3rd Ed.), p. 38.

13. Acquisition time and counts per projection for SPECT studies

Principles:

When developing SPECT protocols you must consider the length of time a patient can lie still, and balance it against the time needed to acquire a sufficient number of counts and projections in order to obtain a high-quality study.

You can determine the acquisition time, time per projection, and counts per projection using the estimated counting rate, the number of projections and total counts desired.

It should be noted that counting rates will vary from one patient to another, even if each receives the same dose. Body attenuation, organ-to-background ratio, pathology, metabolic turnover, excretion rates, etc., will affect the counting rate produced by an individual patient.

---

* Note: When referring to SPECT projections, the terms stops, steps, or frames may also be used.

IV-15 How to calculate total acquisition time for a SPECT study:

$$\text{acquisition time} = (\text{number of projections})(\text{time per projection})$$

OR

$$\text{acquisition time} = \frac{\text{total counts}}{\text{counting rate}}$$

IV-16 How to calculate time per projection for a SPECT study:

$$\text{time per projection} = \frac{\text{total acquisition time}}{\text{number of projections}}$$

IV-17 How to calculate counts per projection for a SPECT study:

$$\text{counts per projection} = \frac{\text{total counts}}{\text{number of projections}}$$

OR

$$\text{counts per projection} = (\text{time per projection})(\text{counting rate})$$

Examples:

A. A 3,000,000-count SPECT study is to be performed on a phantom that produces a counting rate of 200,000 cpm. If the acquisition is to have 64 stops over 360°, what will be the total time of the acquisition, the time per stop, and the counts per stop?

$$\text{acquisition time} = \frac{3,000,000 \text{ counts}}{200,000 \text{ cpm}} = 15 \text{ min}$$

$$\text{time per projection} = \frac{15 \text{ min}}{64 \text{ stops}} = 0.23 \text{ min / stop or} \approx 14 \text{ s/stop}$$

$$\text{counts per projection} = \frac{3,000,000 \text{ counts}}{64 \text{ stops}} \approx 47,000 \text{ counts / stop}$$

B. A 180° SPECT study will be performed using 32 stops for 25 seconds each. If the estimated counting rate is 150,000 cpm, how many counts will be acquired in the study? How many counts will be acquired per stop? How many minutes will be required for the acquisition?

$$\text{acquisition time} = (32 \text{ stops})(25 \text{ s/stop}) = 800 \text{ s or} \approx 13 \text{ min}$$

OR

convert 25 s or 0.42 min, then calculate: (32 stops)(0.42 min) = 13 min

---

* **Note:** To convert 25 seconds to minutes: $\dfrac{25 \text{ s}}{60 \text{ s/min}} = 0.42 \text{ min}$

---

counts per projection = (150,000 cpm)(0.42 min/projection) = 63,000 ct/projection

$$\text{total counts based on acquisition time: } 13 \text{ min} = \frac{x}{150,000 \text{ cpm}} \qquad x = 1,950,000 \text{ ct}$$

OR

$$\text{total counts based on count/projection: } 63,000 \text{ ct/stop} = \frac{x}{32 \text{ stops}} \qquad x = 2,016,000 \text{ ct}$$

---

* **Note:** The difference in total counts for the acquisition using the two methods above is insignificant ($\approx 3\%$). Either method is valid, as you are obtaining a reasonable estimate, not a precise number.

Problems:

1. A SPECT study is to be acquired using 30 s/stop for 30 stops. Approximately 56,000 counts are acquired per stop, what will be the total counts for the acquisition? How much time is required for the acquisition?

2. About 74,000 counts are obtained at each of 62 stops on a 360° SPECT scan. If each step lasts 20 seconds, what is the total imaging time and how many counts will be acquired in the study?

3. A phantom produces a counting rate of 260,000 cpm. A total of 3,000,000 counts is desired for a 32-stop acquisition. Calculate the total acquisition time, the time per projection, and the counts per projection.

4. A 360° SPECT is acquired at 30 s/stop with 60 projections. The counting rate is 73,000 cpm. Calculate the total acquisition time, the counts/stop, and the total counts.

5. A Tl201 SPECT study is to have a total of 1 million counts over 180° and 64 frames. If the patient has an average counting rate of approximately 49,000 cpm, for how long should each frame be acquired? What is the total acquisition time?

6. If a Tc99m RBC liver study produces about 240,000 cpm, how many counts/stop will be acquired when each stop lasts 20 seconds? How many counts will be acquired if the study contains 64 frames? How long will it take to complete the acquisition?

7. A patient is producing a counting rate of 82,000 cpm. How many counts/projection will be acquired if each projection lasts 20 seconds? 30 seconds? What is the total count for each study if 64 projections are used? How many minutes are required for completion of each study?

References:

Powsner & Powsner (2nd Ed.), p. 87–88.
Steves & Wells (3rd Ed.), p. 33.

14. Obtaining desired flood or phantom fill activities

Principles:

Flood sources utilized for various purposes need to produce specific counting rates depending upon their use. You need to be able to estimate the volume of radionuclide that must be added to the phantom to achieve the desired counting rate.

The simplest method would be to determine the activity needed to produce the desired dps. However, geometry, instrument sensitivity, attenuation, deadtime, and other factors will affect both the quantity of incident radiation and the number of events registered. An easy alternative method can be used.

By measuring a small activity in the phantom to determine the counting rate, a reasonable estimate of the total activity needed to produce the desired counting rate can be made. Having counted a small known activity, you can use a direct proportion to calculate the total activity to be used.

IV-18 How to determine the activity needed for flood source or phantom preparation:

1.   Place a known activity in a syringe, flood source, or phantom. Obtain a counting rate by placing the source at the same distance from the camera that the actual flood source or phantom will be used.
2.   Determine the total activity needed to obtain the desired counting rate:

$$\frac{\text{test sample counting rate}}{\text{test sample activity}} = \frac{\text{phantom counting rate}}{\text{phantom activity}}$$

(See Basic Math Skills Section 7.)

---

* Note: Comparable counting rates from sample to phantom will only be achieved if the counting geometry is similar. A measurement using a syringe will be somewhat different from that with a phantom, but it provides a reasonable estimate.

Changes in source to camera distance, however, will make a significant difference in counting rates. A minor difference in distance between the initial measurement and the final product can result in a marked difference in counting rates. (See Radiation Protection Section 4.)

Example:

A. In order to determine the activity needed to produce about 10,000 cpm, how many µCi should be added to the phantom if 1.3 µCi gives a counting rate of 620 cpm?

$$\frac{620\,\text{cpm}}{1.3\,\mu\text{Ci}} = \frac{10,000\,\text{cpm}}{X\,\mu\text{Ci}} \qquad \text{Cross-multiply:}\ (X\,\mu\text{Ci})(620\,\text{cpm}) = (1.3\,\mu\text{Ci})(10,000\,\text{cpm})$$

$$\text{Solve for } X:\ X\,\mu\text{Ci} = \frac{(10,000\,\text{cpm})(1.3\,\mu\text{Ci})}{620\,\text{cpm}} = 21\,\mu\text{Ci}$$

---

* Note: The calculation can also be used to determine the volume needed. Volume is simply used instead of activity.

Problems:

1. If 6 µCi produce 720 cpm in a flood source, how many µCi must be used to obtain approximately 15,000 cpm?

2. If 1.2 mCi produce a counting rate of 1800 cpm in a cylindrical phantom, how many mCi should be used if a total of 30,000 cpm is desired?

3. How many µCi should be added to a phantom to obtain a counting rate of 20,000 cpm if a 520-µCi sample of solution produces 8,740 cpm?

4. A radioactive source is needed which will provide a counting rate of 10,000 cpm. How many µCi are needed if 152 µCi produce 2,430 cpm?

5. If 0.2 ml of solution produces 1,820 cpm, how many ml must be used to spike a phantom for a counting rate of 30,000 cpm?

6. A flood source is needed with a counting rate of 20,000 cpm. If 0.5 ml of eluate produces 5,210 cpm, how many ml must be added to the phantom?

Additional Applications:

7. A thyroid phantom is being prepared which will approximate a normal thyroid uptake of 80,000 counts in 3 minutes. If 1.0 ml of I123 solution produces 7,340 cpm, how many ml should be added to the phantom?

References:

Application of principles from Basic Math Skills Section 5.
Christian & Waterstram-Rich (6th Ed.), p. 5.

15. Total pixels by matrix size

Principles:

Knowing the total number of pixels used when a particular matrix size is selected will help you determine how much storage space will be set aside by the computer and how many images can be placed on the computer screen at a time.

The matrices or formats most commonly used in nuclear medicine are 64×64, 128×128, and 256×256. Other configurations can also be used, such as a 256×128 matrix for a whole body image that utilizes one half of the computer screen.

Most nuclear medicine computer screens are now high resolution, using $1{,}024 \times 1{,}024$ pixels or $2{,}048 \times 2{,}048$ pixels to display images. This area can be divided into multiple images of a smaller matrix size. For example, a dynamic first pass study is displayed as a series of images on the screen, with each image using 64×64 pixels.

IV-19 How to calculate total pixels used based on matrix size:

total pixels = matrix height in pixels × matrix width in pixels

---

IV-20 How to calculate the number of images that can be displayed on a computer screen based on matrix size:

$$\text{number of images displayed} = \frac{\text{total pixels on display screen}}{\text{total pixels per frame}}$$

Examples:

A. If a 128×128 matrix is selected, how many pixels will be included?

128 pixels × 128 pixels = 16,384 pixels.

B. How many 128×128 frames can be simultaneously displayed on a 256×256 computer screen?

$$\frac{256 \text{ pixels} \times 256 \text{ pixels}}{128 \text{ pixels} \times 128 \text{ pixels}} = \frac{65{,}536 \text{ pixels}}{16{,}384 \text{ pixels}} = 4 \text{ frames}$$

Problems:

1.   How many pixels will be used in a 64×64 matrix?

2.   How many 64×64 pixel frames can be displayed on a 256×256 computer screen?

3.   How many pixels are included in a 512×128 matrix?

4.   How many 512×128 frames can be displayed simultaneously on a 512×512 display screen?

5.   How many pixels are used for each frame of a 32×32 pixel matrix?

6.   How many 32×32 pixel frames could be displayed on a 256×256 screen?

References:

Christian & Waterstram-Rich (6th Ed.), p. 117–120.
Early & Sodee (2nd Ed.), p. 224–225.

16. Computer memory requirements based on matrix size and storage mode

Principles:

For most nuclear medicine computer systems a byte is composed of 8 bits and a word is composed of 16 bits or 2 bytes. When data are acquired, each pixel can accumulate and display a predetermined maximum number of events. The maximum is determined by selecting byte or word mode.

The maximum number of events that can be recorded in a pixel is calculated by $2^x - 1$, where x = bits per unit, i.e., a byte or a word.

If byte mode is selected, then each pixel can record a maximum of $2^8 - 1$ or 255 bits of information or events. If word mode is selected, a maximum of $2^{16} - 1$ or 65,535 events can be recorded in each pixel.

> *** Note:** In byte mode, the computer sets aside 255 bits of memory for each pixel and in word mode it sets aside 65,535. This space will be unusable for another study, even if the acquired data did not take up all the memory made available for the study.

Data can be stored in either byte or word mode as well. Because two bytes equal a word, twice as many bytes are required to store the same amount of data as in word mode. Byte data stored as words will require half as many words as compared to byte mode. In each case, however, the same total numbers of bits are used; it is simply the configuration that is different.

> **IV-21 How to calculate the total memory used when data are acquired and stored in the same mode:**
>
> When data are acquired and stored in the same mode (i.e., byte to byte or word to word), use the following equation:
>
> total memory required = (height in pixels)(width in pixels)(frames)

> **IV-22 How to calculate the total memory used when data are acquired in word mode, but stored in byte mode:**
>
> If data are acquired in word mode but stored in byte mode, multiple the memory requirement by 2.
>
> # of bytes of memory required = (height in pixels)(width in pixels)(frames)(2 bytes/word)

IV-23 How to calculate the total memory used when data are acquired in byte mode, but stored in word mode:

If data are acquired in byte mode and stored in word mode, multiply the memory requirement by 1/2.

# of words of memory required = (height in pixels)(width in pixels)(frames)(1/2 word/byte)

which can be rewritten as:

$$\text{\# of words of memory required} = \frac{\text{pixels} \times \text{pixels} \times \text{frames}}{2}$$

Examples:

A.   A 64 × 64 byte matrix is to be used to acquire 30 frames. How much memory will be required if the study is stored in byte mode?

64 pixels × 64 pixels × 30 frames = 122,880 bytes

B.   A study is to be acquired and stored in 128 × 128 word mode. If 60 frames are acquired, how much memory will be used?

128 pixels × 128 pixels × 60 frames = 983,040 words

C.   How much memory will be needed if the study in Example B is stored in byte mode?

128 pixels × 128 pixels × 60 frames × 2 bytes/word = 1,966,080 bytes

D.   How much memory will be required for a series of 8 static images that are collected on a 256 × 256 byte format and stored in word mode?

$$\frac{256 \text{ pixels} \times 256 \text{ pixels} \times 8 \text{ frames}}{2} = 262,144 \text{ words}$$

Problems:

1.   How much memory is required for a 60-frame study using 64 × 64 byte mode if the data are also stored in byte mode?

2.   How much memory is required if the study in Problem 1 is stored in word mode?

3.   If a gated acquisition is acquired in 128 × 128 word mode with 30 frames per cycle, how much memory, in words, will need to be set aside for the study?

4.   How much memory will be reserved if the study in Problem 2 is stored in byte mode?

5.   If daily floods are acquired and saved in 256 × 256 word mode, how much memory will be required to store 90 days' worth of floods?

6.   If resting SPECT myocardial perfusion studies are to be acquired and saved in 128 ×128 byte mode with 64 stops per study, how many bytes of memory will be required?

7.   A gated SPECT myocardial perfusion study is to be acquired for 64 stops with a 64 × 64 matrix. Each stop is divided into 9 bins for the gating (in other words, each R-R interval is divided into 9 segments). How many bytes of memory will be required for the study?

Additional Applications:

8.   If each patient's SPECT myocardial perfusion study is acquired in word mode on a 64 × 64 matrix with 64 stops per study, how many bytes of memory would be needed for each acquisition? If each patient has a gated stress with 9 bins per stop and a non-gated rest study, how many patients can be stored on a 700-MB CD?

References:

Christian & Waterstram-Rich (6th Ed.), p. 117 120.
Early & Sodee (2nd Ed.), p. 224–225.
Harbert & da Rocha, Vol. 1, p. 165–166.

17. Pixel calibration

Principles:

In order to measure organ or lesion volume, or to correct for photon attenuation in SPECT images, pixel size must be known. To determine pixel size in centimeters (cm), use two point sources and a computer-generated activity profile.

Pixel size must be calibrated in both the x- and the y-axis. To assure the accuracy of volume calculations, pixel size must be within 0.5 mm (0.05 cm) when the x-axis dimension is compared to the y-axis dimension.

IV-24 How to calculate pixel size:

1.   Place two point sources about 30 cm apart on the camera surface. Measure the exact distance between the sources.
2.   Acquire an image and generate an activity profile on the computer.
3.   Count the number of pixels between the two sources as represented by the activity peaks.
4.   Apply the data to the following equation:

$$\text{pixel size} = \frac{\text{distance between sources}}{\text{number of pixels between activity profile peaks}}$$

Example:

A.   Two Co57 disk sources are placed exactly 30 cm apart. There are 96 pixels between the peaks. Calculate the pixel size for this 128 × 128 matrix.

$$\text{pixel size} = \frac{30 \text{ cm}}{96 \text{ pixels}} = 0.312 \text{ cm / pixel or } 3.12 \text{ mm / pixel}$$

Problems:

1.   Calculate the pixel size for a 64 × 64 matrix when two sources are placed 25 cm apart and 40 pixels are located between the peaks.

2.   Two sources are placed 30 cm apart on the camera for pixel calibration of a 64 × 64 matrix. What is the pixel size if the peaks on the activity profile are 47 pixels apart?

3.   Calculate the pixel size for a 128 × 128 matrix using the following data.

     distance between sources = 25 cm
     number of pixels between sources = 82

4.   A 64 × 64 matrix on a 2× zoom is to be used for a study that requires pixel calibration. If 2 sources are placed 30 cm apart and 96 pixels are counted between them, what is the size of each pixel?

5. Determine the pixel size when a 2× zoom is used with a 128 × 128 matrix, if 2 sources placed 30 cm apart have 94 pixels between the activity profile peaks.

Additional Applications:

6. Determine if pixel dimensions in the x and the y-axis are within 0.05 cm of one another for a 64 × 64 matrix:

    distance between sources = 25 cm
    number of pixels between activity profile peaks; x-axis = 42
    number of pixels between activity profile peaks; y-axis = 45

7. Two point sources are placed 30 cm apart. In the x-axis there are 101 pixels between the activity profile peaks on a 128 × 128 matrix. In the y-axis there are 97 pixels. Are pixel dimensions within 0.05 cm of each other along the two axes?

References:

Cherry, Sorenson & Phelps (3rd Ed.), p. 364–365.
Early & Sodee (2nd Ed.), p. 225, 298–299.
Harbert & da Rocha, Vol. 1, p. 165 167.
Steves & Wells (3rd Ed.), p. 38.

Chapter V. Radiopharmacy

1. Decay calculation using half-life

Principles:

Because a radionuclide is constantly decaying at a specific rate, the activity is constantly decreasing. The amount of decrease per unit time is dependent upon the half-life of the radionuclide. If you know the activity and half-life of a radionuclide, you can calculate the activity for any time in the future or the past.

V-1 How to calculate activity using the half-life:

$$A_t = A_0 e^{-0.693 \times (t/t_{1/2})}$$

Where: A_t = activity at specified time
A_0 = original activity
e = Euler's number (2.718....), which remains a constant in the equation
t = elapsed time
$t_{1/2}$ = half-life

The exponent 0.693 is the natural log (ln) of 2, which accounts for the halving of activity with each half-life.

The elapsed time and the half-life must be in the same units.

For a detailed explanation of the equation's derivation refer to the references listed at the end of this section.

---

* Note: You may also see the equation in Shadowbox V-1 written as $A_t = A_0 e^{-\lambda t}$, where λ = decay constant. The decay constant (λ) describes the fraction of atoms that are likely to decay per unit time for a particular radionuclide. Typically the unit of time is the second. The decay constant, which is sometimes referred to as the disintegration constant, can also be described as the likelihood that a particular atom will decay per unit time. It is defined as $\lambda = \dfrac{0.693}{t_{1/2}}$, where $t_{1/2}$ = half-life of the radionuclide. Examine the equation in Shadowbox V-1. It can be rewritten as:

$A_t = A_0 e^{-\left(\frac{0.693}{t_{1/2}}\right)(t)}$. If $\lambda = \dfrac{0.693}{t_{1/2}}$, then the equation can be rewritten by substituting λ into the exponent to give $A_t = A_0 e^{-\lambda t}$.

Examples:

A.   A vial of DTPA is reconstituted with 200 mCi of Tc99m. What will its activity be 3 hours later? The half-life of Tc99m is 6.01 hours.

$$A_t = 200 \text{ mCi} \times e^{-0.693 \times (3\,h/6.01\,h)} = 200 \text{ mCi} \times e^{-0.693 \times 0.4992} = 200 \text{ mCi} \times e^{-0.3459}$$

$$A = 200 \text{ mCi} \times 0.7076 = 142 \text{ mCi}$$

> *** Note:** The $e^{-0.693 \times (t/t_{1/2})}$ portion of the equation is calculating the decay factor. As will be seen in Radiopharmacy, Section 2, this factor will be used whenever that particular radionuclide has decayed for that period of time. Therefore, the 3-hour decay factor for Tc99m is 0.7076, which can be rounded to 0.708 without significant loss of accuracy.

B.   If a vial of Ga67 gallium citrate is calibrated to contain 30 mCi at 8:00 am Monday, how many mCi will remain at 8:00 am Wednesday? The half-life of Ga67 equals 78.3 hours. First, determine the elapsed time. Second, convert units of time if necessary, so that the elapsed time and half-life are in identical units.

8:00 am Monday to 8:00 am Wednesday = 2 days or 48 hours

$$A = 30 \text{ mCi} \times e^{-0.693 \times (48\,h/78.3\,h)} = 30 \text{ mCi} \times e^{-0.693 \times 0.6130} = 30 \text{ mCi} \times e^{-0.4248}$$

$$A = 30 \text{ mCi} \times 0.6539 = 19.6 \text{ mCi}$$

> *** Note:** The same equation can be used to determine the amount of activity that must be used when preparing a dose ahead of time to contain a specified activity in the future. In this case A_0 is the unknown, and A_t is the activity desired at a particular time.

C.   A 22-mCi Tc99m HDP dose will be needed at 2:00 pm. It is being prepared 2 hours in advance. What activity must be placed in the syringe at 12:00 noon? $t_{1/2} = 6.01\,h$.

$$22 \text{ mCi} = A_0 \times e^{-0.693 \times (2\,h/6.01\,h)}$$

Simplify the exponent, isolate, and solve for the unknown.

$$22 \text{ mCi} = A_0 \times e^{-0.693 \times 0.3328} \qquad 22 \text{ mCi} = A_0 \times e^{-0.2306} \qquad 22 \text{ mCi} = A_0 \times 0.7940$$

$$\frac{22 \text{ mCi}}{0.7940} = A_0 = 27.7 \text{ mCi}$$

> *** Note:** The $e^{-0.693 \times (t/t_{1/2})}$ portion of the equation gives a decay factor of 0.7940. Since you are looking for an activity now that will decay to a desired amount (called pre-calibration), you divide by the decay factor. (See Radiopharmacy Section 3.)

Problems:

1. A vial of generator eluate contains 432 mCi immediately following elution. How many mCi will remain 8 hours later? The half-life for Tc99m is 6.01 hours.

2. Tl201 has a half-life of 73.1 hours. If a multidose vial contains 12.8 mCi at 9:00 am, how many will it contain at 10:00 am the following day?

3. A vial of Xe133 gas ($t_{1/2}$ = 5.24 d) is calibrated at 22 mCi at 6:00 am on March 1. What is its activity at 6:00 pm on March 8?

4. An I131 sodium iodide capsule was calibrated for 7.3 mCi at 12:00 noon on May 10. If the half-life is 8.05 days, what will be the capsule's activity at noon on May 23?

5. A Cr51 sodium chromate standard solution contained 0.15 µCi/ml when it was produced. What is the activity per milliliter 60 days later? $t_{1/2}$ = 27.7 d.

6. A Mo99/Tc99m generator is calibrated at 2.3 Ci on Friday at 10:00 am. What will the Mo99 activity be when it is eluted at 7:00 am on Monday? Mo99 $t_{1/2}$ = 66.6 h.

7. What will be the Mo99 activity in a 1.6-Ci generator when it is shipped back to the manufacturer 21 days after its calibration date? $t_{1/2}$ = 66.6 h.

8. A multidose vial of Tc99m MDP is being prepared. In order to have an activity of 120 mCi at 10:00 am, how many mCi of Tc99m must be injected into the vial at 5:00 am? $t_{1/2}$ = 6.01 h.

9. If a generator is to contain 1.2 Ci Mo99 ($t_{1/2}$ = 66.6 h) at 8:00 am Thursday, how many Ci must be placed on the column when it is produced at 3:00 pm Tuesday?

Additional Applications:

10. An I123 capsule ($t_{1/2}$ = 13.2 h) contains 320 µCi at calibration time. It is contaminated with 5 µCi of I124 ($t_{1/2}$ = 98 h). How much activity is being produced by each nuclide 24 hours after calibration time? What is the percent I124 contaminant at calibration time and 24 hours later (see Radiopharmacy Section 20)?

11. According to the standard of practice, a dose calibrator constancy check source must contain at least 50 µCi of activity. If a Co57 ($t_{1/2}$ = 270 d) source contains 52 µCi today, will it still be usable in 30 days?

References:

Christian & Waterstram-Rich (6th Ed.), p. 10–13.
Early & Sodee (2nd Ed.), p. 39–40.
Kowalsky & Falen (2nd Ed.), p. 31–38.
Saha (4th Ed.), p. 17–24.

2. Decay calculation using decay charts

Principles:

For convenience most decay problems may be solved using decay charts rather than the half-life equation used in the previous section (Shadowbox V-1). These charts allow quicker problem solving and assure fewer mathematical errors.

The decay factor is also referred to as the post-calibration factor to differentiate it from the pre-calibration factor. (See Radiopharmacy Section 3.)

A series of decay charts for many radionuclides commonly used in nuclear medicine will be found in Appendix A.

V-2 How to calculate activity using a decay factor:

1.   Calculate the time elapsed since the time at which the activity was known (referred to as initial activity, original activity, or A_O).
2.   Refer to the appropriate decay table and select the correct decay factor.
3.   Apply the data to the equation:

$$A_t = A_0 \times DF$$

where: A_t = activity at time t
         A_0 = original activity
         DF = decay factor

Examples:

A.   A vial of Tc99m sodium pertechnetate contains 572 mCi at 8:00 am. What is its activity at 12:30 pm?

Calculate the elapsed time: 8:00 am to 12:30 pm is 4.5 hours
Select the decay factor from Tc99m decay table: 0.595
Calculate the activity at the specified time:

572 mCi × 0.595 = 340 mCi

---

* Note: The decay charts in Appendix A were formulated using the $e^{-0.693 \times (t/t_{1/2})}$ calculation. (See Radiopharmacy, Section 1.) $e^{-0.693 \times (4.5\,h/6.01\,h)} = e^{-0.693 \times 0.7488} = e^{-0.5189} = 0.595$.

B.   A vial of Tl201 contains 6.6 mCi at 8:00 am on Monday. How many mCi remain at 2:00 pm on Tuesday?

Calculate the elapsed time: 30 hours
Select the decay factor from the Tl201 decay table: 0.754
Calculate the activity at the specified time:

6.6 mCi × 0.754 = 5 mCi

---

* **Note:** A mistake frequently made by students and technologists is inaccurate reading of the decay table resulting in selection of the incorrect decay factor. To prevent such errors, the author suggests using a ruler or other straight-edge to read decay tables that do not include gridlines.

V-3 How to calculate decay factors for times that exceed those listed on a decay table:

If a decay table stops short of the time needed, the necessary factor can be calculated by multiplying decay factors for the times that add up to the total desired time.

Examples:

C.   A decay table for Tc99m ends at 4 hours with a decay factor of 0.630, but you need the decay factor for 8 hours post-calibration. What factor should be used?

4 h + 4 h = 8 h
0.630 × 0.630 = 0.397

A check of the Tc99m decay charts shows this is indeed correct. The difference of 1 unit in the thousandths place is due to rounding and is insignificant.

D.   If the 20-hour decay factor for Tl201 is 0.828 and the 30-hour decay factor is 0.754, what is the decay factor for 50 hours?

20 h + 30 h = 50 h
0.828 × 0.754 = 0.624

Problems:

Use the decay charts found in Appendix A to solve the following problems.

1.   A vial of Tc99m MAA contains 54.7 mCi at 7:30 am. What is the activity at 10:15 am?

2.   If Tc99m generator eluate contains 620 mCi activity at 9:00 am, how many mCi will remain at 11:00 am?

3.   A unit dose of Tl201 was calibrated at 2.6 mCi at noon on Monday. What is its activity at noon on Tuesday?

4. If a vial of Ga67 was calibrated to contain 12 mCi at 8:00 am on Tuesday, how many mCi will remain at 8:00 am on Saturday?

5. A vial of P32 contained 25 mCi on June 1. How many mCi will it contain 60 days later?

6. A vial of I125 had an activity of 300 µCi at calibration. How much activity will remain 75 days later?

7. A therapeutic capsule of I131 was made up to contain 120 mCi on August 15. How many mCi remain on August 30?

8. A Co57 source is certified to contain 232 µCi on March 1. What is its activity 262 days later?

9. A unit dose was drawn up to contain 30.8 mCi of Tc99m MDP at 5:00 am. How many mCi will remain at 8:00 am?

10. A capsule containing I123 sodium iodide was calibrated to contain 252 µCi at 8:00 am. How much activity remains when it is administered at 2:00 pm?

References:

Early & Sodee (2nd Ed.), p. 40
Kowalsky & Falen (2nd Ed.), p. 37–38.
Steves & Wells (3rd Ed.), p. 21–22.

3. Pre-calibration calculations

Principles:

When preparing unit doses and bulk kits, you need to determine the amount of activity to be used based on the activity needed at a future time (time t). The time at which the dose is intended for use is referred to as the calibration time. The activity placed in the vial or syringe at preparation time (time 0) will be larger than the actual activity needed at calibration time (time t) in order to account for decay. Pre-calibration factors allow you to determine the activity needed at time 0. For total kit activity calculations, see Radiopharmacy Section 6.

Some decay charts include pre-calibration factors as well as post-calibration factors.

> **∗ Note:** Pre-calibration factors will always be greater than 1, because the activity at preparation time must always be greater than the activity to be used sometime in the future. A larger value can only be produced by multiplying the original activity by a number greater than 1.
>
> Post-calibration or decay factors will always be less than 1, because radioactivity decreases with time. A smaller value can only be produced by multiplying the original activity by a number less than 1.

V-4 How to calculate activity using a pre-calibration factor:

1. Calculate the elapsed time between preparation (A_0) and calibration time (A_t)
2. Refer to the appropriate decay table and select the pre-calibration factor.
3. Apply the equation:

$A_0 = A_t \times$ pre-calibration factor,

where: A_t = activity at time t (calibration time)
         A_0 = activity at time 0 (preparation time)

If pre-calibration factors are not available, decay factors (post-calibration factors) can easily be used by simply rearranging the decay factor equation to solve for A_0 instead A_t.

V-5 How to calculate activity using the decay factor as a pre-calibration factor:

1. Calculate the elapsed time between preparation (A_0) and calibration time (A_t).
2. Refer to the appropriate decay table and select the correct decay factor (DF).
3. Apply the equation:

$A_t = A_0 \times DF$ is rearranged to become $A_o = \dfrac{A_t}{DF}$

where: A_t = activity at time t (calibration time)
         A_0 = activity at time 0 (preparation time)
         DF = decay factor

Examples:

A.   A 22-mCi Tc99m HDP unit dose is needed at 10:00 am. The dose is being prepared at 6:00 am. How many mCi must be placed in the syringe?

   Pre-calibration factor method (see Shadowbox V-4):

      Calculate the elapsed time between preparation and calibration time: 4 hours

      Select the pre-calibration factor from the Tc99m table in Appendix A: 1.587

      Calculate activity to be drawn: 22 mCi × 1.587 = 35 mCi

   Post-calibration decay factor method (see Shadowbox V-5):

      Calculate the elapsed time between preparation and calibration time: 4 hours

      Select the decay factor from the Tc99m table: 0.63

      Calculate the activity to be drawn: $\dfrac{22 \text{ mCi}}{0.63} = 35$ mCi

B.   At 2:00 pm a radiopharmacist is preparing I123 capsules to contain 300 μCi at 10:00 am on the following day. How many μCi of I123 must be placed in each capsule?

   Pre-calibration factor method (see Shadowbox V-4):

      Calculate the elapsed time between preparation and calibration time: 20 hours

      Select the pre-calibration factor from the I123 table in Appendix A: 2.858

      Calculate the activity to be drawn: 300 μCi × 2.858 = 857 μCi

   Post-calibration decay factor method (see Shadowbox V-5):

      Calculate the elapsed time between preparation and calibration time: 20 hours

      Select the decay factor from the I123 table: 0.35

      Calculate the activity to be drawn: $\dfrac{300 \text{ } \mu\text{Ci}}{0.35} = 857 \text{ } \mu\text{Ci}$

---

* Note: The results in the above examples are identical regardless of which of the two methods is used.

V-6 How to calculate pre-calibration factors that exceed the times listed on a table:

A pre-calibration table may not list times far enough into the future to meet your needs. As with decay factors, the necessary pre-calibration factor can be calculated by multiplying factors. (See Radiopharmacy Section 2.)

C. If the 4-hour pre-calibration factor for Tc99m is 1.587 and the 5-hour pre-calibration factor is 1.779, what is the 9-hour pre-calibration factor?

$$4\,h + 5\,h = 9\,h$$
$$1.587 \times 1.779 = 2.823$$

D. Use the following factors to calculate the 21-hour pre-calibration factor for Ga67.

hours	pre-calibration factor
3	1.027
9	1.083

$$9\,h + 9\,h + 3\,h = 21\,h$$
$$1.083 \times 1.083 \times 1.027 = 1.204$$

Problems:

Refer to the decay tables in Appendix A for both decay factors and pre-calibration factors.

Use pre-calibration factors to solve the following problems.

1. A Tc99m sodium pertechnetate dose that is to be drawn up at 8:00 am must be calibrated to contain 10 mCi at 11:00 am. How many mCi must be placed in the syringe?

2. A vial of Tl201 thallous chloride must contain 120 mCi of activity at 8:00 am on Tuesday. If the vial is prepared at 10:00 am on Monday, how many mCi are needed?

3. A 4-mCi unit dose of Tc99m MAA is needed at 4:00 pm. If the dose is being prepared at 2:00 pm, how much activity must be used?

4. If an I131 sodium iodide capsule is to contain 150 mCi on Friday, how many mCi must be used to prepare it on Tuesday?

Use decay factors to solve the following problems.

5. A vial of Ga67 gallium citrate is to contain 8 mCi on Wednesday at 8:00 am. How many mCi must be placed in the vial on Monday at 8:00 am?

6. If I123 capsules are prepared 24 hours prior to the calibration time, how many µCi would be needed to provide 200 µCi at calibration time?

7. An I131 sodium iodide capsule calibrated to contain 7 mCi is needed on Sept. 12. How many mCi must be used to prepare the capsule on Sept. 6?

Use pre-calibration factors to solve the following problems.

8. If 300 mCi of I131 sodium iodide are needed on July 28, how many Ci must be shipped on July 14?

9. A vial of Xe133 is to contain 20 mCi on Oct. 15. How many mCi must be loaded in the vial on Oct. 8?

10. How many Ci would be loaded on to the column at 8:00 am on Friday so that a Mo99 generator would contain 2.0 Ci at 8:00 am on Monday?

References:

Early & Sodee (2nd Ed.), p. 40
Kowalsky & Falen (2nd Ed.), p. 38.
Steves & Wells (3rd Ed.), p. 21–22, 24.

4. Specific concentration

Principles:

The specific concentration of a radiopharmaceutical is the activity per unit volume or unit mass. Because most radiopharmaceuticals are in liquid form, one can usually assume units of volume will be used. Activity is expressed as mCi, µCi, or Ci (or MBq, kBq, or GBq), depending upon convenience or convention.

The specific concentration is commonly referred to as simply the concentration.

You must know the specific concentration in order to calculate the volume of radiopharmaceutical that must be administered in order to provide the patient with the correct dose, or to determine the volume needed to reconstitute a radiopharmaceutical kit to a given activity.

V-7 How to calculate specific concentration:

$$\text{specific concentration} = \frac{\text{activity}}{\text{volume}}$$

Examples:

A. A vial contains 35 mCi of Tl201 thallous chloride in 4.2 ml. What is the concentration?

$$\frac{35\,\text{mCi}}{4.2\,\text{ml}} = 8.3\,\text{mCi/ml}$$

B. A vial of Tc99m MDP contains 175 mCi. Its volume is 5.4 ml. What is the concentration?

$$\frac{175\,\text{mCi}}{5.4\,\text{ml}} = 32.4\,\text{mCi/ml}$$

C. A stock solution contains 1500 µCi in 50 ml. What is the concentration of the solution?

$$\frac{1,500\,\text{µCi}}{50\,\text{ml}} = 30\,\text{µCi/ml}$$

---

* Note: If a decay factor must be applied to the activity, it can be applied either before or after the specific concentration is calculated. The answer will be the same regardless of the sequence used. (See Radiopharmacy Section 2.)

Problems:

1. The eluate from a Mo99/Tc99m generator contains 368 mCi in 5 ml. What is the concentration of the eluate?

2. A Tc99m DTPA kit contains 198 mCi in 7.6 ml. What is the specific concentration of the solution?

3. A syringe of Ga67 citrate contains 12.8 mCi in 4.1 ml. What is the concentration?

4. A vial of Tc99m sulfur colloid contains 63.2 mCi in 5.0 ml at 9:00 am. What is the concentration at 11:00 am?

5. If a vial contains 155 mCi Tc99m sodium pertechnetate in 3 ml at 7:30 am, what is the concentration at 9:00 am?

6. A vial of Tc99m MAA contains 35 mCi in 3.2 ml at 12:00 noon. What is the concentration at 2:15 pm?

7. A vial of Tc99m sodium pertechnetate contains 825 mCi in 18.7 ml at 10:05 am. What is its concentration at 2:25 pm?

8. A vial of Tc99m MDP contains 137.8 mCi at 10:45 am. The volume is 2.1 ml. What is its concentration at 12:20 pm?

References:

Christian & Waterstram-Rich (6th Ed.), p. 12–13.
Kowalsky & Falen (2nd Ed.), p. 35–38.
Steves & Wells (3rd Ed.), p. 20.

5. Dose volume calculations

Principles:

   In order to calculate the volume of a solution needed to provide the desired quantity of radioactivity, the specific concentration of the solution must be known. (See Radiopharmacy, Section 4.)

   The desired dose and the specific concentration must be in the same units of activity. If a mCi dose is needed the specific concentration must be in mCi/ml. If a μCi dose is to be used instead, the concentration must be converted to μCi/ml.

V-8 How to calculate the volume required to provide a desired activity:

$$\text{required volume} = \frac{\text{activity desired}}{\text{specific concentration}} \quad \text{or} \quad ml = \frac{mCi}{mCi/ml}$$

See Shadowbox V-7 for calculating the specific concentration.

∗ **Note:** The dose or activity required represents what you want. The specific concentration represents what you have. An easy way to remember the equation is:

$$\text{volume needed} = \frac{\text{what you want}}{\text{what you have}}$$

Examples:

A. A vial of Tc99m sodium pertechnetate contains 375 mCi in 8.2 ml. If a 20-mCi dose is needed, how many milliliters must be withdrawn from the vial?

   Calculate the concentration: $\dfrac{375\,mCi}{8.2\,ml} = 45\,mCi/ml$

   Calculate the required volume: $\dfrac{20\,mCi}{45\,mCi\,/\,ml} = 0.4\,ml$

∗ **Note:** According to guidelines for significant figures, the answer to the above equation is 0.43 ml. The number is rounded to 0.4 ml, however, because the syringes used to prepare doses and inject patients cannot measure to the hundredths place. As a standard of practice, syringe volumes should be rounded to the tenths place. (See Basic Math Skills Section 1.)

B. An 18-mCi dose of Tc99m MDP is needed. The kit contains 78.3 mCi in 2.8 ml. What volume must be withdrawn to obtain the desired dose?

Calculate the concentration: $\dfrac{78.3 \text{ mCi}}{2.8 \text{ ml}} = 28 \text{ mCi / ml}$

Calculate the required volume: $\dfrac{18 \text{ mCi}}{28 \text{ mCi / ml}} = 0.6 \text{ ml}$

---

* Note: If a decay factor is needed, it can be applied to the original activity before the specific concentration is calculated. An alternative method is to calculate the specific concentration, then apply the decay factor. The answer will be the same regardless of the method used. (See Radiopharmacy Section 2.)

C. A vial of Tc99m sodium pertechnetate contained 325.8 mCi in 5.3 ml at 3:30 pm. At 4:45 pm, a 20-mCi dose is needed. What volume must be withdrawn?

Calculate the current activity using a decay table:
The decay factor for Tc99m for 1 hour 15 minutes is 0.865.

$325.8 \times 0.865 = 281.8 \text{ mCi.}$

Calculate the specific concentration: $\dfrac{281.8 \text{ mCi}}{5.3 \text{ ml}} = 53 \text{ mCi / ml}$

Calculate the required volume: $\dfrac{20 \text{ mCi}}{53 \text{ mCi / ml}} = 0.4 \text{ ml}$

OR

Calculate the concentration, then multiple by the decay factor:

$\dfrac{325.8 \text{ mCi}}{5.3 \text{ ml}} \times 0.865 = 53 \text{ mCi/ml}$

Calculate the required volume: $\dfrac{20 \text{ mCi}}{53 \text{ mCi / ml}} = 0.4 \text{ ml}$

---

* Note: The results are identical regardless of which of the two methods is used.

Problems:

1. A vial of Tc99m DTPA contains 135 mCi in 1.2 ml. A 45-mCi dose is needed for an aerosol ventilation. How many milliliters must be withdrawn?

2. A Tc99m sulfur colloid kit contains 60 mCi in 4.6 ml. If a 4-mCi dose is needed, how many milliliters must be administered?

3. A technologist needs to reconstitute an MDP kit using 100 mCi of Tc99m sodium pertechnetate. If the eluate vial contains 213 mCi in 5.6 ml, what volume must be used for reconstitution?

4. A vial of Ga67 citrate contains 36.8 mCi in 2.7 ml. How many ml are needed for a 10-mCi dose?

5. A vial of Tl201 thallous chloride contains 15.3 mCi in 6.2 ml. What volume is needed for a 3-mCi dose?

6. A 3-mCi dose of Tc99m MAA is to be obtained from a kit containing 45.3 mCi in 4.6 ml. What volume must be used?

7. A vial of Tc99m sodium pertechnetate contained 320 mCi in 2.8 ml at 3:00 pm. What volume is required if an MAA kit is to be reconstituted with 40 mCi at 7:00 pm?

8. At 8:30 am a vial of Tc99m DTPA contained 123 mCi in 2.3 ml. At 9:30 am, a patient requires a 40-mCi aerosol dose. How many ml must be used?

9. A vial of Tc99m sodium pertechnetate contains 287 mCi in 5.3 ml at 1:30 pm. At 3:00 pm an 18-mCi dose is needed. How many ml must be administered?

10. A vial of generator eluate contained 425 mCi in 10 ml at 7:00 am. It is now 4:45 pm and a 40-mCi Tc99m MAA kit is needed. What volume must be used to reconstitute the kit?

11. A vial of Tc99m sodium pertechnetate contained 320 mCi in 4.2 ml at 4:40 pm. How many ml will be needed to reconstitute a DTPA kit to 50 mCi at 9:00 pm?

12. A Tc99m HDP kit was prepared with 173 mCi in 3.2 ml at 9:15 am. A 20-mCi bone scan dose was withdrawn at 10:00 am and another at 11:00 am. How many mCi will be left in the vial after the second dose is withdrawn?

13. A vial of Ga67 citrate contained 25.8 mCi in 3.0 at 8:00 am. What volume is needed for an 8-mCi at 5:00 pm?

Additional Applications:

14. The technologist before you forgot to enter the volume he withdrew from the Tc99m MDP vial the last time a dose was drawn. You must determine the remaining volume so you can accurately calculate your own dose volume. The vial contained 123 mCi in 3.4 ml at the time the dose was drawn. If the dose contained 19.8 mCi, approximately what volume was used?

15. A vial of Tc99m sulfur colloid contains 32 mCi in 2.2 ml. How many ml will be needed for a 5-mCi dose? How many ml will be needed if another 5-mCi dose is required 3.5 hours later? Is there still enough activity for a 5-mCi dose 4.75 hours after the second dose?

16. Three kits must be reconstituted using generator eluate that contains 828 mCi in 10 ml. The kits are to be prepared with the following activities:

MDP   200 mCi → 2.4
DTPA   150 mCi → 1.8
MAA   60 mCi   → 0.72

How many ml will be needed for each kit? What activity and volume will remain in the eluate vial after the kits are prepared?

References:

Kowalsky & Falen (2nd Ed.), p. 35–38.
Steves & Wells (3rd Ed.), p. 21–22, 24.

6. Calculation of total activity needed to provide specific number of kits or doses

Principles:

The total activity needed to reconstitute a radiopharmaceutical kit can be determined when you know the number of doses to be administered and the approximate times the doses will be required. Doses are multiplied by the appropriate pre-calibration factor or divided by a decay factor to determine the activity needed at the time of preparation (See Radiopharmacy Section 3).

Refer to Appendix A for decay factors and pre-calibration factors.

> *** Note:** In reality, a kit will be reconstituted with more than the exact activity calculated. This allows for small volume errors, minor time adjustments, and the fact that not all the activity and volume within a kit's vial can be removed from it.

> **V-9 How to calculate the total activity needed to provide a specific number of kits or doses using pre-calibration factors:**
>
> $$\text{total activity required} = \sum \left[(\text{dose})(\text{pre-calibration factor}) \right]$$
>
> where $\sum$ indicates that the values immediately following the symbol are to be summed.

> **V-10 How to calculate the total activity needed to provide a specific number of kits or doses using decay factors:**
>
> $$\text{total activity required} = \sum \left[\frac{\text{dose}}{\text{decay factor}} \right]$$
>
> where $\sum$ indicates that the values immediately following the symbol are to be summed.

Example:

A.   An MDP kit is being reconstituted to provide one 20-mCi dose at 9:00 am, at 10:00 am, at 11:00 am, and at 12:00 noon. What is the minimum activity that must be placed in the vial when it is being prepared at 7:00 am?

Pre-calibration factor (PFC) method (Shadowbox V-9):

calibration time	elapsed time	dose × PFC = activity needed at 7:00 am
9:00 am	2 h	20 mCi × 1.259 = 25 mCi
10:00 am	3 h	20 mCi × 1.414 = 28 mCi
11:00 am	4 h	20 mCi × 1.587 = 32 mCi
12:00 pm	5 h	20 mCi × 1.779 = 36 mCi

Total minimum activity needed at 7:00 am = 121 mCi

Decay factor method (Shadowbox V-10):

calibration time	elapsed time	dose ÷ DF = activity needed at 7:00 am
9:00 am	2 h	20 mCi / 0.794 = 25 mCi
10:00 am	3 h	20 mCi / 0.707 = 28 mCi
11:00 am	4 h	20 mCi / 0.63 = 32 mCi
12:00 pm	5 h	20 mCi / 0.562 = 36 mCi

Total minimum activity needed at 7:00 am = 121 mCi

---

* Note: The results are identical regardless of which of the two methods is used.

Problems:

Refer to Appendix A for both decay factors and pre-calibration factors.

Use pre-calibration factors to solve the following.

1. A Tc99m DTPA kit is to be used for the following studies. If the kit is to be prepared at 7:00 am, what is the minimum activity needed to reconstitute the kit?

9:00 am	40 mCi	lung aerosol
10:00 am	20 mCi	flow study
10:00 am	8 mCi	pediatric renogram
11:00 am	40 mCi	aerosol

2. A Tc99m MAA kit is to be prepared to perform 4 patient studies of 4 mCi each. One study will be performed at each of the following times: 10:00 am, 11:00 am, 2:00 pm, and 3:00 pm. If the kit is prepared at 8:00 am, what is the minimum activity required?

3. A Tc99m HDP kit must supply the following doses. What is the minimum activity needed when the kit is prepared at 7:00 am?

8:00 am	2 doses × 22 mCi
9:00 am	2 doses × 22 mCi
10:00 am	2 doses × 22 mCi

Use decay factors to solve the following.

4. A Tc99m disofenin kit is needed for 3 studies. The patients are scheduled at 10:00 am, 12:00 noon, and 2:00 pm, and the required dosage is 10 mCi. What is the minimum activity needed when the kit is prepared at 7:00 am?

5. At 4:00 am on Monday, a bulk vial of Ga67 gallium citrate is being prepared to provide doses for a department throughout the week. The calibration times and doses are listed below. What is the minimum activity that must be placed in the vial?

Monday noon	6 mCi
Tuesday 7:00 am	6 mCi
Wednesday noon	4 mCi

6. Three Tc99m HMPAO brain studies are to be performed using 15 mCi each. What is the minimum activity required to prepare the kit at 8:00 am, if the studies are to be performed at 10:00 am, 11:30 am, and 1:30 pm?

7. What is the minimum activity needed to reconstitute a Tc99m DTPA kit at 8:30 am, if it is to supply doses for the following studies?

9:00 am	20 mCi	brain flow
9:30 am	20 mCi	renogram
11:30 am	20 mCi	renogram
1:30 pm	8 mCi	pediatric renogram
2:00 pm	15 mCi	flow study

8. Three I123 thyroid scans are to be performed using liquid sodium iodide. If the following doses are required, what is the minimum activity needed at 5:00 am when the solution is prepared?

9:00 am	200 μCi
11:00 am	50 μCi
3:00 pm	300 μCi

Reference:

Kowalsky & Falon (2nd Ed.), p. 35–38.

7.   Total volume to be added to kit considering volume and activity limits

Principles:

The manufacturer of each radiopharmaceutical kit sets minimum and maximum activity, and volume limits for each product. These limits are based on the quantity of various chemicals in the kit. In some kits, such as MAA, the number of particles that will be present in a dose determines the volume limits. (See Radiopharmacy Section 14.)

If Tc99m generator eluate must be diluted in order to meet the minimum volume limit, preservative-free sodium chloride injection USP (physiological saline or 0.9% NaCl) must be used. The use of diluents containing bacteriostatic preservatives can interfere with the tagging process of many Tc99m-labeled radiopharmaceuticals.

V-11 How to determine the total volume to be added to a kit considering volume limits:

To determine if the volume limits are met:

1.   Calculate the specific activity.
2.   Calculate the volume to be added.
3.   Compare the volume to the manufacturer's range.
4.   Dilute eluate if minimum volume is not met.

minimum volume diluent to be added = minimum kit volume – calculated kit volume

5.   Prepare the kit for fewer doses if the maximum volume will be exceeded.

Example:

A.   The package insert for a Tc99m-labeled radiopharmaceutical kit recommends 1-5 ml volume. The technologist plans to reconstitute the kit with 30 mCi of eluate. The eluate contains 150 mCi in 2 ml. Determine the volume to be added. If it fails to meet the manufacturer's recommended minimum, determine the volume of physiological saline that must be added.

Calculate the eluate concentration: $\dfrac{150 \text{ mCi}}{2 \text{ ml}} = 75 \text{ mCi / ml}$

Calculate the volume of eluate to be used: $\dfrac{30 \text{ mCi}}{75 \text{ mCi / ml}} = 0.4 \text{ ml}$

Calculate the minimum volume of saline to be added: 1.0 ml – 0.4 ml = 0.6 ml

In order to meet the minimum volume requirement, at least 0.6 ml of preservative-free saline must be added.

V-12 How to determine the total volume to be added to a kit considering activity limits:

To determine if the activity requirements are met:

1.	Determine the total activity needed using pre-calibration or decay factors. (See Radiopharmacy Section 6.)
2.	Sum the doses.
3.	Compare the activity to the manufacturer's range.
4.	Add activity if the minimum is not met.
5.	Prepare the kit for fewer doses if the maximum activity will be exceeded.

Example:

A.	According to the package insert, a particular MDP kit should be reconstituted with a maximum of 200 mCi of eluate. If 3 20-mCi doses are needed at 9:00 am and 3 more are needed at 11:00 am, will the activity limit be exceeded when the kit is prepared at 7:00 am?

9:00 doses:	2-hour pre-calibration factor = 1.259, so 3 × 20 mCi × 1.259 = 76 mCi
11:00 doses:	4-hour pre-calibration factor = 1.587, so 3 × 20 mCi × 1.587 = 95 mCi
											Total = 171 mCi

No, the activity limit will not be exceeded.

Problems:

The activity and volume ranges used in this section are examples. When preparing kits always follow the directions on the package insert supplied with the kit.

1.	An MAA kit can be prepared using 20 to 50 mCi in 2 to 8 ml. The eluate has an activity of 830 mCi in 10 ml. If 50 mCi are used to reconstitute the vial, will further dilution be necessary to meet the volume requirements?

2.	A vial of generator eluate has an activity of 485 mCi in 8.3 ml. A DTPA kit is to be prepared with 50 mCi of eluate. If the volume limits for the kit are 2 to 8 ml, will additional saline be needed, and if so, how much?

3.	An HMPAO kit is to be reconstituted with 30 mCi of eluate having an activity of 276 mCi in 5 ml. If the volume requirement for the kit is 5 ml, how many ml of preservative-free saline must be added?

4.	The package insert for a mertiatide kit recommends a volume of 4 to 10 ml. If the kit is prepared with 80 mCi of eluate that has an activity of 246 mCi and a volume of 4.3 ml, how many ml of saline must be added?

5.	The eluate used to prepare an HDP kit has an activity of 714 mCi in 9.2 ml. The kit should have a volume of 3 to 7 ml. How much saline should be added if the kit is reconstituted with 180 mCi of eluate?

Use decay factors to solve the following problem.

6. The package insert for a DTPA kit recommends using 3 to 160 mCi to prepare the radiopharmaceutical. Will the kit provide the following doses if it is prepared at 8:00 am?

9:30 am	20 mCi for a renogram
10:30 am	40 mCi for an aerosol ventilation scan
12:30 pm	40 mCi for an aerosol ventilation scan
1:00 pm	20 mCi for a flow study

Use pre-calibration factors to solve the following problems.

7. An HDP kit is being reconstituted at 8:00 am. Four scans are scheduled with one each at 10:00 am, 11:00 am, 12:00 noon, and 1:00 pm. If a 20-mCi dose is to be used for each study, can all four be obtained from the same kit? The activity limit for this kit is 200 mCi.

8. An MDP kit is to be prepared at 8:00 am. How much activity is needed to provide the following doses? If the package insert sets the maximum activity at 200 mCi, can a single kit be used for all the doses?

9:00 am	2 doses of 20 mCi each
10:00 am	2 doses of 20 mCi each
11:00 am	1 dose of 10 mCi
12:00 pm	2 doses of 20 mCi each
1:00 pm	2 doses of 20 mCi each

9. Determine the minimum activity needed at 9:00 am to prepare a mertiatide kit for the following doses. If the activity limit for the kit is 100 mCi, can all the doses be obtained from one kit?

10:00 am	10 mCi	1:00 pm	5 mCi
11:00 am	5 mCi	2:00 pm	10 mCi
12:00 pm	10 mCi		

References:

Application of principles from Radiopharmacy, Sections 3 and 5.
Kowalsky & Falen (2nd Ed.), p. 35–38.

8. Dose calculation based on activity per unit weight

Principles:

The doses of some radiopharmaceuticals and many of the interventional drugs used in nuclear medicine are calculated according to the patient's weight. The recommended dose is expressed as mCi/kg, mg/kg, mCi/lb, or mg/lb. (For weight conversions see Basic Math Skills Section 12.)

A direct proportion is used to calculate the patient dose: $\dfrac{\text{dose}}{1 \text{ kg}} = \dfrac{\text{patient dose}}{\text{patient weight in kg}}$.

The patient dose is the unknown. The equation can be rearranged to isolate the unknown:

$$\text{patient dose} = \frac{(\text{dose})(\text{patient weight in kg})}{1 \text{ kg}}$$

Since the denominator will always be 1, the calculation process can be simplified by ignoring it. So the final, quick equation is shown in the Shadowbox below.

V-13 How to calculate a dose based on activity per unit weight:

patient dose = (dose/kg)(patient weight in kg)

* Note: The equation can also be worked in pounds if both the dose rate and the patient's weight are expressed in pounds.

Examples:

A. A 35-kg pediatric patient is scheduled for a Meckels scan. The protocol requires a Tc99m sodium pertechnetate dose of 75 µCi/kg. What dose should be administered?

$$(75 \,\mu\text{Ci/kg})(35 \text{ kg}) = 2,625 \,\mu\text{Ci or } 2.6 \text{ mCi}$$

B. Calculate the dipyridamole dose needed for a 92-kg patient who is undergoing a pharmacological stress test. The recommended dose is 0.57 mg/kg.

$$(0.57 \text{ mg/kg})(92 \text{ kg}) = 52 \text{ mg}$$

Problems:

---

* Note: Be sure the units match within a problem. Convert between lb and kg as needed.

---

1. An MAA lung scan protocol recommends 25 µCi/lb for pediatric patients. What dose would be administered to a 40-lb patient?

2. A furosemide dose of 1.0 mg/kg is recommended for a pediatric diuretic renogram, with a maximum dose of 20 mg. How many mg would be administered to an 18-kg patient?

3. A furosemide dose of 0.5 mg/kg is needed for a diuretic renogram for an adult. How many mg would be administered to an 85-kg patient if the maximum dose to be administered is 40 mg?

4. If 200 μCi/lb are recommended for a pediatric testicular scan, how many mCi of Tc99m sodium pertechnetate should be administered to a 52-lb patient?

5. The recommended dose of dipyridamole is 0.57 mg/kg. How many mg should a 185-lb patient receive?

6. If 0.02 mcg/kg of sincalide (synthetic cholecystokinin) is to be administered, how many mcg should be prepared for a 138-lb patient?

7. A protocol for a pediatric liver/spleen study calls for 25 μCi/lb of Tc99m sulfur colloid. How many μCi would be administered to a 12-kg child?

8. Enalapril is needed for an ACE inhibitor renogram for a 220-lb patient. The standard dose is 40 mcg/kg. How much enalapril should the patient receive?

9. The 6-minute protocol for an adenosine stress test uses 140 mcg/kg/min of the drug. How much adenosine is given to a 167-lb patient?

References:

Adenoscan® adenosine injection package insert.
Christian & Waterstram-Rich (6th Ed), p. 628 629.
Dipyridamole Injection USP package insert.
Kinevac® Sincalide for injection package insert.
O'Connor, p. 356, 362, 378, 398.
Steves & Wells (3rd Ed.), p. 50, 86, 96, 98.

9. Unit dose adjustments

Principles:

When using unit doses, the activity may need to be adjusted. An adult dose may need to be decreased for use as a pediatric dose, or a dose may be used at an earlier hour than that for which it was calibrated. You must apply the appropriate decay factors or pre-calibration factors to determine the activity and concentration at the time of use. The volume to be retained in the syringe is then calculated, followed by the volume to be discarded.

To prevent wasting of long-lived radiopharmaceuticals, such as Tl201 thallous chloride and Ga67 gallium citrate, unused doses can be combined at a later date, so long as their expiration times have not been exceeded. When injected through an IV, a butterfly, or a heparin lock, the relatively large volume involved should not pose a problem.

V-14 How to determine the volume to be discarded when adjusting unit doses:

Calculate the current concentration:

If the dose is to be used prior to its calibration time:

$$\text{current concentration} = \frac{(\text{calibrated activity})(\text{pre - calibration factor})}{\text{volume in syringe}}$$

If the dose is to be used after its calibration time:

$$\text{current concentration} = \frac{(\text{calibrated activity})(\text{decay factor})}{\text{volume in syringe}}$$

Calculate volume to be retained in syringe (i.e., volume for required dose):

$$\text{volume to be retained in syringe} = \frac{\text{desired dose}}{\text{current concentration}}$$

Calculate volume to be discarded, so only the desired dose remains in the syringe:

volume to be discarded = actual volume − volume to be retained.

∗ Note: If 2 unit doses are to be combined for an individual patient, use the entire dose from one syringe, then calculate the portion needed from the second syringe to complete the dose. This method is more desirable than using a portion from each syringe, because it requires manipulation of only 1 radioactive dose as opposed to 2. This is a good example of putting the ALARA philosophy into practice.

Examples:

A.   A unit dose of Tc99m sodium pertechnetate was calibrated for 9:30 am to contain 3.0 mCi in 1.8 ml. At 11:00 it is to be used as a 2-mCi dose. How many ml must be discarded?

Calculate the current concentration:
The decay factor for 1.5 hours for Tc99m is 0.841.

$$\frac{(3.0 \text{ mCi})(0.841)}{1.8 \text{ ml}} = 1.4 \text{ mCi / ml}$$

Calculate the volume to be administered (the volume to be retained in the syringe):

$$\frac{2.0 \text{ mCi}}{1.4 \text{ mCi / ml}} = 1.4 \text{ ml to be retained}$$

Calculate the volume to be discarded from the syringe:

1.8 ml actual volume – 1.4 ml to be retained = 0.4 ml to be discarded

B.   A unit dose of Tc99m DTPA is calibrated for 30 mCi at noon. A 20-mCi dose is needed at 10:00 am. The syringe contains 1.5 ml. How many ml must be discarded so the desired dose remains in the syringe?

Calculate the current concentration:
The pre-calibration factor for 2 hours for Tc99m is 1.259.

$$\frac{(30 \text{ mCi})(1.259)}{1.5 \text{ ml}} = 25.2 \text{ mCi / ml}$$

Calculate the volume to be administered (the volume to be retained in the syringe):

$$\frac{20 \text{ mCi}}{25.2 \text{ mCi / ml}} = 0.8 \text{ ml to be retained}$$

Calculate the volume to be discarded from the syringe:

1.5 ml actual volume – 0.8 ml to be retained = 0.7 ml to be discarded

Problems:

1.   A unit dose of Tl201 thallous chloride contains 3.2 mCi in 1.2 ml. How many ml must be removed so a 2.5-mCi dose remains in the syringe?

2.   If a 10-mCi dose is needed, how many ml must be discarded from a unit dose of Ga67 gallium citrate that contains 12.8 mCi in 3.4 ml? The dose to be administered remains in the syringe.

3. A unit dose of Tc99m sodium pertechnetate is calibrated to contain 20 mCi in 1.2 ml at 2:00 pm. A 20-mCi dose is needed at 10:00 am. How many ml must be discarded so the correct dose remains in the syringe?

4. A unit dose syringe containing 25 mCi of Tc99m HDP in 1.5 ml was calibrated for 1:00 pm. At 3:00 pm a 16-mCi dose is needed. How many ml must be discarded so the unit dose can be used?

5. A unit dose syringe containing 40 mCi of Tc99m DTPA in 3 ml is calibrated for 10:00 am. The unit is to be used for a 30-mCi dose at 11:10 am. How many ml must be discarded so the correct dose is retained in the syringe?

6. A 20-mCi dose of Tc99m sodium pertechnetate is needed at 9:20 am. A unit dose containing 30 mCi in 2 ml at 8:00 am is to be adjusted to provide the dose. How many ml must be discarded from the syringe?

7. A 2-mCi Ga67 gallium citrate dose is needed for a pediatric patient. The unit dose available contained 8 mCi in 2.3 ml at its calibration time 96 hours earlier. How many ml must you discard to obtain the desired dose in the syringe?

8. A unit dose of Tc99m sodium pertechnetate is calibrated to contain 20 mCi in 0.5 ml at 2:00 pm. At 12:00 noon a 10-mCi dose is needed. How many ml must be discarded from the syringe so the correct dose remains?

9. A 2.2-mCi dose of thallium was calibrated for 2:00 pm on Wednesday. It is to be used as a 1-mCi reinjection dose at 10:00 am on Thursday. What volume must be retained in the syringe if it contains 1.2 ml?

Additional Applications:

10. Two unit doses of Ga67 gallium citrate were calibrated as 6 mCi in 2 ml at 8:00 am on Monday. At 8:00 am on Thursday, a 5-mCi dose is needed. How can it be provided using the two existing doses?

11. Two Tc99m HDP doses were calibrated to contain 20 mCi each in 0.4 ml at 8:00 am. It is now 1:00 pm and a 20-mCi dose is needed. How can it best be provided using the available unit doses?

References:

Application of principles from Radiopharmacy Sections 2 to 5.

10. Pediatric dose calculations using Clark's formula

Principles:

Clark's formula allows calculation of pediatric doses by comparing the child's weight to an average adult weight of 150 lb. The standard adult dose is adjusted accordingly.

V-15 How to calculate pediatric doses using Clark's formula:

$$\text{Clark's formula:}\quad \text{child's dose} = \frac{(\text{child's weight in lb})(\text{adult dose})}{150\ \text{lb}}$$

---

* Note: Clark's formula may NOT provide an accurate determination for doses for children with very low body weights or with excessive weight. Calculations using body surface area are more accurate. (See Radiopharmacy Sections 11, 12, and 13.)

Examples:

A.   A 40-lb child needs a bone scan. What dose should be given if the adult dose is 20 mCi?

$$\frac{(40\ \text{lb})(20\ \text{mCi})}{150\ \text{lb}} = 5\ \text{mCi}$$

B.   If the adult dose for a salivary gland scan is 10 mCi, what would be the dose for an 85-lb child?

$$\frac{(85\ \text{lb})(10\ \text{mCi})}{150\ \text{lb}} = 6\ \text{mCi}$$

Problems:

* Note: Be sure the units match within a problem. Convert between lb and kg as needed. (See Basic Math Skills Section 12.)

1.   A 90-lb boy is scheduled for a MUGA scan. The average adult dose for this study is 20 mCi. How many mCi should this child receive?

2.   A 120-lb child needs a gallium scan. The usual adult dose at the facility is 6 mCi. How many mCi should be administered?

3.   How many mCi of Tc99m DTPA should be administered to a 45-lb child if the standard adult renogram dose is 20 mCi?

4.   If the adult dose for a bone scan is 22 mCi, what dose should be given to a 50-lb child?

5.   If the adult dose for a GI bleeding scan is 20 mCi, how many mCi should be administered to a 75-lb child?

6. A 140-lb child needs a DTPA renogram. How many mCi should be administered if the adult dose is 20 mCi?

7. If the standard adult dose for an hepatobiliary scan is 8 mCi, how many mCi would be administered to a 20-lb child?

8. If 300 μCi of I123 are given to adult patients, how many would be given to a 60-lb child?

Additional Applications:

9. A 32-kg child needs a gallium scan. If the standard adult dose for your facility is 4 mCi, how many mCi should the child receive? If a vial of Ga67 gallium citrate contains 6.8 mCi in 3.2 ml, how many ml must be administered to the child?

10. At 2:00 pm a vial of Tc99m MDP contains 92.8 mCi in 4.7 ml. The facility's adult dose is 20 mCi. At 4:30 pm a dose is needed for a 53-lb child. What dose must be used? What volume must be administered?

11. A 36-kg child needs a Tc99m mertiatide scan. If the usual adult dose is 10 mCi, what dose should the child be given? The mertiatide vial contained 53 mCi in 4.2 ml at 12:00 noon. It is now 1:45 pm. How many ml must be withdrawn to obtain the correct dose?

References:

Steves & Wells (3rd Ed.), p. 25.

11. Pediatric dose calculations using body surface area

Principles:

A child's organs are proportionally larger than those of an adult when compared to body mass. Organ mass, metabolic rates, and blood fluid volumes are more closely related to body surface area (BSA) than to body weight. The BSA is therefore a more accurate method for calculating pediatric doses as compared to Clark's formula, which uses body weight. (See Radiopharmacy Section 10.)

Body surface area can be estimated using the formula below. To save time, tables have been developed listing patient weight, the calculated body surface area, and the fraction of the adult dose that should be used. The standard adult dose is based on the "reference man." The reference man has a weight of 70 kg or 154 lb, and a body surface area of 1.779 m². The reference man is used to determine standard radiopharmaceutical dose ranges and the predicted radiation doses to organs and to the total body.

---
* Note: A survey of literature found a number of BSA tables that used an adult reference of 1.73 m² BSA, which is equivalent to 148 lb or 67 kg, or a 1.7 m² BSA, which is equivalent to 144 lb or 66 kg.

The BSA is calculated as follows: $\text{body surface area in m}^2 = \dfrac{\left(\text{body weight in kg}\right)^{0.7}}{11}$

---
* Note: To calculate (body weight)$^{0.7}$ on a calculator use the x^y function with the body weight as x and 0.7 as y. For the proper key sequence, refer to the instrument's instruction book.

The fraction of the adult dose to be used based on BSA is calculated as follows:

$$\text{fraction of adult dose} = \frac{\text{child's BSA in m}^2}{1.779 \text{ m}^2}$$

The two equations can be combined into a single equation:

$$\text{fraction of adult dose} = \frac{\left(\text{body weight in kg}\right)^{0.7}}{\left(11\right)\left(1.779 \text{ m}^2\right)}$$

V-16 How to calculate pediatric doses using the body surface area (BSA) equation:

1. Calculate the fraction of the adult dose to be used:

$$\text{fraction of adult dose} = \frac{\left(\text{body weight in kg}\right)^{0.7}}{\left(11\right)\left(1.779 \text{ m}^2\right)}$$

2. Calculate the child's dose: pediatric dose = (adult dose)(fraction of adult dose)

Example:

A. If a 4-mCi dose of Tc99m MAA is given to an adult, how much should be administered to a 24-kg child?

$$\frac{(24)^{0.7}}{(11)(1.779)} = \frac{9.25}{19.569} = 0.47 \qquad\qquad (4\ \text{mCi})(0.47) = 1.9\ \text{mCi}$$

A body surface area table can be created using the equations listed in the Principles section. Such a table eliminates some of the calculations, and therefore saves time and decreases possible errors.

Body Surface Area Table

Weight kg	lb	Body Surface Area in m^2 *	Fraction of Adult Dose ✦	Weight kg	lb	Body Surface Area in m^2 *	Fraction of Adult Dose ✦
2	4.4	0.15	0.08	14	30	0.58	0.32
3	6.6	0.20	0.11	15	33	0.61	0.34
4	8.8	0.24	0.13	20	44	0.74	0.42
5	11	0.28	0.16	25	55	0.87	0.49
6	13	0.32	0.18	30	66	0.98	0.55
7	15	0.35	0.20	35	77	1.10	0.62
8	18	0.39	0.22	40	88	1.20	0.68
9	20	0.42	0.24	45	99	1.31	0.73
10	22	0.46	0.26	50	110	1.41	0.79
11	24	0.49	0.27	55	121	1.50	0.84
12	26	0.52	0.29	60	132	1.60	0.90
13	29	0.55	0.31	65	143	1.69	0.95

* Calculated from body surface area in m^2 $= \dfrac{(\text{body weight in kg})^{0.7}}{11}$

✦ Calculated from fraction of adult dose $= \dfrac{(\text{body weight in kg})^{0.7}}{(11)(1.779\ \text{m}^2)}$

(Adapted from O'Connor M, ed. *The Mayo Clinic manual of nuclear medicine*. New York: Churchill Livingstone; 1996:569. Reprinted with permission.)

V-17 How to calculate a pediatric dose using a body surface area table:

1. Locate the child's weight in either the kg or lb column.
2. Read across to the fraction of adult dose column.
3. Calculate the child's dose: pediatric dose = (adult dose)(fraction of adult dose)
4. If the patient's weight falls between the values listed, use the nearest weight or estimate the fraction by extrapolation. Although the fraction is not exactly correct, the small difference is insignificant in regards to the quality of the study and the radiation dose to the patient.

Examples:

A. If a 4-mCi dose of Tc99m MAA is given to an adult, how much should be administered to a 24-kg child?

Estimate the fraction from the table: 0.48
(4 mCi)(0.48) = 1.9 mCi

---

* Note: This is the same example that was used to demonstrate the equation in Shadowbox V-16, Example A. Notice that the answers are identical.

B. A 15-kg child needs a bone scan. If the adult dose is 20 mCi, how many mCi should be administered?

Fraction of adult dose from table: 0.34
(20 mCi)(0.34) = 6.8 mCi

Problems:

1. A 6-kg child needs a GI bleeding scan. If 20 mCi of Tc99m sodium pertechnetate is used to tag the red blood cells, how much should be used for the child?

2. If the adult dose for Tc99m MAG3 is 8 mCi, how many mCi should be used for a 35-kg child?

3. The adult dose for a Tc99m sulfur colloid liver/spleen scan is 5 mCi. How many µCi should be administered to a 3-kg infant?

4. Calculate the pediatric dose for a 42-kg patient if the adult dose for a Tc99m MDP is 20 mCi.

5. If a protocol recommends 6 mCi of Ga67 gallium citrate for adult patients, how much activity should be administered to a 37-kg child?

6. A 4-kg infant is to be examined for ectopic thyroid tissue using I123 sodium iodide. If the adult dose is 300 µCi, how many µCi should be administered to the baby?

7. If the adult dose for Tc99m HMPAO brain imaging is 12 mCi, what is the appropriate dose for an 11-kg child?

8. Determine the dose of Tc99m sodium pertechnetate to be given to a 52-kg child if the standard dose for a testicular scan is 10 mCi.

Problems 9 to 16 are the same as problems 1 to 8 in Radiopharmacy, Sections 10 and 12. Compare the results to Clark's and Talbot's methods.

9. A 90-lb boy is scheduled for a MUGA scan. The average adult dose for this study is 20 mCi. How many mCi should this child receive?

10. A 120-lb child needs a gallium scan. The usual adult dose at the facility is 6 mCi. How many mCi should be administered?

11. How many mCi of Tc99m DTPA should be administered to a 45-lb child if the standard adult renogram dose is 20 mCi?

12. If the adult dose for a bone scan is 22 mCi, what dose should be given to a 50-lb child?

13. If the adult dose for a GI bleeding scan is 20 mCi, how many mCi should be administered to a 75-lb child?

14. A 140-lb child needs a DTPA renogram. How many mCi should be administered if the adult dose is 20 mCi?

15. If the standard adult dose for an hepatobiliary scan is 8 mCi, how many mCi would be administered to a 20-lb child?

16. If 300 μCi of I123 are given to adult patients, how many would be given to a 60-lb child?

References:

Christian & Waterstram-Rich (6th Ed.), p. 628 629.
O'Connor, p. 569.
Steves & Wells (3rd Ed.), p. 25.

12. Pediatric dose calculations using Talbot's nomogram

Principles:

A nomogram is a graph or table representing the relationship between variables—in this case, weight or body surface area and the fraction of the adult dose.

Talbot's nomogram was calculated using body surface area, which was then correlated with body weight. For simplicity of use, the child's weight can now be used to determine the dose.

Talbot's Nomogram

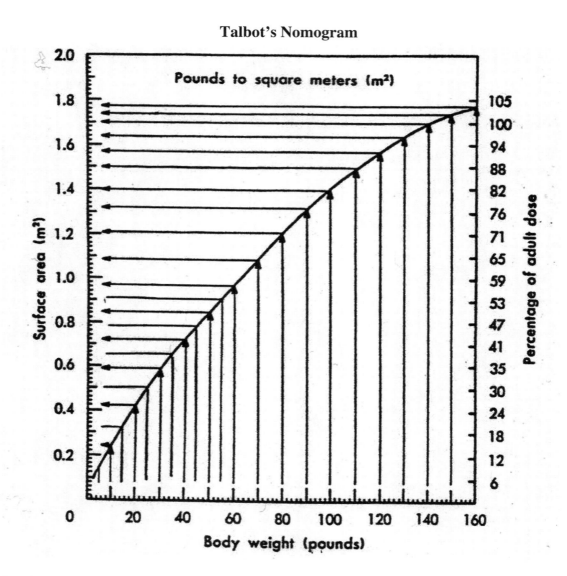

(Reprinted with permission from Talbot N, Richie R. The advantages of surface area of the body as a basis for calculating pediatric dosages. *Pediatrics* 1959;24:495–498.)

V-18 How to calculate pediatric doses using Talbot's nomogram:

1. Use a straightedge to read from the patient's "Body weight" on the bottom line to the arching line that crosses the table diagonally. Now read from the arching line to the "Percentage of adult dose" on the right-hand side of the table.
2. Change the whole number to a decimal and apply it to the calculation:

pediatric dose = (fraction of adult dose)(adult dose)

Examples:

A. A 20-lb child needs a hepatobiliary scan. If the standard adult dose is 10 mCi, how many mCi should the child receive?

According to Talbot's nomogram, the child should receive about 26% of the adult dose. (0.26)(10 mCi) = 2.6 mCi

* **Note:** Do not be surprised by small variations between the percentage doses listed in the answers below and those you chose. There is always some personal judgment involved when making estimates. Your answers should be reasonably close; for example, you may see a 20-lb child as receiving 25% of the adult dose, while the author selected 26%. These are not significant differences.

If, however, you find the percentage you selected is markedly different from that chosen by the author, check the nomogram again.

B. An I123 thyroid scan is to be performed on a 40-lb child. How many μCi should be administered if the adult dose in 200 μCi?

According to Talbot's nomogram, 43% of the adult dose should be administered. (0.43)(200 μCi) = 86 μCi

Problems:

* **Note:** Be sure the units match within a problem. Convert between lb and kg when needed. (See Basic Math Skills Section 12.)

Problems 1 to 8 are the same as problems 1 to 8 in Radiopharmacy Section 10. They are also the same as problems 9 to 16 in Radiopharmacy Section 11. Compare the results to Clark's and the BSA methods.

1. A 90-lb boy is scheduled for a MUGA scan. The average adult dose for this study is 20 mCi. How many mCi should this child receive?

2. A 120-lb child needs a gallium scan. The usual adult dose at the facility is 6 mCi. How many mCi should be administered?

3. How many mCi of Tc99m DTPA should be administered to a 45-lb child if the standard adult renogram dose is 20 mCi?

4. If the adult dose for a bone scan is 22 mCi, what dose should be given to a 50-lb child?

5. If the adult dose for a GI bleeding scan is 20 mCi, how many mCi should be administered to a 75-lb child?

6. A 140-lb child needs a DTPA renogram. How many mCi should be administered if the adult dose is 20 mCi?

7. If the standard adult dose for an hepatobiliary scan is 8 mCi, how many mCi would be administered to a 20-lb child?

8. If 300 μCi of I123 are given to adult patients, how many would be given to a 60-lb child?

9. A 4.5-kg child needs a bone scan. If the adult dose is 20 mCi, how many mCi will be administered to the child?

10. If the adult dose for a Tc99m sodium pertechnetate thyroid scan is 10 mCi, what dose should be given to a 45-lb child?

11. A 9-kg child needs a DMSA renal scan. How many mCi are administered if the adult dose is 5 mCi?

12. If an adult receives 6 mCi of Ga67 gallium citrate, how many mCi should a 70-lb child receive?

13. A 45-kg child is to have a Tc99m DTPA renogram. What dose should the child receive if an adult is given 20 mCi?

14. A 30-lb child needs a liver/spleen scan. If the standard adult dose is 4 mCi, what activity should be administered to the child?

Additional Applications:

15. If the adult dose for a liver/spleen scan is 4 mCi of Tc99m sulfur colloid, what dose should be given to a 50-kg child? How many ml should be administered if the Tc99m sulfur colloid kit contains 42 mCi in 3.8 ml? (See Radiopharmacy Section 5.)

16. The adult dose for a hepatobiliary scan is 5 mCi. Calculate the dose for a 15-lb child. If the disofenin vial contains 25 mCi in 5.2 ml, how many ml should the child receive?

17. An 18-kg child needs a GI bleeding scan. The usual adult dose is 20 mCi of Tc99m tagged red blood cells. What dose should the child receive? If the Tc99m sodium pertechnetate vial contains 20 mCi in 1.4 ml, how many ml must be used to tag the red blood cells with the correct dose?

18. A 60-lb child needs a bone scan at 9:00 am. A unit dose is calibrated to contain the standard adult dose of 22 mCi in 0.8 ml at 11:00 am. How many ml must be discarded from the syringe so it holds the correct pediatric dose for the child? (See Radiopharmacy Section 9.)

References:

Christian & Waterstram-Rich (6th Ed.), p. 629.
Talbot & Richie, p. 497.

13. Minimum and maximum pediatric doses

Principles:

In order to obtain a valid scan, the photon flux produced in the organ or area of interest must be sufficiently high to produce a diagnostic study. Although we want to minimize the absorbed radiation dose, we cannot compromise the quality of the study. For newborns and infants the calculated radiopharmaceutical dose may provide too low a photon flux.

Minimum doses have been determined for most studies. If the calculated dose falls below the recommended minimum, then the minimum dose should be used instead.

Maximum doses should also be set for pediatric patients.

---

* Note: Any facility that performs studies on children should have a list of minimum and maximum pediatric doses that have been approved by the authorized user. (See the references at the end of this section.)

V-19 How to determine pediatric doses based on minimum and maximum dose standards:

1. Determine the pediatric dose using one of the pediatric dose determination methods as shown in Radiopharmacy, Sections 8, 10, 11, and 12.
2. Compare the calculated dose to the minimum and maximum dose list.
3. If the calculated dose is smaller than the minimum dose, the minimum dose must be used. If the calculated dose is larger than the maximum dose, the maximum dose is used.

Examples:

Use the BSA table in Radiopharmacy Section 11 to solve examples A and B.

A. The adult dose for Tc99m HMPAO brain imaging is 10 mCi. What dose would be given to a 6-kg infant if the minimum dose is 2 mCi?

   Using the BSA table, determine the fraction of the adult dose to be used: 0.18.
   Calculate the dose: 0.18 × 10 mCi = 1.8 mCi.
   Since 1.8 mCi is below the minimum dose of 2 mCi, the minimum dose should be used.

B. Calculate the Tc99m MDP dose for an 11-lb infant. The adult dose is 20 mCi and the minimum dose is 5 mCi.

   Using the BSA table, determine the fraction of the adult dose to be used: 0.16.
   Calculate the dose: 0.16 × 20 mCi = 3.2 mCi.
   Since 3.2 mCi is below the minimum dose of 5 mCi, the minimum dose should be used.

C.   If the pediatric dose for a perfusion lung scan is 25 µCi/lb with a maximum of 2 mCi, how many mCi should be administered to a 60-lb child? (See Radiopharmacy Section 8.)

Calculate the dose: (25 µCi/lb)(60 lb) = 1,500 µCi or 1.5 mCi. This does NOT exceed the 2 mCi maximum, so it can be used.

Problems:

* **Note:** Be sure the units match within a problem. Convert between lb and kg as needed. (See Basic Math Skills Section 12.)

Use the BSA table in Radiopharmacy Section 11 to calculate the following.

1.   A 3-kg infant is being evaluated for biliary atresia. What dose of Tc99m disofenin should be given if the adult dose is 10 mCi and the minimum dose is 1 mCi?

2.   If 3 mCi are needed for a standard adult liver dose, how many µCi must be administered to a 10-lb infant? The minimum dose is 500 µCi.

3.   An 11-kg baby needs a gallium study. If a protocol gives the adult dose as 10 mCi and the minimum dose as 3 mCi, how much should the child receive?

4.   A Tc99m DMSA study is to be performed on a 6-kg infant. The adult dose is 5 mCi and the minimum dose is 500 µCi. How many µCi should the infant be given?

5.   A newborn baby weighing 7 lbs needs a perfusion lung scan. If the adult dose is 4 mCi and the minimum dose is 500 µCi, what dose should be administered to the infant?

6.   A 13-lb infant is to receive I123 sodium iodide. The adult dose is 200 µCi and the recommended minimum dose is 30 µCi. What dose should be given?

For the following questions calculate the pediatric dose based on activity per pound of body weight. (See Radiopharmacy, Section 8.)

7.   A 70-lb child is scheduled for a gated cardiac study. How much activity should the child receive if the recommended dose is 350 µCi/lb and the maximum dose is 20 mCi?

8.   If the pediatric dose for bone imaging is set at 300 µCi/lb with a maximum of 20 mCi, how many mCi should be administered to an 85-lb child?

9.   Calculate the dose to be administered to a 55-lb child who is to have a Meckel's scan. The dose rate is 100 µCi/lb and the maximum is not to exceed 15 mCi.

10. A 110-lb child needs a testicular scan. Determine the activity that should be administered if the dose rate is 200 µCi/lb, with a total dose not to exceed 15 mCi.

11. What dose should be administered to an 18-kg child who is having a liver scan? The dose rate is to be 25 µCi/lb with a maximum of 2 mCi.

12. If the recommended dose for a Meckel's scan is 100 μCi/lb with a minimum of 2.5 mCi, what dose should be administered to a 10-kg child?

13. An MAA lung perfusion protocol recommends 25 μCi/lb with a minimum of 500 μCi for pediatric patients. If a 32-lb child needs a lung scan, how many μCi should be given?

14. A Tc99m mertiatide protocol calls for the use of 50 μCi/kg for pediatric patients. What activity should be used for a 33-lb child if the minimum dose is 1 mCi?

References:

Christian & Waterstram-Rich (6th Ed.), p. 628–629. (Includes recommended pediatric dose rates, plus minimum and maximum doses.)
O'Connor, p. 566–568. (Includes a list of minimum pediatric doses.)

14. Lung perfusion radiopharmaceutical particle calculations

Principles:

In order to assure an adequate distribution of the macroaggregates or microspheres used for lung perfusion imaging, a patient should receive a specific number of particles. The manufacturer's package inserts for various MAA kits recommend ranges from 200,000 to 1,200,000 particles per patient dose, with a recommended average of 100,000 to 500,000 particles. An inadequate number of particles could result in decreased scan sensitivity. Doses containing quantities greater than 1,200,000 do not appear to improve the quality of the study and are therefore unnecessary.

A minimum number of particles, usually 60,000, is administered to adults with right-to-left cardiac shunts or pulmonary hypertension. A maximum dose of only 50,000 particles is recommended for newborns and 150,000 particles for children up to 1 year old.

---

* Note: Once a kit is reconstituted, the specific radioactive concentration decreases with time. The MAA particle concentration, however, does not. Therefore, as a larger and larger kit volume is required to obtain a given patient dose, a greater number of MAA particles is administered.

V-20 How to calculate the particles per dose for lung perfusion agents:

1. Determine the volume dose to be administered to the patient:

    $$\text{specific concentration} = \frac{\text{activity}}{\text{volume}} \quad \text{(See Shadowbox V-7.)}$$

    $$\text{required volume} = \frac{\text{activity desired}}{\text{specific concentration}} \quad \text{or} \quad ml = \frac{mCi}{mCi/ml} \quad \text{(See Shadowbox V-8.)}$$

2. Calculate the particle concentration of the reconstituted kit:

    $$\frac{\text{total particles in kit}}{\text{ml added to kit}} = \text{particles} / ml$$

3. Calculate the particles per dose:

    A direct proportion can be used: $\dfrac{\text{particles}}{1 \; ml} = \dfrac{\text{particles in patient dose}}{\text{ml of patient dose}}$

    The equation can be rearranged and simplified as follows:
    (particle concentration in particles/ml)(ml dose volume) = particles in patient dose.

Examples:

A. An MAA kit produced by company XYZ contains an average of 4,000,000 particles. If the kit is reconstituted with 5.0 ml, what is the particle concentration?

$$\frac{4,000,000 \text{ particles}}{5.0 \text{ ml}} = 800,000 \text{ particles} / \text{ml}$$

B. If a kit has a particle concentration of 1,200,000 particles/ml, how many particles will be contained in a 0.4-ml dose?

$$(1,200,000 \text{ particles/ml})(0.4 \text{ ml}) = 480,000 \text{ particles}$$

Problems:

1. A protocol recommends that an MAA kit be reconstituted with 50 mCi Tc99m pertechnetate in 5 ml. What will be the particle concentration if a kit contains an average of 14 million particles?

2. The MAA kits from Company XIX contain an average of 8,000,000 particles. If a kit is prepared with 6 ml of eluate, what is the particle concentration?

3. An MAA kit has a concentration of 800,000 particles/ml. How many particles will be administered in a 0.3-ml dose?

4. How many particles are contained in a 0.7-ml dose if an MAA has a concentration of 500,000 particles per ml?

5. An MAA kit containing an average of 5,500,000 particles is reconstituted with 40 mCi and 6 ml. How many particles will be administered in a 4-mCi dose?

6. If an MAA kit containing 3 million particles is prepared with 20 mCi in 2 ml, how many particles will be present in a 3-mCi dose?

7. A given manufacturer's MAA kit contains an average of 8 million particles. A kit is prepared with 40 mCi and 5 ml at 9:00 am. How many particles are contained in a 4-mCi dose at the time of reconstitution?

8. How many particles will be contained in a 4-mCi dose drawn from the vial in problem #7 at 12:00 noon?

---

* Note: In problems 7 and 8, observe that the number of particles in the 4-mCi doses drawn at different times from the same kit contain variable numbers of particles.

As the radioactivity decreases due to decay, a larger volume must be used to obtain the same dose activity. Particle concentration, however, does not change. Therefore, the total number of particles withdrawn for the same activity dose will increase with time.

---

9. An MAA kit containing 12 million particles is prepared with 90 mCi in 5 ml at 7:00 am. How many particles will be administered when a 4-mCi dose is given at 11:00 am?

Additional Applications:

10. If an MAA kit contains an average of 5,000,000 particles, what volume should be used to prepare the kit so a 0.5-ml dose will contain 400,000 particles? (See Basic Math Skills Section 7.)

11. In order to obtain 300,000 particles in a 0.4-ml dose, how many ml would be needed to reconstitute an MAA kit that averages 8 million particles?

12. An average of 2,500,000 particles are found in a brand of MAA. What volume must be used to dilute the kit if a maximum dose volume of 1.0 ml is used and no more than 1,200,000 particles are to be administered?

References:

Application of principles from Basic Math Skills Section 7.
Application of principles from Radiopharmacy Sections 1 to 6.
DraxImage™ MAA Kit package insert.
Kowalsky & Falen (2nd Ed.), p. 564 565, 578.
Pulmolite ® Kit package insert.

15. Generator yield based on efficiency

Principles:

When eluting a radionuclide generator, it is never possible to remove all the daughter nuclide, because of channeling, variations in thickness of the Mo99 coating on the alumina beads, radiolysis, etc. The ratio of the average amount that can be eluted (actual yield) versus the amount of daughter actually on the column (theoretical yield) is referred to as the elution_efficiency or generator efficiency. This is a useful number, as it will give a reasonable estimate of the amount of Tc99m that will actually be obtained from a generator.

V-21 How to calculate generator efficiency:

A simple percentage equation is used to determine percent elution efficiency.

$$\text{elution efficiency} = \frac{\text{actual yield}}{\text{theoretical yield}} \times 100\%$$

where: theoretical yield =   Tc99m present on column
              actual yield   =   Tc99m removed during elution

---

Example:

A.   If a Mo99/Tc99m generator contains 820 mCi of Tc99m, but only 680 mCi can be eluted, what is the efficiency of the generator?

$$\frac{680 \text{ mCi}}{820 \text{ mCi}} \times 100 = 83\%$$

V-22 How to estimate generator yield based on theoretical yield and elution efficiency:

If you know the elution efficiency, you can estimate the activity that will be eluted by rearranging the equation in Shadowbox V-21. The actual yield becomes the estimated yield.

$$\text{If elution efficiency} = \frac{\text{estimated yield}}{\text{theoretical yield}} \times 100\% \text{ ,}$$

$$\text{then estimated yield} = \frac{\text{elution efficiency}}{100\%} \times \text{theoretical yield} \text{ , which can be simplified to:}$$

estimated yield = (theoretical yield)(elution efficiency as a decimal)

Example:

A. If a generator regularly yields 85% of the Tc99m activity on its column, how many mCi will be eluted when 710 mCi are present on the column?

Convert 85% to its decimal form: 0.85

(710 mCi)(0.85) = 604 mCi

Problems:

1. If a generator yields 550 mCi when 600 mCi of technetium are actually present on the column, what is its percent efficiency?

2. When 1 Ci is available in the generator, 830 mCi were actually eluted. What is the percent efficiency of the generator?

3. If 375 mCi are eluted from the generator when the column actually contains 480 mCi, what is the elution efficiency?

4. If a column has 265 mCi of Tc99m available but only 190 mCi are eluted, what is the elution efficiency?

5. The expected yield from a generator is 430 mCi and the actual elution activity is 380 mCi. What is the elution efficiency?

6. Estimate the activity that will be eluted from a generator with an elution efficiency of 87% when 880 mCi are present on the column.

7. If a generator is 82% efficiency and 1.2 Ci are present, how many mCi should be eluted?

8. If 260 mCi are on a column and a generator has a known efficiency of 89%, how many mCi can be obtained?

9. A generator has a 93% elution efficiency. Estimate the eluate activity when there are 540 mCi of technetium on the column.

References:

Saha (4th Ed.), p. 71–73.
Steves & Wells (3rd Ed.), p. 20.

16. Mo99/Tc99m generator yield based on decay

Principles:

A Mo99/Tc99m generator operates in transient equilibrium. About 86% of the Mo99 decays directly into Tc99m, with the remainder decaying into Tc99. When equilibrium is reached at about 48 hours post-elution, the quantity of Tc99m on the column is approximately 95% of the Mo99 activity. That proportion remains essentially constant from the time equilibrium is reached until the generator is eluted.

Prior to reaching equilibrium, the ratio of Tc99m to Mo99 (or the fraction of activity in the form of Tc99m as compared to Mo99 activity) increases with time from the point of elution. The following table lists the activity of Tc99m present on the column as a fraction of the Mo99 activity for a given time post-elution. The fractions were calculated using the ratio of Tc99m activity divided by Mo99 activity.

Tc99m/Mo99 Activity Table
Fraction Tc99m radioactivity (as compared to Mo99 radioactivity)

$$= \frac{A_2}{A_1} = \frac{0.860\lambda_2 \left(e^{-\lambda_1 t} - e^{-\lambda_2 t}\right)}{\left(\lambda_2 - \lambda_1\right)\left(e^{-\lambda_1 t}\right)}$$

Time (t) (h)	$\dfrac{A_2}{A_1}$	Time (t) (h)	$\dfrac{A_2}{A_1}$	Time (t) (h)	$\dfrac{A_2}{A_1}$
0.5	0.048	10.0	0.614	27	0.890
1.0	0.094	10.5	0.631	28	0.896
1.5	0.138	11.0	0.647	29	0.901
2.0	0.179	11.5	0.662	30	0.905
2.5	0.218	12.0	0.677	32	0.913
3.0	0.255	13.0	0.704	34	0.919
3.5	0.290	14.0	0.728	36	0.924
4.0	0.324	15.0	0.750	38	0.929
4.5	0.356	16.0	0.769	40	0.932
5.0	0.386	17.0	0.787	44	0.937
5.5	0.414	18.0	0.803	48	0.940
6.0	0.441	19.0	0.817	54	0.943
6.5	0.467	20.0	0.830	60	0.944
7.0	0.492	21.0	0.841	66	0.945
7.5	0.515	22.0	0.852	72	0.946
8.0	0.537	23.0	0.861	78	0.946
8.5	0.558	24.0	0.870	84	0.946
9.0	0.578	25.0	0.877	90	0.946
9.5	0.596	26.0	0.884	96	0.946

(Reprinted with permission from Chilton H, Wotcofski R. *Nuclear pharmacy: an introduction to the clinical application of radiopharmaceuticals*. Philadelphia: Lea & Febiger; 1986:59.)

* Note: Note the rapid increase in Tc99m activity versus Mo99 activity in the first 12 hours. After this time, the change in the fraction per unit time begins to slow and eventually levels off, becoming a constant after 72 hours post-elution.

V-23 How to determine the theoretical yield of a Mo99/Tc99m generator at a specified time post-elution:

1.   Calculate the elapsed time from the last elution and select the appropriate Mo99 decay factor. (See Radiopharmacy Sections 2 and 3.)
2.   Select the Tc99m/Mo99 fraction for the elapsed time.
3.   Determine the theoretical yield of Tc99m for the specified time:

theoretical yield = (Mo99 activity × decay factor)(Tc99m/Mo99 ratio as fraction).

Examples:

A.   A generator calibrated for 4,100 mCi of Mo99 at 12:00 noon on Wednesday is to be eluted at 8:00 am on Thursday. Assuming the generator was last eluted at calibration time, what is the theoretical yield of Tc99m at 8:00 am?

Calculate the time between elutions: 20 hours.

Select decay factor for Mo99 (see Appendix A): 0.812
Select fraction from Tc99m/Mo99 the table: 0.830
(4,100 mCi × 0.812)(0.830) = 2,763 mCi Tc99m

B.   At 10:00 am a generator containing 850 mCi Mo99 was eluted. How many mCi of Tc99m will be present on the column when the generator is eluted 3 hours later?

Mo99 decay factor: 0.969
Tc99m/Mo99 fraction for 3 hours: 0.255
(850 mCi × 0.969)(0.255) = 210 mCi Tc99m

∗ **Note:** The estimated yield equation from Shadowbox V-22 can be combined with the theoretical yield equation from Shadowbox V-23 to form a single equation that allows estimation of Mo99/Tc99m generator yield at a specified time post-elution.

V-24 How to estimate Mo99/Tc99m generator yield at a specified time post-elution:

estimated yield = (Mo99 activity × decay factor)(Tc99m/Mo99 ratio as fraction)(efficiency).

Example:

A.   A generator column containing 522 mCi Mo99 was eluted at 2:00 pm. It is eluted again at 10:00 pm. Estimate the yield if the generator has an 85% elution efficiency.

Elapsed time: 8 hours
Mo99 decay factor: 0.911
Tc99m/Mo99 fraction: 0.537

(522 mCi × 0.911)(0.537)(0.85) = 217 mCi

Problems:

1.   A 6.6-Ci generator is calibrated at 7:00 pm Friday. It is eluted for the first time on Monday at 7:00 am. What is the theoretical yield of Tc99m?

2.   After elution, a generator retains 610 mCi Mo99 on its column. What is the theoretical yield when the unit is eluted 6 hours later?

3.   If 495 mCi of Mo99 are present at 4:00 pm Tuesday, how many mCi of Tc99m are on the column at 8:00 am Wednesday?

4.   A generator containing 1.2 Ci of Mo99 was eluted at 6:00 am. How many mCi of Tc99m are available on the column at 6:00 am the following day?

5.   At 2:00 pm 270 mCi Mo99 were present in the generator after elution. If the unit is not eluted again until 9:00 pm, how much Tc99m is theoretically available?

6.   A generator with an 80% efficiency is eluted, leaving 315 mCi of Mo99 on the column. What will be the estimated yield of Tc99m 18 hours later?

7.   A generator containing 720 mCi Mo99 that was eluted at 7:00 am is to be eluted at 10:00 am. If the standard elution efficiency is 87%, how many mCi of Tc99m could be expected?

8.   If 690 mCi of Mo99 remained in a generator after elution at 3:00 pm on Friday, how many mCi of Tc99m should be eluted at 1:00 pm on Saturday? The generator has an 80% efficiency.

9.   How many mCi of Tc99m would be eluted from the generator in Problem 8 if it is not eluted until 4:00 pm on Saturday?

10. How many mCi of Tc99m would be eluted from the generator in Problem 8 if it is not eluted until 11:00 pm on Saturday?

> *** Note:** Compare the results of Problems 8, 9, and 10. As a generator reaches its maximum activity post-elution (23 h), a delay in elution does not increase the yield. Even though the Tc99m/Mo99 fraction slowly increases during this period, the Mo99 activity decreases due to decay. Waiting a long period before eluting the generator does not increase the Tc99m activity obtained and eventually the amount will actually begin to decrease. This is typical of a generator that operates in transient equilibrium.

11. A generator has an activity of 1,540 mCi Mo99 on the column after elution at 7:00 am. How many mCi of Tc99m can be eluted at 10:00 am if the generator has an efficiency of 80%?

12. How many mCi of Tc99m can be eluted if the generator in Problem 11 is not eluted until 12:00 noon?

13. How many mCi of Tc99m can be eluted if the generator in Problem 11 is not eluted until 2:00 pm?

> *** Note:** Compare the results of Problems 11, 12, and 13. Note that a relatively small increase in time (a few hours) results in a significant increase in Tc99m yield. This occurs only in the first 7 hours post-elution; growth then slows until it reaches a maximum at 23 hours post-elution. Early, rapid growth is typical of both transient and secular equilibrium generators.

References:

Christian & Waterstram-Rich (6th Ed.), p. 168–170.
Kowalsky & Falen (2nd Ed.), p. 219–221.
O'Connor, p. 74–77.
Saha (4th Ed.), p. 71–73.

17. Allowable Mo99 content in generator eluate

Principles:

All Tc99m is produced in a Mo99-Tc99m ion exchange generator. Although the Mo99 is carefully loaded into the generators and should remain bound to the supporting aluminum trioxide beads, small amounts of Mo99 can become dislodged. Any unbound Mo99 will be washed out during elution to become part of the Tc99m generator eluate.

Because of its high energy, relatively long half-life, and beta production, the presence of Mo99 in eluate is undesirable. Since Mo99 would expose a patient to unnecessary radiation, the NRC has placed limits on the level of Mo99 contaminant that can be present in radiopharmaceuticals.

➤ **Regulations:** According to NRC 10CFR35, Tc99m generator eluate cannot contain more than 0.15 μCi of Mo99 per mCi of Tc99m at the time of administration. This is commonly written as 0.15 μCi Mo99/mCi Tc99m. The NRC only requires eluate obtained from the first elution after receipt of the generator to be checked for Mo99 content. As with all regulations concerning the practice of nuclear medicine, state and local government requirements may differ from the NRC.

For every 1 mCi of Tc99m, you can have a maximum of 0.15 μCi of Mo99. This is a direct relationship or direct proportion.

$$\frac{0.15\,\mu\text{Ci Mo99}}{1\,\text{mCi Tc99m}} = \frac{X\,\mu\text{Ci Mo99}}{\text{activity of Tc99m in mCi}}$$

To find the maximum Mo99 activity allowed for the Tc99m dose, isolate and solve for X.

$$\frac{(0.15\,\mu\text{Ci Mo99})(\text{activity of Tc99m in mCi})}{1\,\text{mCi Tc99m}} = X\,\mu\text{Ci Mo99}$$

Notice that the equation can be simplified. The 1 in the denominator can be ignored and the equation simplified to:

(0.15 μCi Mo99/mCi Tc99m)(activity of Tc99m in mCi) = X μCi Mo99

To determine if a particular concentration of Mo99 in Tc99m generator eluate is within limits, the direct proportion is again used. A different element of the equation becomes the unknown.

$$\frac{X\,\mu\text{Ci Mo99}}{1\,\text{mCi Tc99m}} = \frac{\text{activity of Mo99 in }\mu\text{Ci}}{\text{activity of Tc99m in mCi}}$$

Notice that you are actually simplifying the ratio of Mo99 to Tc99m to the lowest denominator possible, in this case 1. The 1 in the denominator can again be ignored so the equation becomes:

$$X \text{ μCi Mo99/mCi Tc99m} = \frac{\text{activity of Mo99 in μCi}}{\text{activity of Tc99m in mCi}}$$

V-25 How to calculate the Mo99 limit for a particular activity of Tc99m:

X μCi Mo99 = (0.15 μCi Mo99/mCi Tc99m)(activity of Tc99m in mCi)

* Note: The answer is NOT expressed as μCi Mo99/mCi Tc99m because this is the total amount permitted in a stated activity of Tc99m. It is NOT the concentration. Read questions concerning allowable limits carefully to determine what information is requested.

---

* Note: In all of the following calculations, μCi and mCi are mixed within the equation. Although this is not normally an acceptable practice in mathematics, it is required here. The NRC has defined the limits in these terms; therefore, by definition, the units are mixed in the equation.

If the Mo99 activity is expressed in mCi, it must to be converted to μCi. Likewise, the Tc99m must be expressed as mCi.

Examples:

A. A vial of generator eluate contains 450 mCi Tc99m. What is the maximum activity of Mo99 allowed for this activity?

(0.15 μCi Mo99/mCi Tc99m)(450 mCi Tc99m) = 67.5 μCi Mo99

B. How many μCi of Mo99 would be allowed in 800 mCi of Tc99m generator eluate?

(0.15 μCi Mo99/mCi Tc99m)(800 mCi Tc99m) = 120 μCi Mo99

V-26 How to determine if a specific concentration of Mo99 is within NRC limits:

$$X \text{ μCi Mo99/mCi Tc99m} = \frac{\text{activity of Mo99 in μCi}}{\text{activity of Tc99m in mCi}}$$

* Note: In this case, the answer IS expressed as μCi Mo99/mCi Tc99m because you are dealing with the concentration.

Examples:

A. What is the concentration of Mo99 in a vial containing 310 mCi Tc99m and 20 μCi Mo99? Is it within NRC limits?

$$\frac{20\,\mu Ci\;Mo99}{310\;mCi\;Tc99m} = 0.06\,\mu Ci\;Mo99/mCi\;Tc99m$$

Since 0.06 μCi is less than the 0.15 μCi limit, the eluate can be used on patients.

B. If an elution vial contains 168 mCi Tc99m and 32 μCi of Mo99, can it be used for patient doses or radiopharmaceutical kit preparation?

$$\frac{32\,\mu Ci\;Mo99}{168\;Tc99m} = 0.19\,\mu Ci\;Mo99/mCi\;Tc99m$$

Since 0.19 μCi is greater than the 0.15 μCi limit, the eluate cannot be used on patients or to prepare kits.

Problems:

1. Determine the maximum Mo99 activity allowed in 748 mCi Tc99m.

2. If a vial of generator eluate contains 237 mCi Tc99m, how many μCi of Mo99 is it permitted to contain?

3. What is the maximum activity of Mo99 permitted in 1246 mCi Tc99m?

4. Calculate the permissible activity of Mo99 if a vial of Tc99m generator eluate is found to contain 87 mCi.

5. A vial of Tc99m contains 513 mCi. At what activity of Mo99 must the vial be discarded?

6. If a vial of Tc99m eluate reads 136 mCi in the dose calibrator, what is the maximum activity of Mo99 allowed?

7. How many μCi of Mo99 are allowed when Tc99m eluate activity is 822 mCi?

8. If a vial of generator eluate contains 727 mCi Tc99m and 93 μCi of Mo99, can it be used for patients?

9. What is the concentration of Mo99 in the Tc99m generator eluate if 916 mCi of Tc99m and 182 μCi of Mo99 are present? Is the Mo99 concentration within acceptable limits?

10. Determine if the generator eluate is within acceptable limits:

    Tc99m = 314 mCi.
    Mo99 = 38 μCi.

11. If there are 41 µCi of Mo99 in 539 mCi of Tc99m generator eluate, can it be used for patient doses or kit preparation at the time of elution?

12. Dose calibrator readings show that a vial contains 457 mCi of Tc99m and 66 µCi of Mo99. Does the Mo99 contamination fall within acceptable limits?

13. A vial of eluate contains 80 mCi Tc99m and 9 µCi Mo99. Is the Mo99 concentration within NRC limits?

Additional Applications:

14. A vial of Tc99m contained 380 mCi Tc99m and 53 µCi Mo99 at 8:00 am. Can the eluate be used to prepare a patient dose at 12:00 noon?

---

* Note: Observe how much more quickly the Tc99m activity decreases as compared to the Mo99 activity. The Mo99 concentration, therefore, increases with time.

---

15. Can a vial of generator eluate that contained 189 mCi of Tc99m and 13 µCi of Mo99 at noon be used to prepare a radiopharmaceutical kit at 6:00 pm?

16. A vial contains 65 mCi Tc99m and 9.0 µCi of Mo99 at 2:00 pm. Will it still be usable for a patient dose at 5:00 pm?

References:

Early & Sodee (2nd Ed.), p. 96–97.
Kowalsky & Falen (2nd Ed.), p. 222–223.
Steves & Wells (3rd Ed.), p. 20–21.
US NRC 10CFR35.204.

18. Eluate expiration time based on Mo99 content

Principles:

Because Mo99 has a longer half-life (66.6 h) than Tc99m (6.01 h), Mo99 contamination increases as the activity of the Tc99m in the generator eluate decreases.

Even though Mo99 contamination levels are acceptable at the time of elution, they may exceed allowable limits before all the eluate can be used. The time at which contamination levels are exceeded must be calculated. This becomes the eluate expiration time and the eluate cannot be administered to patients or used to prepare kits after this time.

➤ **Regulations:** According to NRC 10CFR35, Tc99m generator eluate cannot contain more than 0.15 µCi of Mo99 per mCi of Tc99m at the time of administration. (See Radiopharmacy Section 17.)

V-27 How to determine Tc99m eluate or kit expiration time based on Mo99 activity:

To determine the time at which Mo99 levels exceed the limit, the following calculation is used.

$$t = \frac{-\ln Mo_0/Tc_0}{0.1052} - 18.03$$

where: t = number of hours after the elution that the eluate expires
Mo_0 = initial Mo activity in µCi
Tc_0 = initial Tc99m activity in mCi

* Note: To determine the negative natural log (-ln), press the ln key on the calculator, followed by the sign change key (+/-).

Examples:

A. At the time of elution a vial contains 150 mCi of Tc99m and 18.3 µCi of Mo99. Determine when the eluate will exceed the NRC limits.

$$t = \frac{-\ln(18.3\,\mu Ci/150\,mCi)}{0.1052} - 18.03 = \frac{-\ln(0.122)}{0.1052} - 18.03 = \frac{2.1037}{0.1052} - 18.03$$

$t = 19.997 - 18.03 = 1.97$ hours or 1 hour & 58 minutes

B. A generator was eluted at 7:00 am to produce 632 mCi Tc99m and 51.9 µCi Mo99. What is the expiration time of the eluate?

$$t = \frac{-\ln(51.9\,\mu Ci/632\,mCi)}{0.1052} - 18.03 = \frac{-\ln(0.082)}{0.1052} - 18.03 = \frac{2.4996}{0.1052} - 18.03$$

$t = 23.76 - 18.03 = 5.7$ hours or about 5 hours and 40 minutes

The expiration time would therefore be 12:40 pm.

Problems:

1. How many hours can a vial of generator eluate be used if it contains 573 mCi Tc99m and 74 μCi Mo99 at the time of elution?

2. A vial of eluate contains 188 mCi of Tc99m and 12 μCi of Mo99. How long can it be used?

3. There are 6μCi of Mo99 in 130 mCi of Tc99m of generator eluate. When does the solution expire?

4. Eluate obtained at 12:00 noon contains 340 mCi Tc99m and 35 μCi Mo99. What is the expiration time?

5. Determine the expiration time for eluate that has an activity of 95 mCi Tc99m and 8 μCi of Mo99 at 5:30 pm.

6. At 2:15 pm a vial of eluate has an activity of 267 mCi Tc99m and 38 μCi Mo99. What is its expiration time?

7. A generator elution yielded 442 mCi Tc99m and 52 μCi Mo99 at 7:30 am. Can the eluate be used to prepare a kit at 10:00 am?

8. If eluate contained 210 mCi Tc99m and 15 μCi Mo99 at 1:00 pm, can it be used at 9:00 pm?

9. At 4:00 pm a vial of eluate contained 159 mCi Tc99m and 20 μCi of Mo99. Can the eluate be used for a patient dose at 5:15 pm?

10. Can a vial of eluate be used at 1:30 pm if it contained 348 mCi Tc99m and 37 μCi Mo99 at 10:30 am?

References:

Kowalsky & Falen (2nd Ed.), p. 222 223.
Steves & Wells (3rd Ed.), p. 21.
US NRC 10CFR35.204.

19. Chromatography calculations

Principles:

Many radiopharmaceuticals are tested for purity using thin layer chromatography (TLC). Tc99m labeled radiopharmaceuticals are usually tested for unbound Tc99m O_4^- (commonly referred to as Free Tc99m) and hydrolyzed-reduced Tc99m (called H-R Tc or R-Tc). Both of these impurities result in increased background activity, changes in radionuclide biodistribution, and an undesirable radiation dose to the patient.

Limits for radiochemical impurities, those in which the correct radionuclide is in the incorrect chemical state, are established by the United States Pharmacopedia (USP). The percent minimum purity for the more common Tc99m-labeled radiopharmaceuticals are listed below.

Radiopharmaceutical	*USP % Minimum Purity*
Tc99m sodium pertechnetate	95
Tc99m tetrophosmin	90
Tc99m sestamibi (MIBI)	90
Tc99m pyrophosphate (PYP)	90
Tc99m exametazime (HMPAO)	80
Tc99m bicisate (ECD)	90
Tc99m MAA	90
Tc99m disofenin	90
Tc99m mebrofenin	90
Tc99m medronate (MDP)	90
Tc99m oxidronate (HDP)	90
Tc99m mertiatide (MAG3™)	90
Tc99m pentetate (DTPA)	90
Tc99m succimer (DMSA)	85
Tc99m sulfur colloid	92

> *** Note:** Although the standards of good practice dictate the performance of quality control on radiopharmaceuticals, neither FDA nor NRC regulations require hospitals and clinics to perform such tests when they reconstitute kits. The manufacturers of several new radiopharmaceuticals clearly state in their package inserts that radiochemical purity tests must be done and that solutions that fail to meet minimum tagging efficiencies must not be administered to patients.
>
> Some states and local agencies may require testing.

Refer to the manufacturer's package insert for individual radiopharmaceutical kits to find the correct assay method recommended for each.

After a TLC strip has been incubated and dried, if required, for the designated period of time, it is cut in two. The upper portion contains the solvent front (SF) and the lower portion contains the point of origin (O). Which chemical form is located on each portion depends upon the radiopharmaceutical being measured, the impurities, the composition of the strip, and the solvents being used.

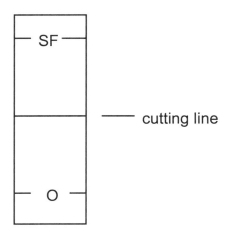

cutting line

The sections of the chromatography strip can be measured in either a dose calibrator or well counter, depending upon the level of activity involved. A high activity must be measured in a dose calibrator, and a low activity in a well counter. A background count is also acquired when a well counter is used. If the dose calibrator is used, the background should read zero before the strip sections are measured.

Apply the data to the following equations to determine either the percent purity of the radiopharmaceutical or percent impurity of a specific impurity.

V-28 How to determine the percent radiochemical _purity_ of a radiopharmaceutical:

$$\% \text{ purity} = \frac{\text{activity of radionuclide in desired form}}{\text{total activity}} \times 100\%$$

Example:

A. Calculate the percent purity of a Tc99m MAA kit. The TLC strip has been measured in a dose calibrator.

Tc99m Tc99mO$_4^-$ _____
5 µCi

Tc99m MAA _____
65 µCi

$$\frac{65 \text{ mCi}}{65 \text{ mCi} + 5 \text{ mC}i} \, x100 = 93\% \text{ Tc99m MAA}$$

V-29 How to determine the percent radiochemical <u>impurity</u> of a radiopharmaceutical:

$$\% \text{ impurity} = \frac{\text{activity of radionuclide in specific undesirable form}}{\text{total activity}} \times 100\%$$

B. Calculate the percent $Tc99mO_4^-$ in a Tc99m DTPA kit. The $Tc99mO_4^-$ has migrated to the SF section of the strip and the Tc99 DTPA remains on the O section. The strip sections have been counted in a well counter.

SF   6,200 cpm
O   884,000 cpm
background   120 cpm

$$\frac{6,200 \text{ cpm} - 120 \text{ cpm}}{\left(884,000 \text{ cpm} - 120 \text{ cpm}\right) + \left(6,200 \text{ cpm} - 120 \text{ cpm}\right)} \times 100 = 0.7\% \ Tc99mO_4^-$$

Problems:

1. A chromatography strip for generator eluate gives a count of 49,270 cpm for pertechnetate and 525 cpm for HR-Tc. The well counter has a background count of 102 cpm. What is the percent purity for the pertechnetate?

2. A Tc99m DTPA kit has been tested with TLC, giving 87,920 cpm for the Tc99m DTPA section of the strip and 2,450 cpm for the free Tc99m section. Background equals 620 cpm. What is the percent purity?

3. Calculate the percent purity of a Tc99m HDP kit. The Tc99m HDP remains at the point of origin and the $Tc99mO_4^-$ migrates to the solvent front. The strip has been measured in a well counter.

SF   2,246 cpm
O   125,000 cpm
background   135 cpm

4. Calculate the percent purity of a Tc99m DMSA kit. The $Tc99mO_4^-$ migrates to the solvent front and the Tc99m DMSA remains at the point of origin. The SF section gives a count of 4,150 cpm and the origin section gives a count of 962,800 cpm. The background count for the well counter is 492 cpm.

5. A Tc99m sulfur colloid kit is being tested for free Tc99m content. What is the percent impurity if the point of origin, which contains the Tc99m sulfur colloid, reads 86 µCi and the solvent front, containing the free Tc99m, reads 2 µCi?

6. Generator eluate can contain hydrolyzed, reduced Tc99m (HR-Tc), which is in a chemical state that prevents it from binding to most pharmaceuticals. When TLC is performed using acetone as a solvent, the HR-Tc remains at the point of origin and the $Tc99mO_4^-$ migrates to the solvent front. Calculate the percent HR-Tc in the following eluate.

SF	19,620 cpm
O	758 cpm
background	234 cpm

7. To test for HR-Tc in Tc99m DTPA, a strip of ITLC-SG media is developed with distilled water. The HR-Tc will remain at the point of origin, while the Tc99m DTPA migrates to the solvent front. What is the HR-Tc content for the following kit?

SF	68.3 µCi
O	4.72 µCi

8. To determine the $Tc99mO_4^-$ content in Tc99m GH, Whatman 31ET paper is developed with acetone. The $Tc99mO_4^-$ will migrate while the Tc99m GH remains stationary. What is the percent $Tc99mO_4^-$ impurity in this kit?

SF	29.2 µCi
O	157.8 µCi

* **Note:** When testing a radiopharmaceutical for 2 impurities using 2 separate test strips, calculate the percent impurity for each strip, add the results, then subtract the sum from 100%. This will give you the percent purity.

9. Both free Tc99m and HR-Tc may occur as impurities in some kits. Each impurity is measured using specific assay techniques. Calculate the percent purity for the following Tc99m MDP kit.

Strip 1   Whatman 31ET paper; acetone solvent

O	253 µCi Tc99m MDP
SF	23.9 µCi $Tc99mO_4^-$

Strip 2   ITLC-SG media; H_2O solvent

O	6.4 µCi Tc99m HR-Tc
SF	147 µCi Tc99m MDP

10. A Tc99m DISIDA kit is being tested for radiochemical impurities giving the following results. What is the percent purity?

Strip 1   ITLC-SA media; 20% NaCl solvent

O   97.5 µCi Tc99m DISIDA
SF   8.2 µCi $Tc99mO_4^-$

Strip 2   ITLC-SG media; H_2O solvent

O   6.4 µCi Tc99m HR-Tc
SF   122.6 µCi Tc99m DISIDA

References:

Christian & Waterstram-Rich (6th Ed.), p. 184–188.
Early & Sodee (2nd Ed.), p. 98–99.
Kowalsky & Falen (2nd Ed.), p. 409–423.
Saha (4th Ed.), p. 150–162.
Steves & Wells (3rd Ed.), p. 22–24.

Chapter VI. Clinical Procedures

1. Left ventricle ejection fraction

Principles:

The ejection fraction (EF) is the percentage of blood ejected from the heart during each contraction. It is most commonly calculated for the left ventricle (LVEF), but can also be determined for the right ventricle (RVEF). During planar equilibrium gated blood pool imaging, the LVEF can be determined by comparing the counts in the left ventricle at end diastole (ED) to the counts at end systole (ES). This study is commonly called an equilibrium radionuclide angiogram or ERNA. It is also known as a multiple gated acquisition or MUGA.

The left ventricle ejection fraction must be calculated using the left anterior oblique (LAO) image that provides maximum septal separation, usually an LAO between 30^0 and 45^0.

> *** Note:** Using a view that does not sufficiently separate the left ventricle from other chambers could result in an erroneous LVEF. For this reason, the ejection fraction cannot be accurately determined from other standard views, such as anterior, left lateral, or LAO 70^0. Nor can the right ventricle ejection fraction be determined using planar equilibrium imaging. Only a first pass dynamic study can be used because it allows the individual chambers to be momentarily visualized.

A background region drawn near the left ventricle, usually between 3 and 6 o'clock, is used by the computer program to correct for activity in the tissues overlying the heart.

> *** Note:** Including areas with activity above background levels, such as the spleen or great vessels, or extending the background region outside of the body margin, will change the EF.

Some computer programs require the technologist to draw irregular regions around the left ventricle blood pool at end diastole and/or end systole. Even with automated region selection programs, the technologist must be certain that all the regions are correctly drawn and adjust them when necessary.

> *** Note:** Drawing a region of interest (ROI) that is too small or too large can also result in erroneous ejection fractions.

A normal LVEF is 50% to 80%.

VI-1 How to calculate the left ventricle ejection fraction:

$$\%EF = \frac{\text{net ED counts} - \text{net ES counts}}{\text{net ED counts}} \times 100\%$$

Net counts are calculated using a background (Bkgd) ROI drawn near the left ventricle. The average counts per pixel in the Bkgd ROI are subtracted from the cardiac ROI, and adjusted for the size of the region.

$$\text{net cardiac ROI counts} = \text{cardiac ROI counts} - \left(\frac{\text{Bkgd ROI counts}}{\text{Bkgd ROI pixels}} \times \text{cardiac ROI pixels} \right).$$

* Note: While planar equilibrium gated blood pool imaging uses counts from an ROI on a single plane, gated SPECT myocardial perfusion imaging uses an elaborate automated algorithm to determine the EF. Because SPECT produces three-dimensional images that are sliced along multiple planes, an automated program can compute the change in left ventricle chamber volume from end diastole (EDV) to end systole (ESV). These data are used to calculate the LVEF, the stroke volume (SV), and the cardiac output (CO). (See Clinical Procedures Section 2.)

Examples:

A. Calculate the LVEF using the following data:

ES = 24,560 net counts
ED = 62,240 net counts

$$\frac{62,240 - 24,560}{62,240} \times 100\% = 60\%$$

B. Given the following data, calculate the LVEF.

ES   = 28,100 counts in 422 pixels
ED   = 44,800 counts in 634 pixels
Bkgd =   1,750 counts in   88 pixels

$$\text{net ES counts} = 28,100 \text{ counts} - \left(\frac{1,750 \text{ counts}}{88 \text{ pixels}} \times 422 \text{ pixels} \right) = 19,700 \text{ counts}$$

$$\text{net ED counts} = 44,800 \text{ counts} - \left(\frac{1,750 \text{ counts}}{88 \text{ pixels}} \times 634 \text{ pixels} \right) = 32,200 \text{ counts}$$

$$\frac{32,200 \text{ counts} - 19,700 \text{ counts}}{32,200 \text{ counts}} \times 100\% = 39\%$$

Problems:

Calculate the LVEF for each of the following sets of data:

1. net ES = 30,770 counts
    net ED = 69,510 counts

2. net ES = 20,170 counts
    net ED = 28,900 counts

3. net ES =   6,730 counts
    net ED = 19,280 counts

4. net ES = 42,300 counts
    net ED = 70,520 counts

5. net ES = 20,190 counts
    net ED = 35,660 counts

6. net ES = 14,380 counts
    net ED = 49,690 counts

7. ES   = 29,300 counts in 520 pixels
    ED   = 34,570 counts in 612 pixels
    Bkgd =   1,220 counts in 46 pixels

8. ES   = 23,610 counts in 237 pixels
    ED   = 50,140 counts in 449 pixels
    Bkgd =   2,180 counts in 114 pixels

Additional Applications:

9. Use the following data to determine the effects of poorly selected background regions. Does the EF increase or decrease as background activity increases or decreases?

    ES = 25,170 counts in 360 pixels
    ED = 48,630 counts in 596 pixels
    correctly positioned background region = 1,800 counts in 60 pixels
    background region including portion of spleen = 2,900 counts in 60 pixels
    background region extending outside the body margin = 120 counts in 60 pixels

10. Use the following data to determine the effects of poorly drawn end diastole regions. Does the EF increase or decrease as the ED ROI increases or decreases? Assume background has already been subtracted from each value.

    ES = 23,670 counts
    correctly drawn ED = 47,130 counts
    ED drawn too large = 50,130 counts
    ED drawn too small = 43,130 counts

11. Use the following data to determine the effects of poorly drawn end systole regions. Does the EF increase or decrease as the ES ROI increases or decreases? Assume background has already been subtracted from each value.

ED = 47,130 counts
correctly drawn ES = 23,670 counts
ES drawn too large = 26,670 counts
ES drawn too small = 20,670 counts

References:

Christian & Waterstram-Rich (6th Ed.), p. 502–507.
Crawford & Husain, p. 80–82.
Early & Sodee (2nd Ed.), p. 391–393.
Faber, et al., p. 650–651.
Scheiner, et al., p. 4–5.
Steves & Wells (3rd Ed.), p. 59–60.

2. Cardiac Output and Stroke Volume

Principles:

Gated SPECT myocardial perfusion studies produce three-dimensional images that are sliced along multiple planes. Various automated analytical programs use the short-axis slices to compute the change in left ventricle chamber volume from end diastole to end systole. This data can be used to calculate the end diastolic volume (EDV), the end systolic volume (ESV), the left ventricle ejection fraction (LVEF), the stroke volume (SV), and the cardiac output (CO).

---

* Note: With gated blood pool imaging, the counts in the ROI are obtained from the radionuclide within the ventricle chamber. With SPECT myocardial perfusion, the radionuclide is within the myocardial wall, not the chamber, so the LVEF algorithm uses the inside edge of the myocardium to determine the size of the chamber, or its volume. Therefore, ROI counts are used for the calculation of the LVEF in equilibrium gated blood pool imaging while chamber volumes are used in gated SPECT myocardial perfusion imaging.

EF calculation for gated blood pool imaging: $\%EF = \dfrac{net\ ED\ counts - net\ ES\ counts}{net\ ED\ counts} \times 100\%$

EF calculation for SPECT myocardial perfusion imaging: $\%EF = \dfrac{EDV - ESV}{EDV} \times 100\%$

The stroke volume (SV) is the amount of blood pumped by the ventricle with each contraction. It is calculated by subtracting the end-systolic volume (ESV) from the end-diastolic volume (EDV). The end-systolic volume is the volume contained within the ventricle when it is fully contracted, i.e., its minimum volume. The end-diastolic volume is the volume contained within the ventricle at maximum dilation.

VI-2 How to calculate the stroke volume:

$SV = EDV - ESV$

where SV = stroke volume in ml
         EDV = end-diastolic volume in ml
         ESV = end-systolic volume in ml

Example:

A. Calculate the stroke volume if the EDV is 94 ml and the ESV is 24 ml.

94 ml – 24 ml = 70 ml

The cardiac output (CO) is the amount of blood pumped by the left ventricle per minute. It is calculated by multiplying the stroke volume (SV) by the heart rate (HR).

VI-3 How to calculate the cardiac output:

CO = (SV)(HR),

where CO = cardiac output in ml/min or L/min
          SV = stroke volume in ml
          HR = heart rate in beats/min

Example:

A. Calculate the cardiac output for a patient with a heart rate of 65 bpm and a stroke volume of 70 ml.

(70 ml)(65 bpm) = 4,550 ml/min or about 4.6 L/min

Problems:

Calculate the stroke volume and cardiac output for each of the following:

1. EDV = 108 ml
     ESV = 39 ml
     HR = 60 bpm

2. EDV = 127 ml
     ESV = 42 ml
     HR = 65 bpm

3. EDV = 151 ml
     ESV = 58 ml
     HR = 55 bpm

4. EDV = 84ml
     ESV = 26 ml
     HR = 75 bpm

5. EDV = 147 ml
     ESV = 95 ml
     HR = 70 bpm

6. EDV = 101 ml
     ESV = 27 ml
     HR = 75 bpm

Calculate the stroke volume, ejection fraction (see Clinical Procedures Section 1), and cardiac output for each of the following:

7.   EDV   =   108 ml
      ESV   =   39 ml
      HR   =   78 bpm

8.   EDV   =   55 ml
      ESV   =   19 ml
      HR   =   92bpm

9.   EDV   =   205 ml
      ESV   =   173 ml
      HR   =   70 bpm

10.   EDV   =   141 ml
      ESV   =   82 ml
      HR   =   81 bpm

References:

Christian & Waterstram-Rich (6th Ed.), p. 483.
Early & Sodee (2nd Ed.), p. 376.
Faber, et al., p. 650 651.

3. Gallbladder ejection fraction

Principles:

The gallbladder ejection fraction (GBEF) is a useful measure of gallbladder function in patients with chronic cholecystitis whose other diagnostic studies appear normal. Neither nuclear medicine imaging nor ultrasound can accurately diagnose biliary diseases, such as chronic acalculous cholecystitis and cystic duct syndrome, because gallstones are not present and duct patency varies with time.

An abnormally low gallbladder ejection fraction is a positive indicator for these types of disease states. A normal gallbladder ejection fraction, as reported by various authors, is 35 to 40% or greater.

The gallbladder ejection fraction is determined by injecting the patient with an hepatobiliary imaging agent, such as Tc99m disofenin or mebrofenin. When the gallbladder reaches maximum filling, the patient is given cholecystikinin (CCK) or sincalide (synthetic CCK), which causes the gallbladder to contract. Serial computer images are obtained until the gallbladder reaches minimal content. Regions of interest (ROI) are drawn around the gallbladder on the maximum and minimum images. A background region of interest is drawn within the liver, just to the right of the gallbladder. The counts and the number of pixels for each region are obtained from the computer and applied to the ejection fraction equation.

VI-4 How to calculate the gallbladder ejection fraction:

$$\%GBEF = \frac{\text{net maximum GB counts} - \text{net minimum GB counts}}{\text{net maximum GB counts}} \times 100\%$$

Net counts are calculated using the background (Bkgd) ROI. The average counts per pixel in the Bkgd ROI are subtracted from the gallbladder ROI, adjusted for the size of the region.

$$\text{net GB ROI counts} = \text{GB ROI counts} - \left(\frac{\text{Bkgd ROI counts}}{\text{Bkgd ROI pixels}} \times \text{GB ROI pixels} \right)$$

* Note: These calculations are identical to those used to determine the left ventricle ejection fraction. (See Clinical Procedures Section 1.)

Examples:

A. The net counts for the gallbladder prior to CCK administration are 63,800. The net counts post-administration are 37,200. What is the patient's ejection fraction?

$$\frac{63,800 \text{ counts} - 37,200 \text{ counts}}{63,800 \text{ counts}} \times 100\% = 42\%$$

B.   Calculate the GBEF using the following data.

GB maximum   = 254,000 counts in 241 pixels
Bkgd maximum   =   11,000 counts in 125 pixels
GB minimum   =   92,000 counts in 84 pixels
Bkgd minimum   =   3,000 counts in 62 pixels

$$\text{net minimum GB counts} = 254{,}000 \text{ counts} - \left(\frac{11{,}000 \text{ counts}}{125 \text{ pixels}} \times 241 \text{ pixels} \right) = 233{,}000 \text{ counts}$$

$$\text{net minimum GB counts} = 92{,}000 \text{ counts} - \left(\frac{3{,}000 \text{ counts}}{62 \text{ pixels}} \times 84 \text{ pixels} \right) = 88{,}000 \text{ counts}$$

$$\frac{233{,}000 \text{ counts} - 88{,}000 \text{ counts}}{233{,}000 \text{ counts}} \times 100\% = 62\%$$

Problems:

Calculate the GBEF for each set of data.

1.   net maximum counts = 235,000 counts
     net minimum counts = 174,000 counts

2.   net maximum counts = 142,800 counts
     net minimum counts =   84,310 counts

3.   net maximum counts =   97,290 counts
     net minimum counts =   73,180 counts

4.   net maximum counts = 295,000 counts
     net minimum counts =   57,000 counts

5.   net maximum counts = 312,500 counts
     net minimum counts = 187,300 counts

6.   net maximum counts = 126,900 counts
     net minimum counts =   87,200 counts

7.   net maximum counts = 235,000 counts
     net minimum counts = 174,000 counts

8.   net maximum counts = 195,900 counts
     net minimum counts =   48,700 counts

9.   maximum GB counts   = 268,000 counts in 269 pixels
     maximum Bkgd counts =   14,000 counts in 191 pixels
     minimum GB counts   = 193,000 counts in 186 pixels
     minimum Bkgd counts =   4,100 counts in 102 pixels

10. maximum GB counts   =   84,320 counts in 284 pixels
     maximum Bkgd counts =   5,760 counts in   96 pixels
     minimum GB counts   =   53,140 counts in 220 pixels
     minimum Bkgd counts =   1,420 counts in   79 pixels

11. maximum GB counts   = 224,000 counts in 487 pixels
     maximum Bkgd counts =   12,400 counts in 142 pixels
     minimum GB counts   = 117,000 counts in 193 pixels
     minimum Bkgd counts =   2,430 counts in   57 pixels

References:

Balon, Brill, et al.
Christian & Waterstram-Rich K (6th Ed.), p. 540–542.
Steves & Wells (3rd Ed.), p. 85–86.

4. Gastroesophageal reflux

Principles:

Radiolabeled liquids can be used to detect and quantitate gastroesophageal reflux. The patient drinks the liquid, then images are acquired over a period of time and/or with increasing pressure on the abdomen.

Regions of interest (ROI) are drawn for each image. The ROIs include the esophagus, a background (Bkgd) region lateral to the esophagus, and the stomach and duodenum combined.

The percent reflux or reflux index is calculated for each time period or at each pressure.

Various authors have reported reflux of 4 to 5% or greater is abnormal.

VI-5 How to calculate the percent esophageal reflux:

$$\text{reflux index as a percent} = \frac{\text{esophagus counts} - \text{esophagus background counts}}{\text{maximum stomach counts}} \times 100\%$$

$$\text{esophagus background counts} = \left(\frac{\text{Bkgd ROI counts}}{\text{Bkgd ROI pixels}} \times \text{esophagus ROI pixels} \right)$$

Example:

A. Given the data below, calculate the esophageal reflux index in percent. The background data has already been corrected for ROI size.

ROI	counts per 30 seconds
esophagus	4,050
esophagus background	170
maximum stomach	45,700

$$\frac{4,050 \text{ counts} - 170 \text{ counts}}{45,720 \text{ counts}} \times 100\% = 8.5\%$$

Problems:

Calculate the percent esophageal reflux based on the following ROIs. The background data has already been corrected for ROI size.

1.

ROI	counts per 30 seconds
esophagus	1,090
esophagus background	110
maximum stomach	18,300

2.

ROI	counts per 30 seconds
esophagus	984
esophagus background	44
maximum stomach	32,800

3.

ROI	counts per 30 seconds
esophagus	872
esophagus background	38
maximum stomach	55,400

4. A gastroesophageal reflux study is performed with images acquired at increasing abdominal pressure for 30 seconds per image. Computer analysis yields the following data. Determine the percent of esophageal reflux at each pressure.

Pressure in mm Hg	Esophagus	Esophagus Background	Stomach & Bowel
20	193	20	21,969
40	285	71	22,847
60	658	56	22,544
80	1,343	83	21,835

5. A patient with known esophageal reflux has a baseline study followed by drug therapy and a repeat study. The studies are performed 1 day apart to assure non-interference. Determine the reflux index in percent before and after drug therapy.

	Esophagus	Esophagus Background	Stomach & Bowel
		(all counts acquired for 30 seconds)	
before therapy	2,783	34	30,923
after therapy	2,032	48	42,776

6. A patient is imaged upright after ingestion of radiolabeled liquid. He is then imaged supine. Using the following data, determine if the patient is experiencing positional reflux.

	Esophagus	Esophagus Background	Stomach & Bowel
		(all counts acquired for 30 seconds)	
upright	1,919	120	61,355
supine	4,287	199	61,002

References:

Christian & Waterstram-Rich K (6th Ed.), p. 524–526.
Early & Sodee (2nd Ed.), p. 525–528.
Steves & Wells (3rd Ed.), p. 89–90.

5. Gastric emptying half-time

Principles:

In order to evaluate the time required for food to pass through the stomach, the patient is fed solid food and/or liquid labeled with a radionuclide. When only the solid phase is used, Tc99m sulfur colloid is the radionuclide of choice. If both solid and liquid phases are desired, the solid is labeled with Tc99m sulfur colloid and the liquid with In111 DTPA. A dual window can then be used to measure the radionuclides simultaneously.

Although many protocols specify anterior imaging, a higher degree of accuracy is achieved if both anterior and posterior images are acquired. The data obtained when regions of interest (ROI) are drawn around the stomach is combined to produce a geometric mean.

Either the percent remaining or the percent emptied can be used to calculate the half-emptying time. Both methods are shown below. The percent emptied is often provided for 1 hour and 2 hours post-ingestion intervals.

Gastric function can also be expressed as the half-emptying time. Data can be graphed to allow a reasonable estimation of actual half-emptying times. Emptying of solid food follows a linear pattern, so data is graphed on linear graph paper. Liquid emptying, however, demonstrates an exponential pattern, so semilogarithmic paper must be used to produce a straight line.

Normal values are dependent upon the meal and the imaging protocol used for the study.

VI-6 How to calculate gastric emptying as the percent activity remaining in the stomach:

The percent remaining in the stomach is calculated by comparing region of interest counts at a given time (time T) to maximum counts obtained immediately following radionuclide ingestion (time 0).

In order to assure accuracy when Tc99m is being used, a decay factor must be applied to the count for each time the percent remaining is calculated.

1. Determine the geometric mean for the given time (time T) and for the time at which maximum counts were obtained from the stomach ROI (time 0).

$$\text{Geometric mean} = \sqrt{\text{anterior ROI counts} \times \text{posterior ROI counts}}$$

2. $\% \text{ remaining at time } T = \dfrac{\text{geometric mean at time } T}{\text{geometric mean at time } 0 \times \text{decay factor for time } T} \times 100\%$

* Note: If only anterior images are used, insert the anterior ROI counts in place of the geometric mean.

Example:

A. Immediately after ingestion of Tc99m-labeled scrambled eggs, gastric ROI counts equal 79,700 cpm for the anterior image and 75,800 cpm for the posterior image. At 30 minutes post-ingestion (time T), ROIs provide 69,500 cpm for the anterior and 68,200 cpm for the posterior. What is the percent activity remaining? (30-min decay factor: 0.944.)

$$\frac{\sqrt{(69{,}500\,\text{cpm})(68{,}200\,\text{cpm})}}{\sqrt{(79{,}700\,\text{cpm})(75{,}800\,\text{cpm})}\times 0.944}\times 100\% = \frac{68{,}800\,\text{cpm}}{77{,}700\,\text{cpm}\times 0.944}\times 100\% = 94\%$$

VI-7 How to determine the gastric half-emptying time using graphed data:

1. Determine the percent remaining in the gastric ROI for various time intervals.
2. Graph the data with percent remaining on the y-axis and time on the x-axis. Use linear graph paper for studies using solid food and semi-logarithmic paper for studies using liquids.
3. Draw a line from the 50% remaining point on the y-axis to where it intercepts with the graphed line.
4. Drop a line directly to the x-axis to find the time at which the stomach contained 50% of the maximum count.

Example:

A. The percent activity remaining in the stomach after oral administration of Tc99m sulfur colloid labeled solid meal is measured over a 2-hour period. Graph the results to determine the half-emptying time.

Time in Minutes	% Remaining	Time in Minutes	% Remaining
15	91	75	37
30	80	90	25
45	72	105	17
60	55	120	5

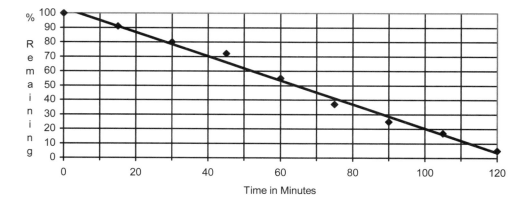

To find the half-emptying time draw a line from the 50% mark on the y-axis to the graphed line. Drop a line from the intercept point down to the x-axis to find the time at which 50% of the activity remained in the stomach. The half-emptying time is about 65 minutes.

VI-8 How to calculate gastric emptying as the percent emptied at a given time:

$$\% \text{ emptying at time T} = \frac{\text{geometric mean at time 0} - \text{geometric mean at time T}}{\text{geometric mean at time 0}} \times 100\%$$

where the geometric mean at time 0 is corrected for decay: (geometric mean)(decay factor)

Example:

A. A patient consumes Tc99m sulfur colloid-labeled oatmeal. The counts from the stomach ROI immediately post-ingestion are 55,200 cpm on the anterior image and 53,100 cpm on the posterior image. One hour later the counts are 36,800 cpm and 35,900 cpm, respectively. Calculate the percent gastric emptying at 1 hour. (1-h decay factor: 0.891.)

geometric mean at time 0 = $\sqrt{55,200 \times 53,100}$ = 54,100

geometric mean at time 0 corrected for 1 hour decay = (54,000)(0.891) = 48,200

geometric mean at 1 hour = $\sqrt{36,800 \times 35,900}$ = 36,300

$$\% \text{ gastric emptying at 1 hour} = \frac{48,200 - 36,300}{48,200} \times 100\% = 25\%$$

---

* Note: Observe the error that occurs when the mean for time 0 is not corrected for decay:

$$\frac{54,100 - 36,300}{54,100} \times 100\% = 33\%.$$

Check the expected value using the % remaining equation: $\dfrac{36,300}{54,100 \times 0.891} \times 100\% = 75\%.$

Problems:

Calculate the percent activity remaining for each set of data.

1. initial anterior stomach ROI   59,300 cpm
    initial posterior stomach ROI   57,900 cpm
    30-min anterior stomach ROI   43,200 cpm
    30-min posterior stomach ROI   40,800 cpm
    30-min decay factor   0.944

2. initial anterior stomach ROI   41,600 cpm
    initial posterior stomach ROI   37,100 cpm
    45-min anterior stomach ROI   23,500 cpm
    45-min posterior stomach ROI   19,600 cpm
    45-min decay factor   0.917

3. initial anterior stomach ROI   78,400 cpm
    initial posterior stomach ROI   73,300 cpm
    90-min anterior stomach ROI   33,600 cpm
    90-min posterior stomach ROI   30,200 cpm
    90-min decay factor   0.841

4. initial anterior stomach ROI   66,400 cpm
    initial posterior stomach ROI   65,500 cpm
    15-min anterior stomach ROI   53,100 cpm
    15-min posterior stomach ROI   51,900 cpm
    15-min decay factor   0.972

5. A patient eats a Tc99m-labeled solid meal and is imaged in the anterior and posterior projection at intervals for 2 hours. For each of the following times, calculate the percent remaining activity in the stomach. Graph the results and determine the half-emptying time.

| | Counts in CPM | | |
Time in Minutes	Anterior ROI	Posterior ROI	Decay Factor
0	63,600	61,900	
15	57,800	53,200	0.972
30	51,800	48,400	0.944
60	40,500	39,300	0.891
90	25,700	23,500	0.841
120	10,900	9,800	0.794

6. The data listed below has been acquired during a Tc99m solid food gastric emptying study. Calculate the half-emptying time using a graph.

Time in Minutes	% Remaining
15	90
30	62
45	35
60	19

7. A Tc99m solid food gastric emptying study provided the following values. Using a graph, calculate the half-emptying time.

Time in Minutes	% Remaining
15	98
30	92
45	86
60	82
90	68
120	62

* Note: Because the half-emptying time has not been reached at 2 hours post-ingestion, the data can be plotted and the actual half-emptying time can be estimated by extrapolation.

8. Region of interest data for a Tc99m sulfur colloid–labeled scrambled egg gastric emptying study is listed below. What is the percent gastric emptying at 2 hours post-ingestion? (2-h decay factor: 0.794.)

Time	Anterior	Posterior
0 minutes	79,300 cpm	77,500 cpm
2 hours	44,600 cpm	42,800 cpm

9. In111 DTPA–tagged orange juice is used for a gastric emptying study. The counts over the stomach immediately after the patient drinks are 15,200 cpm on the anterior view and 13,900 cpm on the posterior view. What is the percent gastric emptying 1 hour later when the same areas produce 3,800 cpm and 2,500 cpm, respectively?

---

* Note: Because the half-life of In111 is 2.8 days, a decay factor does not have to be used at 1 or 2 hours post-administration intervals.

---

10. A gastric emptying study using Tc99m produced the following data. Calculate the percent emptying at 2 hours post-ingestion. (2-h decay factor: 0.794.)

Time	Anterior	Posterior
0 minutes	65,400 cpm	63,700 cpm
2 hours	25,600 cpm	24,800 cpm

11. Determine the percent gastric emptying at 1 and 2 hours post-ingestion for a patient suspected of gastric dumping.

Time in Hours	Counts in CPM Anterior ROI	Posterior ROI	Decay Factor
0	43,700	45,200	
1	11,400	13,200	0.891
2	9,670	9,940	0.794

References:

Christian & Waterstram-Rich (6ᵗʰ Ed.), p. 526–532.
Donohoe, et al., p. 2–3.
Early & Sodee (2ⁿᵈ Ed.), p. 522–525.
Steves & Wells (3ʳᵈ Ed.), p. 90.

6. Calculation of expected bladder capacity for voiding cystogram

Principles:

When performing a voiding cystogram it is useful to have an estimate of the child's bladder capacity. A standard formula is available that provides a reasonable estimate for children less than 9 years of age. The figures become less reliable above that age.

It should be noted that children with bladder pathologies may have capacities that differ greatly from the expected volume. The capacity estimate is, therefore, only a guideline. The technologist must use good judgment to determine if maximum bladder filling has been accomplished during the study.

VI-9 How to estimate urinary bladder capacity in the pediatric patient:

For children under the age of 9, the following equation will provide a reasonable estimate of normal bladder capacity.

expected bladder capacity = (age + 2)(30 ml)

Example:

A. What would be the expected capacity of a 2-year-old child's bladder?

(2 + 2)(30 ml) = 120 ml

Problems:

1. Calculate the expected bladder capacity for a 6-year-old child.
2. What is the normal capacity for a 1-year-old child's bladder?
3. How much saline can a technologist expect to infuse into a 4-year-old child's bladder during a voiding cystogram?
4. Calculate the normal bladder capacity for a 3-year-old child.
5. Will a 250-ml bag of saline be sufficient to fill an 8-year-old child's bladder during a voiding cystogram?

References:

Christian & Waterstram-Rich (6th Ed.), p. 637.
Early & Sodee (2nd Ed.), p. 614.

7. Quantitation of total bladder volume, residual bladder volume and reflux with a voiding cystogram

Principles:

A voiding cystogram is performed to determine if reflux from the urinary bladder into the ureters is occurring. In addition to identifying reflux, the test allows quantitation of ureteral reflux, total bladder volume, and urine retention in the bladder after voiding.

In order to perform these calculations all urine voided during the test must be collected. Any loss of urine invalidates the quantitation. The activity in the bladder and ureters is determined both pre- and post-void by acquiring gamma camera images and creating regions of interest.

VI-10 How to calculate residual bladder volume:

$$\text{residual volume} = \frac{(\text{voided volume})(\text{post - void count})}{\text{pre - void count} - \text{post - void count}}$$

Example:

A. A 4-year-old child is being evaluated for ureteral reflux. Visualization of reflux into one ureter and kidney is evident on the full-bladder images of the voiding cystogram. Use the following data to determine the residual bladder volume.

pre-void counts	113,253 counts	volume saline instilled	105 ml
post-void counts	23,373 counts	volume urine voided	94 ml
reflux ROI counts	7,559 counts		

$$\text{residual volume} = \frac{(94\,\text{ml})(23,373\,\text{counts})}{113,253\,\text{counts} - 23,373\,\text{counts}} = 24\,\text{ml}$$

VI-11 How to calculate total bladder volume:

total volume = voided volume + residual volume.

Example:

A. Use the data from Example A (Shadowbox VI-10) to calculate the total bladder volume.

total volume = 94 ml + 24 ml = 118 ml

VI-12 How to calculate the actual volume of refluxed urine:

A region of interest (ROI) is drawn around the pre-void bladder and around the area of reflux. The counts in each ROI are determined by the computer and the data is applied to the following equation.

$$\text{reflux volume} = \text{reflux ROI counts} \times \frac{\text{total bladder volume}}{\text{pre - void bladder ROI counts}}$$

Example:

A.   Use the data from the Examples in Shadowboxes VI-10 and VI-11 to calculate the reflux volume.

$$\text{reflux volume} = 7{,}559 \text{ counts} \times \frac{118 \text{ ml}}{113{,}253 \text{ counts}} = 8 \text{ ml}$$

VI-13 How to calculate bladder volume at the time of reflux:

1.   Because some urine remains in the bladder after catheterization and prior to the saline instillation, the initial bladder volume must be calculated:

     initial volume = total volume – total saline instilled

2.   bladder volume at reflux = initial volume + saline reflux volume,

     where saline reflux volume is the volume of saline that has been instilled into the bladder at the time reflux occurs.

Example:

A.   Use the data from the Examples in Shadowboxes VI-10 and VI-11 to calculate the initial bladder volume and the bladder volume at reflux.

     initial volume = 118 ml – 105 ml = 13 ml

     reflux bladder volume = total volume in this instance or 118 ml

Problems:

1.   Calculate the residual volume for a child who has had a voiding cystogram. The pre-void bladder contained 95,571 counts and the post-void bladder contained 12,605 counts. The child voided 190 ml during the test.

2.   If the voided volume during a cystogram is 95 ml, the pre-void bladder contained 105,449 counts, and the post-void bladder contained 18,983 counts, what is the residual volume in the bladder?

3.   A child has had a voiding cystogram that was positive for reflux. What volume has been refluxed if the ureter ROI gives 3,826 counts and the pre-void bladder ROI gives 96,244 counts? The total bladder volume is 180 ml.

4.   Calculate the bladder volume at reflux using the following data.

total volume of saline instilled	260 ml
volume of saline instilled at time of reflux	240 ml
total bladder volume	285 ml

5.   Calculate the residual volume and reflux volume for a patient who has undergone a voiding cystogram.

pre-void counts	121,903 counts
post-void counts	24,451 counts
reflux ROI counts	
right kidney	6,850 counts
left kidney	1,372 counts
volume urine voided	132 ml

6.   Calculate the residual bladder volume, the total bladder volume, the bladder volume at reflux, and the volume of reflux for a child who has undergone a voiding cystogram. Reflux first appeared after 105 ml of saline had been instilled.

pre-void counts	164,368 counts
post-void counts	70,347 counts
reflux ROI counts	9,880 counts
volume saline instilled	170 ml
volume urine voided	110 ml

7.   The following results were obtained from a voiding cystogram. Determine the residual bladder volume, the total bladder volume, the bladder volume at reflux, and the volume of reflux. Reflux became evident upon instillation of 190 ml saline.

pre-void counts	134,507 counts
post-void counts	27,941 counts
reflux ROI counts	
right kidney	1,523 counts
left kidney	3,554 counts
volume saline instilled	235 ml
volume urine voided	190 ml

8. A child who had a voiding cystogram showed no reflux, but demonstrated significant bladder retention, with 80 ml of urine remaining in the bladder after voiding. A repeat study is performed 6 months later. Has the child's condition improved?

pre-void counts	164,495 counts
post-void counts	72,631 counts
volume urine voided	118 ml

References:

Christian & Waterstram-Rich (6th Ed.), p. 636–637.
Early & Sodee (2nd Ed.), p. 612–615.
O'Connor, p. 416–417.

8. Lung quantitation

Principles:

In some studies it is useful to determine the percentage of activity found in each region of interest (ROI) as compared to the total activity in all the ROIs. Lung quantitation allows the physician to determine the percentage of perfusion and ventilation occurring in each lung or portion of a lung.

This type of analysis is most likely to be used for patients who are to undergo resection for lung cancer. It is not employed when lung scans are performed to rule out pulmonary embolus.

The number of regions to be drawn varies with protocol and physician preference. One entire lung may be compared to the other, or each lung may be divided into 2 or 3 segments.

VI-14 How to determine the percent activity in a particular ROI:

$$\% \text{ activity in ROI} = \frac{\text{counts ROI}}{\text{total counts in all ROIs}} \times 100\%$$

* Note: This equation can be used any time you want to determine the percent function or percent uptake in one ROI, as compared to other ROIs.

Examples:

A. Because of the normal size difference between the left and the right lung, the left lung usually receives 45% of perfusion, while the right lung receives 55%. Determine if a patient with 186,011 counts from the left lung and 359,548 counts from the right lung has a normal distribution.

left lung $\qquad \dfrac{186,011 \text{ counts}}{186,011 \text{ counts} + 359,548 \text{ counts}} \times 100\% = 34\%$

right lung $\qquad \dfrac{359,548 \text{ counts}}{186,011 \text{ counts} + 359,548 \text{ counts}} \times 100\% = 66\%$

The patient does not have a normal distribution.

B.   A patient has had a xenon ventilation study. Each lung has been divided into three segments for quantitation. Calculate the percent ventilation for each segment.

Lung Segment	Right Lung	Left Lung
upper segment	10,403 counts	18,269 counts
middle segment	23,203 counts	27,120 counts
lower segment	42,382 counts	4,715 counts

Calculate the total activity in both lungs: 126,092 counts

right upper segment $\dfrac{10,403 \text{ counts}}{126,092 \text{ counts}} \times 100\% = 8\%$

right middle segment $\dfrac{23,203 \text{ counts}}{126,092 \text{ counts}} \times 100\% = 18\%$

right lower segment $\dfrac{42,382 \text{ counts}}{126,092 \text{ counts}} \times 100\% = 33\%$

left upper segment $\dfrac{18,269 \text{ counts}}{126,092 \text{ counts}} \times 100\% = 14\%$

left middle segment $\dfrac{27,120 \text{ counts}}{126,092 \text{ counts}} \times 100\% = 22\%$

left lower segment $\dfrac{4,715 \text{ counts}}{126,092 \text{ counts}} \times 100\% = 4\%$

Problems:

1.   Calculate the percent perfusion to each lung using the following data.

right lung	319,203 counts
left lung	515,977 counts

2.   Calculate the perfusion to each lobe of lungs.

right apical lobe	86,757 counts
right middle lobe	76,647 counts
right basal lobe	138,805 counts
left apical lobe	81,513 counts
left basal lobe	122,358 counts

3.   What percentage of air circulation will be lost if the right lung is removed from a patient with lung cancer?

right lung	16,643 counts
left lung	21,150 counts

4.   What percentage of perfusion capacity will be lost when the right apical lobe is removed?

right apical lobe	2,347 counts
right middle lobe	10,656 counts
right basal lobe	15,138 counts
left apical lobe	7,403 counts
left basal lobe	15,947 counts

5.   Determine the percent perfusion to each lung.

right lung	184,537 counts
left lung	336,246 counts

6.   Determine the percent ventilation to each portion of the lung.

right upper segment	9,120 counts
right middle segment	25,100 counts
right lower segment	13,800 counts
left upper segment	25,500 counts
left middle segment	53,900 counts
left lower segment	18,600 counts

References:

Christian & Waterstram-Rich (6th Ed.), p. 475.
Early & Sodee (2nd Ed.), p. 457–459.
O'Connor, p. 464 465.
Steves & Wells (3rd Ed.), p. 104.

9. Thyroid uptake with and without decayed standard

Principles:

The ability of the thyroid to trap iodine is readily quantified using orally administered I123 or I131 sodium iodide. The thyroid uptake value is particularly useful for evaluating the severity of Grave's disease and the amount of I131 needed to partially ablate the hyperactive thyroid.

The 24-hour post-administration uptake value is determined, with some facilities using 2-, 4-, or 6-hour uptakes as well. At the time of the uptake test, counts are acquired over the thyroid and, as a background area, over the thigh.

The capsule that is administered to the patient can be used for the standard. The standard is counted with the uptake probe prior to being given to the patient. A decay factor is applied to the original count at the time the uptake value is calculated. An alternative method uses a capsule of identical dose for a standard, which is counted at the time of the uptake.

Normal range values vary somewhat by region and institution. In general, the normal range for the 24-hour uptake is about 7 to 30%. There is a gray area at either end of the normal range where it is difficult to determine if a patient's thyroid function is normal (euthyroid) or abnormal. A survey of literature found hypothyroidism was usually diagnosed below 5% and hyperthyroidism above 35 to 40%.

VI-15 How to calculate the thyroid uptake using an identical capsule for the standard:

$$\% \text{ uptake} = \frac{\text{thyroid counts} - \text{thigh counts}}{\text{capsule counts} - \text{background}} \times 100\%$$

Example:

A. A patient receives a 200-µCi capsule of I123 sodium iodide. At 24 hours post-administration the following data are obtained. What is the patient's uptake value?

200 µCi standard	325,482 cpm
background	119 cpm
thyroid	47,973 cpm
thigh	1,178 cpm

$$\frac{47,973 \text{ cpm} - 1,178 \text{ cpm}}{325,482 \text{ cpm} - 119 \text{ cpm}} \times 100 = 14\%$$

---

* Note: When the standard dose is so much larger than the background, the background becomes insignificant. The same answer would be obtained without it. The background should always be counted, however, and compared to the expected background value. Inappropriate background values could indicate malfunction, incorrect settings, or contamination.

> *** Note:** It is reasonable to express the uptake in whole numbers because the diagnosis is not affected by the tenths place. If the diagnosis is not changed as the result of an increase or decrease of one percentage point, such as 20% to 21%, then there is certainly no need to express an uptake as 20.2% or 21.3%.

VI-16 How to calculate the thyroid uptake using the patient's capsule for the standard:

$$\% \text{ uptake} = \frac{\text{thyroid counts} - \text{thigh counts}}{(\text{capsule counts} - \text{background})(\text{decay factor})} \times 100\%$$

Background is counted when the capsule is counted.

Example:

A. A patient is given 285 μCi of I123 sodium iodide. Using the original dose as the standard calculate the 24-hour uptake value.

capsule count prior to administration	1,425,916 cpm
uptake probe background	88 cpm
thyroid	193,046 cpm
thigh	473 cpm
24-hour decay factor	0.284

$$\frac{193,046 \text{ cpm} - 473 \text{ cpm}}{(1,425,916 \text{ cpm} - 88 \text{ cpm})(0.284)} \times 100\% = 48\%$$

> *** Note:** The same results will be obtained if the numbers are rounded to three significant figures when possible. The background has been dropped because of its insignificant size.
>
> $$\frac{193,000 \text{ cpm} - 473 \text{ cpm}}{(1,420,000 \text{ cpm})(0.284)} \times 100\% = 48\%$$
>
> Rounding numbers is a worthy time-saving device, but care must be taken when deciding when to round. Accuracy must not be affected. (See Basic Math Skills Section 2.)

Problems:

For the following problems the standard is an identical capsule counted at the time of uptake.

Use the following data to calculate the percent uptake.

1.	thyroid	245,000 cpm
	thigh	1,200 cpm
	standard	1,142,000 cpm
	background	56 cpm

2   thyroid   376,750 cpm
     thigh   436 cpm
     standard   755,060 cpm
     background   121 cpm

3.   thyroid   27,540 cpm
     thigh   597 cpm
     standard   1,382,000 cpm
     background   59 cpm

4.   Calculate the uptake for a patient with a thyroid count of 79,240 cpm and a thigh count of 874 cpm. The capsule count at the time of uptake is 1,284,766 cpm and the room background is 168 cpm.

5.   The count over a patient's thyroid is 174,448 cpm and 692 cpm over the thigh. What is the uptake value if the capsule count is 992,241 cpm and the background is 83 cpm?

6.   What is the 4-hour uptake for a patient with a count rate of 350,163 cpm over the thyroid and 2,145 cpm over the thigh? The standard counts are 1,167,210 cpm and background is 77 cpm.

7.   Determine the percent uptake.
     standard capsule   854,000 cpm
     background   91 cpm
     thyroid   219,000 cpm
     thigh   1,800 cpm

For the following problems the standard is the capsule that was administered to the patient.

Use the following data to calculate the percent uptake.

8.   4-hour uptake: 4-hour decay factor = 0.810
     capsule   734,915 cpm
     background   103 cpm
     thyroid   29,760 cpm
     thigh   683 cpm

9.   6-hour uptake: 6-hour decay factor = 0.73
     capsule   805,312 cpm
     background   65 cpm
     thyroid   52,905 cpm
     thigh   438 cpm

10. 24-hour uptake: 24-hour decay factor = 0.284
     capsule   969,140 cpm
     background   87 cpm
     thyroid   167,136 cpm
     thigh   374 cpm

11. Calculate the 24-hour uptake. The capsule produced 637,777 cpm prior to administration. Background was 105 cpm. The patient's thyroid is producing 56,528 cpm and the thigh count is 367 cpm. (24-hour decay factor = 0.284.)

12. Do the following results suggest hyperthyroidism?

original capsule count	1,414,000 cpm
background	96 cpm
24-hour thyroid count	226,700 cpm
24-hour thigh count	520 cpm

13. What is the 24-hour uptake if the capsule produced 1,267,000 cpm with a background of 117 cpm, and the patient's thyroid produced 49,400 cpm and the thigh 450 cpm?

References:

Balon H, Silberstein E, et al, p. 3.
Christian & Waterstram-Rich (6th Ed.), p. 424–427.
Early & Sodee (2nd Ed.), p. 628–630.
Steves & Wells (3rd Ed.), p. 77–78.

10. Calculation of concentration of a solution

Principles:

The concentration of a solution is the amount of dissolved substance per unit volume of solution. The dissolved material, or solute, may be measured in moles, in units of weight, or in units of radioactivity.

In nuclear medicine, the activity per unit volume is referred to as the specific concentration. (see Radiopharmacy Section 4). Occasionally activity per unit weight is used, when a solid form of radionuclide is utilized.

---

* **Note:** Specific concentration is NOT the same as specific activity, although these terms are sometimes used interchangeably. The specific activity is the activity per unit mass of a particular radionuclide. It is used to describe the purity of a radionuclide (i.e., the higher the specific activity, the greater the purity).

VI-17 How to calculate the concentration of a radioactive solution:

$$\text{concentration} = \frac{\text{activity of solute}}{\text{volume of solution}}$$

Examples:

A. A 200-μCi I123 capsule is diluted in 100 ml of water. What is the specific concentration of the solution?

$$\frac{200 \ \mu Ci}{100 \ ml} = 2 \ \mu Ci \ / \ ml$$

VI-18 How to determine the volume of solution or the activity needed to produce a specific concentration:

The equation from Shadowbox VI-17 is rearranged so that the "volume of solution" or the "activity of solute" becomes the unknown.

$$\text{volume of solution} = \frac{\text{activity of solute}}{\text{concentration}}$$

activity of solute = (concentration)(volume of solution).

* **Note:** You do not need to memorize three equations. If you know one, you know the others because they are simply three arrangements of the same equation.

Example:

A. A 100-μCi I123 capsule needs to be diluted to produce a solution with a concentration of 0.5 μCi/ml. To what volume must the activity be diluted?

$$\frac{100\ \mu Ci}{0.5\ \mu Ci/ml} = 200\ ml$$

---

* Note: This problem could also be solved using the equation in Shadowbox VI-16.

$$0.5\ \mu Ci/ml = \frac{100\ \mu Ci}{X\ ml}.\ \text{Isolate and solve for } X.\ \ X = \frac{100\ mCi}{0.5\ mCi/ml} = 200\ ml$$

Problems:

1. What is the concentration of a solution which was prepared with 50 μCi diluted to 10 ml?

2. A solution is prepared with 12.5 μCi in 50 ml. What is the concentration?

3. If 10 μCi is diluted to a volume of 1,000 ml, what is the concentration?

4. Calculate the concentration of a solution containing 20 μCi in 5 ml.

5. What is the concentration of a 20-ml solution which contains 100 μCi?

6. A standard is to be prepared which has a concentration of 0.1 μCi/ml. If 5 μCi are to be used, how many ml of water are required?

7. How many ml are needed to dilute 20 μCi if a 0.5-μCi/ml solution is desired?

8. What volume of solvent is needed to dilute 150 μCi to a concentration of 0.3 μCi/ml?

9. A study calls for a standard with a concentration of 10 μCi/ml. If 100 ml are needed, how many μCi will be needed to produce the standard?

10. A phantom with a 50-ml volume is to be filled with solution having a 0.02 μCi/ml concentration. How many μCi are to be used?

11. Calculate the activity needed to provide 4 ml of 0.5 μCi/ml solution.

References:

Christian & Waterstram-Rich (6th Ed.), p. 13.
Steves & Wells (3rd Ed.), p. 20 21, 24–25.

11. Preparing standards from bulk solution (dilutions)

Principles:

There are a number of situations in nuclear medicine in which a solution of a known concentration is used to make another solution of a lesser concentration. For instance, a bulk stock solution may be used to prepare a more dilute standard.

The standard is often described as having a given percent of the administered dose. For example, the standard that is prepared for a red cell mass study may contain 1% of the dose that the patient received. It is therefore referred to as a 1% solution.

The solution would be prepared by diluting an equivalent dose in 100 ml of water. One ml of the solution would contain 1/100th or 1% of the dose.

The solution could also be expressed as a ratio: a 1:100 dilution. This ratio can be rewritten as $\dfrac{1}{100}$, which equals 0.01 or 1%.

Dilution calculations are inverse proportions because as one variable increases, the second variable decreases. As volume increases, the concentration decreases. (See Basic Math Skills Section 7.)

VI-19 How to prepare a dilute solution from a stock solution:

$$C_1 V_1 = C_2 V_2$$

where: C_1 = original concentration or stock solution concentration
V_1 = original volume or the volume of bulk solution to be used
C_2 = concentration of the final solution
V_2 = volume of the final solution

The concentration can be expressed as either a percent or a decimal, such as 1% or 0.01, so long as the chosen form is used consistently within a problem.

Any element in the equation can be the unknown. Isolate the unknown by rearranging the equation, then solve for the unknown.

Examples:

A. A 500-ml solution of 5% Cr51 is desired. The stock solution has a 20% concentration. How many ml of stock will be needed?

$(20\%)(X \text{ ml}) = (5\%)(500 \text{ ml})$

Isolate and solve for X: $X \text{ ml} = \dfrac{(5\%)(500 \text{ ml})}{20\%} = 125 \text{ ml}$

The 125 ml of stock would be placed in a volumetric flask and diluted to 500 ml to produce the 5% solution.

---

* Note: The equation can also be solved with the concentration written in decimal form. The same answer will be obtained. $(0.2)(X \text{ ml}) = (0.05)(500 \text{ ml})$.

B. If 2 ml of 10% stock solution are placed in a volumetric flask and diluted to 100 ml, what is the concentration of the new solution?

$(10\%)(2 \text{ ml}) = (X \%)(100 \text{ ml})$

Isolate and solve for X: $X \% = \dfrac{(10\%)(2 \text{ ml})}{100 \text{ ml}} = 0.2\%$

C. If 5 ml of a stock solution having a 10% concentration of I131 is to be used to prepare a 1% standard, to what volume should the 5 ml of stock be diluted?

$(5 \text{ ml})(10\%) = (X \text{ ml})(1\%)$.

Isolate and solve for X: $X \text{ ml} = \dfrac{(5 \text{ ml})(10\%)}{1\%} = 50 \text{ ml}$

Problems:

1. A 100-ml standard of 1% Cr51 is needed. How many ml of a 10% stock solution will be required?

2. A stock solution contains 10% Cr51. In order to prepare 100 ml of a 0.5% Cr51 standard, how many ml of stock will be used?

3. One liter of solution is needed containing 1% I125. The stock solution has a 25% concentration. How many ml will be needed?

4. A 100-ml solution containing 0.05% Cr51 is desired. How many ml of 0.5% stock will be needed?

5. A stock solution contains 10% Cs137. How many ml of stock will be used to produce 50 ml of 5% solution?

6. A 1-liter standard with a concentration of 5% is to be prepared from a 20% stock solution. How many ml of stock are needed?

7. If 10 ml of 0.5% stock solution are placed in a volumetric flask and diluted to 50 ml, what will be the concentration of the new solution?

8. A 10-ml aliquot of 0.25% stock solution is placed in a volumetric flask and diluted to 50 ml. What is the concentration of the solution?

9. A standard is to be prepared using 2 ml of a 10% I123 solution. If the 2-ml aliquot is diluted to 10 ml, what is the concentration of the standard?

10. What will be the concentration of a standard that was prepared by diluting 2 ml of 5% stock to 100 ml?

11. A 10-ml aliquot of 20% solution is to be used to produce a 2% solution. To what volume must the aliquot be diluted?

12. If 5 ml of 5% I125 solution is to be used to make a 0.1% standard, what will be the final volume of the standard?

13. A 0.05% Cr51 standard is to be prepared using 10 ml of 5% stock. Determine the final volume of the standard.

Additional Applications:

14. A 200-µCi capsule of I123 is diluted in 100 ml of water. If 1 ml of the solution is placed in a flask and diluted to 100 ml, what will be the percent concentration of the final solution?

15. A 200-µCi capsule of I123 is diluted in 50 ml of water. If 1 ml of the solution is placed in a flask and diluted to 100 ml, what will be the percent concentration of the final solution?

16. A stock solution of Cr51 is prepared by diluting 10 µCi to 100 ml. What is the percent concentration of a standard that is prepared by diluting 10 ml of stock to 100 ml? What is the percent concentration if 10 ml of stock solution are diluted to 50 ml? What is the percent concentration if 50 ml of stock solution are diluted to 100 ml?

References:

Christian & Waterstram-Rich (6th Ed.), p. 4–5.

12. Plasma volume

Principles:

Plasma volume is determined using a dilution study. A known volume and activity of I125 radio-iodinated serum albumin (RISA) is administered to the patient. After the radiopharmaceutical has reached a state of equilibrium within the vascular compartment, blood samples are drawn. By measuring the activity per milliliter of plasma, the technologist can determine to what degree the original activity has been diluted. This will provide an accurate measure of how much plasma is contained in the patient's vascular system.

When counting the patient samples, the data is compared to a standard. The standard would ideally be the same activity as the patient dose. However, this activity would be too high for the well counter to detect without coincidence loss. When the count rate is very high, numerous photons may strike the crystal while the instrument is in deadtime. Deadtime, or resolving time, occurs when the instrument is processing one event and is therefore blind to any photons that strike the crystal during that time. These coincidental events cannot be registered by the instrument and the information is lost. The standard is, therefore, usually 1/1,000th or 1/4,000th of the actual patient dose.

A dilution factor is added to the equation to compensate for diluting the standard.

The basic dilution equation is an inverse proportion. (See Basic Math Skills Section 7.)

$$A_1 V_1 = A_2 V_2,$$

where: A_1 = original activity
           V_1 = original volume
           A_2 = sample activity
           V_2 = calculated volume

You are solving for V_2 so the equation is rearranged as follows: $V_2 = \dfrac{A_1 V_1}{A_2}$

Because a diluted standard is used as A_1, a dilution factor (DF) must be added to the numerator. The plasma volume equation is therefore:

$$V_2 = \frac{A_1 \times DF \times V_1}{A_2}$$

This equation is usually written as shown in Shadowbox VI-19.

VI-20 How to determine the plasma volume:

$$\text{plasma volume} = \frac{\left(\text{net standard activity in cpm / ml}\right)\left(\text{DF}\right)\left(\text{injected volume}\right)}{\text{net patient plasma activity in cpm / ml}}$$

If the standard is 1/1,000th of the original activity or patient dose, the DF equals 1,000. The DF equals 4,000 if the standard is 1/4,000th of the original dose.

The net counts are obtained by subtracting background counts from each value.

Examples:

A.   A patient is injected with 2 ml of I125 RISA. The patient plasma sample gives a count rate of 651 cpm/ml and an equivalent standard provides 456,100 cpm/ml. What is the patient's plasma volume?

$$\frac{\left(456,100 \text{ cpm / ml}\right)\left(2 \text{ ml}\right)}{651 \text{ cpm / ml}} = 1,401 \text{ ml}$$

* Note: Notice the large difference between the standard counts and the patient sample counts when the standard is not diluted. A solution with such a high activity is likely to produce coincidence loss.

B.   Calculate the plasma volume for a patient who receives a 1-ml dose of RISA. The patient's plasma sample produces 1,550 cpm/ml. The standard was prepared by diluting an activity equivalent to the patient dose to 1,000 ml. The standard produces 3,766 cpm/ml.

$$\frac{\left(3,766 \text{ cpm/ml}\right)\left(1000\right)\left(1 \text{ ml}\right)}{1,550 \text{ cpm/ml}} = 2,430 \text{ ml}$$

* Note: Because the standard was diluted to 1/1,000th of the patient dose activity, a dilution factor of 1,000 is used in the numerator.

Problems:

1.   Calculate the plasma volume using a standard diluted to 1/4,000th of the patient dose. The patient was injected with 1 ml. The standard gives 1,490 cpm/ml and the patient sample gives 3,221 cpm/ml.

2.   A patient receives a 2-ml dose of RISA. The patient's plasma samples are compared to a standard that is 1/1,000th of the dose. What is the plasma volume if the standard produces a count rate of 2,946 cpm/ml and the patient's samples a count rate of 2,343 cpm/ml?

3.   A RISA standard is a 1/4,000th dilution of the patient dose. Standard counts equal 390 cpm/ml. Patient sample counts equal 891 cpm/ml. A 1-ml dose was administered to the patient. What is the plasma volume?

4. Calculate the plasma volume using the following data. The standard is equal to 1/1,000th of the patient dose. The sample and standard have been counted for 5 minutes each.

patient dose volume	1 ml
patient sample counts	18,210 counts
standard counts	52,335 counts

5. Calculate the plasma volume for a patient who receives a 1 ml dose of RISA. The standard is equal to 1/1,000th of the patient's dose. All counts are acquired for 3 minutes each.

patient sample counts	12,324 counts
standard counts	18,768 counts

---

* Note: Good laboratory technique requires samples and standards to be prepared in duplicate. Poor pipetting technique can be readily identified by differences of greater than 5% between duplicates. Duplicates are averaged and the average values are applied to the equation.

---

6. Using the following data, calculate the plasma volume.

patient dose volume	1 ml
standard concentration	1/1,000th dose
patient sample counts	1,634 cpm/ml
	1,602 cpm/ml
standard counts	3,628 cpm/ml
	3,589 cpm/ml

7. Using the following data, calculate the plasma volume.

patient dose volume	1 ml
standard concentration	1/4,000th dose
patient sample counts	15,668 cpm/ml
	16,059 cpm/ml
standard counts	16,470 cpm/ml
	16,964 cpm/ml

8. Use the following data to calculate the plasma volume.

patient dose volume	1 ml
standard concentration	1/4,000th dose
patient sample counts	4,658 cpm/ml
	4,844 cpm/ml
standard counts	4,658 cpm/ml
	4,821 cpm/ml

9.   Use the following data to calculate the plasma volume.

Patient dose volume	1 ml
Standard concentration	1/4,000th dose
Patient sample counts	16,832 cpm/ml
	16,766 cpm/ml
Standard counts	10,402 cpm/ml
	10,632 cpm/ml

References:

Christian & Waterstram-Rich (6th Ed.), p. 599.
Early & Sodee (2nd Ed.), p. 726–728.
Harbert & da Rocha, Vol. 2, p. 564–565
International Atomic Energy Agency, p. 363.
International Committee for Standardization in Haematology, p. 797.
Steves & Wells (3rd Ed.), p. 124–125.

13. Red cell mass

Principles:

As with plasma volumes, red cell mass or red cell volume (RCV) determinations use a dilution method. A known volume and activity of Cr51-tagged red blood cells is administered to the patient. After equilibrium has been reached within the vascular compartment, blood samples are drawn. The activity per milliliter of whole blood is measured in order to calculate the degree to which the original activity has been diluted.

The patient's hematocrit (Hct) must be known to account for the portion of blood that consists of red cells.

> *** Note:** The Hct is expressed either as a percentage, such as 48%, or as a decimal, 0.48. In equations, the hematocrit is always expressed in its decimal form.

A plasma count is also obtained and subtracted as background activity, because the Cr51 that failed to bind to red blood cells will remain suspended in the plasma.

Typically a standard is produced at the same time the patient's blood is being tagged in vitro. A portion of the tagged blood is retained to prepare a whole blood standard. Some of the remaining blood is centrifuged and the resultant plasma is used to obtain the background counts of the standard. The hematocrit of the standard solution must also be determined.

The equation used to calculate red cell mass appears to be complicated. In reality, it is the basic dilution equation.

$$V_2 = \frac{A_1 \times DF \times V_1}{A_2}$$

where: A_1 = original activity
V_1 = original volume
A_2 = sample activity
V_2 = calculated volume
DF = dilution factor (See Clinical Procedures Section 12.)

The additional components seen in the equation Shadowbox VI-21 account for background activity from unbound radionuclide (plasma counts) and for the fact that only a portion of the blood is actually composed of red blood cells (hematocrit or Hct) or plasma (plasmacrit or Pct).

The standard is usually prepared using 1/100th of the dose administered to the patient, in which case the dilution factor would be 100.

VI-21 How to calculate the red cell volume:

$$RCV = \frac{\left[(\text{net Std whole blood cpm} \times DF) - (\text{net Std plasma cpm} \times \text{std Pct})\right]\text{injected volume}}{\text{net patient whole blood cpm} - (\text{net patient plasma cpm} \times \text{patient Pct})} \times Hct,$$

where: Std   = standard
         DF   = dilution factor
         Hct   = hematocrit in decimal form
         Pct   = plasmacrit in decimal form; Pct = 1 − Hct
         net counts = gross counts − background

* Note: The component enclosed in brackets is actually A_1 from the basic dilution equation. The plasma counts are subtracted to account for background activity resulting from unbound Cr51. The injected volume element is V_1. The whole denominator is actually A_2 with unbound Cr51 background activity being subtracted. As noted above, the Hct and Pct elements account for the fraction of blood being measured.

Example:

A. Using the following data calculate the red cell volume. A 10-ml dose was administered to the patient. The standard was diluted to 1/100th, so the dilution factor is 100.

Net Std whole blood	6,416 cpm
Net Std plasma	394 cpm
Std hematocrit	0.37
Net patient whole blood	1,257 cpm
Net patient plasma	174 cpm
Patient hematocrit	0.44

First calculate the plasmacrits:

Std Pct	$1 - 0.37 = 0.63$
Patient Pct	$1 - 0.44 = 0.56$

Determine the RCV:

$$RCV = \frac{\left[(6{,}416\,\text{cpm} \times 100) - (394\,\text{cpm} \times 0.63)\right](10\,\text{ml})}{1{,}257\,\text{cpm} - (174\,\text{cpm} \times 0.56)} \times 0.44$$

$$RCV = \frac{(641{,}600\,\text{cpm} - 248\,\text{cpm})(10\,\text{ml})}{1{,}257\,\text{cpm} - 97\,\text{cpm}} \times 0.44$$

$$RCV = 2{,}433\,\text{ml}$$

Problems:

Use the following data to calculate the red cell volume. In each case a 10-ml dose was administered to the patient. The standard was diluted to 1/100th, so the dilution factor is 100.

1. Net Std whole blood   10,055 cpm
    Net Std plasma   312 cpm
    Std hematocrit   0.27

    Net patient whole blood   2,098 cpm
    Net patient plasma   436 cpm
    Patient hematocrit   0.47

2. Net Std whole blood   4,498 cpm
    Net Std plasma   360 cpm
    Std hematocrit   0.26

    Net patient whole blood   970 cpm
    Net patient plasma   63 cpm
    Patient hematocrit   0.43

3. Net Std whole blood   15,352 cpm
    Net Std plasma   498 cpm
    Std hematocrit   0.30

    Net patient whole blood   3,035 cpm
    Net patient plasma   233 cpm
    Patient hematocrit   0.54

4. Net Std whole blood   7,686 cpm
    Net Std plasma   280 cpm
    Std hematocrit   0.28

    Net patient whole blood   1,689 cpm
    Net patient plasma   148 cpm
    Patient hematocrit   0.51

5. Net Std whole blood   9,657 cpm
    Net Std plasma   347 cpm
    Std hematocrit   0.29

    Net patient whole blood   1,822 cpm
    Net patient plasma   185 cpm
    Patient hematocrit   0.56

6.   Net Std whole blood   14,991 cpm
     Net Std plasma   1,027 cpm
     Std hematocrit   0.26

     Net patient whole blood   3,881 cpm
     Net patient plasma   252 cpm
     Patient hematocrit   0.49

7.   Net Std whole blood   11,456 cpm
     Net Std plasma   526 cpm
     Std hematocrit   0.30

     Net patient whole blood   1,918 cpm
     Net patient plasma   422 cpm
     Patient hematocrit   0.52

References:

Christian & Waterstram-Rich (6th Ed.), p. 599–600.
Early & Sodee (2nd Ed.), p. 728–733.
Harbert & da Rocha Vol. 2, p. 563–564.
International Atomic Energy Agency, p. 363–364.
International Committee for Standardization in Haematology, p. 794–796.
Steves & Wells (3rd Ed.), p. 124–127.

14. Whole blood volume with dual nuclide method

Principles:

The most accurate method for determining the whole blood volume is to use the dual nuclide method, in which the plasma volume is measured with I125 RISA and the RBC mass is calculated using Cr51.

Some protocols provide mathematical formulas for determining the RBC mass and total blood volume using I125 RISA, and for determining plasma and total blood volume using Cr51. These formulas merely provide estimates.

The peripheral venous hematocrit (Hct_v) is used in blood volume calculations. The peripheral venous hematocrit is higher than the hematocrit in the large central vessels of the body (Hct_b). This is due to the smaller size of peripheral veins. The relationship between the venous hematocrit and whole body hematocrit is expressed as the F_{cell} ratio.

$$F_{cell} \text{ ratio} = \frac{Hct_b}{Hct_v}$$

In normal individuals the ratio is 0.89 to 0.92. In patients with polycythemia vera or other blood diseases, the ratio may increase and even exceed 1. In this case the venous hematocrit or plasmacrit cannot be used in conjunction with a single radionuclide to determine the patient's blood volume. Since most patients having a nuclear medicine blood volume study are suspected of having a blood abnormality that would affect the F_{cell} ratio, use of the dual nuclide method for measuring plasma volume and red cell mass separately should be the standard of practice.

---

* Note: The following is an example of the error inherent in the single nuclide method of determining blood volumes. The patient had both an I125 RISA study and a Cr51 red cell mass study. The computer program provided the direct measurements for plasma using I125 RISA and RBC mass using Cr51, as well as the estimated volumes using the hematocrit. Note the difference between the directly measured values and the estimates.

Directly measured values are in bold text, indirectly measured values are in normal text. The percent error for each indirect measurement appears in parentheses after the value.

	plasma volume	red cell mass	whole blood volume
I125 RISA study	**4,145 ml**	3,704 ml (39%)	7,849 ml (15%)
Cr51 study	3,625 ml (12%)	**2,658 ml**	6,283 ml (8%)
Combined study			**6,803 ml**

VI-22 How to calculate the total blood volume using the dual nuclide method:

total blood volume = plasma volume + red cell mass.

Example:

A.   Using RISA, a patient has been found to have a plasma volume of 3,079 ml. A Cr51-tagged RBC study gives a red cell mass of 2,843 ml. What is the patient's total blood volume?

3,079 ml + 2,843 ml = 5,922 ml total blood volume

Problems:

1.   Calculate the patient's total blood volume from a dual nuclide study using the following data.

     red cell mass   1,862 ml
     plasma volume   2,299 ml

2.   According to a Cr51 red cell mass study a patient has 1,531 ml of red cells. A RISA study performed on the same day gives a plasma volume of 2,114 ml. What is the patient's total blood volume?

3.   A patient with a hematocrit of 52% has a red cell mass of 3,230 ml according to a red cell study. A plasma volume study demonstrates a plasma volume of 2,981 ml. What is the patient's total blood volume?

References:

Christian & Waterstram-Rich (6th Ed.), p. 599–600.
Early & Sodee (2nd Ed.), p. 733–734.
Harbert & da Rocha, Vol. 2, p. 562–563.
International Committee for Standardization in Haematology, p. 798.
Steves & Wells (3rd Ed.), p. 124–127.

Appendix A. Decay Charts

Several different decay chart formats are used here to give you experience with various models. Some charts include pre-calibration factors.

Answers to problems may vary slightly depending upon the method you use to determine activity at a specified time. For example, an answer may differ by a percentage point when you multiply by a pre-calibration factor versus dividing by a decay factor. Multiplying decay factors to provide factors that exceed the charts may give a slightly different answer than using the half-life equation (see Shadowbox V.1). For our purposes, these variations are insignificant.

For instructions on using decay factors see Radiopharmacy Section 2. For instructions on using pre-calibration factors see Radiopharmacy Section 4.

* **Note:** A survey of references found that many radionuclides have been assigned half-lives that vary from one author to another. For instance, the half-life of Tc99m may be listed as 6.007, 6.01, 6.0, or 6.02. Decay factors will, of course, vary depending upon which half-life is used, so answers to problems may also be affected. The level of variations is usually insignificant.

The following half-lives were used to create the decay charts used in this book.

barium	Ba133	10.66 years or 127.9 months
cesium	Cs137	30.0 years or 360 months
chromium	Cr51	27.7 days
cobalt	Co57	270 days
	Co60	5.26 years or 63.1 months
fluorine	F18	1.8 hours or 109.7 minutes
gallium	Ga67	78.3 hours or 3.26 days
indium	In111	2.83 days or 67.9 hours
iodine	I123	13.2 hours
	I131	8.05 days or 193.2 hours
molybdenum	Mo99	66.7 hours or 2.78 days
nitrogen	N13	9.97 minutes
phophorus	P32	14.28 days
rubidium	Rb82	1.25 minutes or 75 seconds
samarium	Sm153	1.93 days or 46.3 hours
strontium	Sr89	50.5 days
technetium	Tc99m	6.01 hours
thallium	Tl201	73.1 hours or 3.04 days
xenon	Xe133	5.24 days or 125.8 hours
yttrium	Y90	2.67 days or 64.1 hours

Abbreviations used with the Decay Charts:

PCF = Pre-Calibration Factor
DF = Decay Factor

The charts for the radionuclides listed above appear in alphabetical order on the following pages.

Barium   Ba133   10.66 years or 127.9 months

Months	DF
1	0.994
2	0.989
3	0.984
4	0.978
5	0.973
6	0.968
7	0.963
8	0.958
9	0.952
10	0.947
11	0.942
12	0.937

Years	DF
2	0.878
3	0.823
4	0.771
5	0.722
6	0.677
7	0.634
8	0.594
9	0.557
10	0.522

Cesium   Cs137   30.0 years or 360 months

* **Note:** To read this table, select the years that have elapsed from the left hand column and the months from the top of the chart. Read across from the left and down from the top. The decay factor appears where the two intersect.

Example: If 1 year and 6 months have elapsed since a Cs137 source was calibrated, the decay factor would be 0.966.

Years	Months 0	1	2	3	4	5	6	7	8	9	10	11
		0.998	0.996	0.994	0.992	0.990	0.988	0.987	0.985	0.983	0.981	0.979
1	0.977	0.975	0.973	0.972	0.97	0.968	0.966	0.964	0.962	0.960	0.958	0.957
2	0.955	0.953	0.951	0.949	0.948	0.946	0.944	0.942	0.940	0.938	0.937	0.935
3	0.933	0.931	0.929	0.928	0.926	0.924	0.922	0.920	0.919	0.917	0.915	0.914
4	0.912	0.91	0.908	0.907	0.905	0.903	0.901	0.899	0.898	0.896	0.894	0.893
5	0.891	0.889	0.888	0.886	0.884	0.882	0.881	0.879	0.877	0.876	0.874	0.872
6	0.871	0.869	0.867	0.866	0.864	0.862	0.861	0.859	0.857	0.856	0.854	0.852
7	0.851	0.849	0.847	0.846	0.844	0.842	0.841	0.839	0.838	0.836	0.834	0.832
8	0.831	0.83	0.828	0.826	0.825	0.823	0.822	0.820	0.818	0.817	0.815	0.814
9	0.812	0.811	0.809	0.808	0.806	0.804	0.803	0.801	0.8	0.798	0.797	0.795
10	0.794	0.792	0.791	0.789	0.788	0.786	0.785	0.783	0.782	0.78	0.779	0.777

Chromium   Cr51   27.7 days

Days	DF		Days	DF
1	0.975		20	0.606
2	0.951		25	0.535
3	0.928		30	0.472
4	0.905		40	0.368
5	0.882		50	0.286
6	0.861		60	0.223
7	0.839		70	0.173
8	0.819		80	0.135
9	0.798		90	0.105
10	0.779		100	0.082
15	0.687		200	0.007

Cobalt   Co57   270 days

Days	DF		Days	DF
1	0.997		50	0.880
2	0.995		60	0.857
3	0.992		70	0.836
4	0.990		80	0.814
5	0.987		90	0.794
10	0.975		100	0.774
20	0.95		200	0.598
30	0.926		300	0.463
40	0.902		365	0.392

Cobalt   **Co60**   **5.26 years or 63.1 months**

Months	DF
1	0.989
2	0.978
3	0.968
4	0.957
5	0.946
6	0.943
7	0.926
8	0.916
9	0.906
10	0.896
11	0.886
12	0.876

Years	DF
2	0.768
3	0.674
4	0.590
5	0.517
6	0.454
7	0.398
8	0.348
9	0.306
10	0.268

Fluorine   **F18**   **1.8 hours or 109.7 minutes**

Minutes	PCF	DF
15	1.1	0.909
30	1.209	0.827
45	1.328	0.753
60	1.462	0.684
75	1.605	0.623
90	1.764	0.567
110	2	0.500
220	4	0.250
440	16	0.063

Gallium   Ga67   78.3 hours or 3.26 days

Hours	PCF	DF
1	1.008	0.991
2	1.018	0.982
3	1.027	0.974
4	1.036	0.965
5	1.045	0.957
6	1.055	0.948
7	1.064	0.94
8	1.073	0.932
9	1.083	0.923
10	1.093	0.915
11	1.102	0.907
12	1.112	0.899
18	1.173	0.853
24	1.237	0.808
30	1.304	0.767
36	1.375	0.727
42	1.450	0.689
48	1.529	0.654

Days	PCF	DF
3	1.892	0.529
4	2.339	0.427
5	2.890	0.346
6	3.584	0.279
7	4.425	0.226
8	5.495	0.182
9	6.757	0.148
10	8.403	0.119

Indium   In111   2.83 days or 67.9 hours

Hours	PCF	DF
1	1.010	0.99
2	1.021	0.98
3	1.031	0.97
4	1.042	0.960
5	1.053	0.950
6	1.063	0.941
7	1.074	0.931
8	1.084	0.922
9	1.096	0.912
10	1.107	0.903
11	1.118	0.894
12	1.130	0.885
18	1.202	0.832
24	1.278	0.783
30	1.358	0.736
36	1.444	0.693
42	1.535	0.651
48	1.632	0.613

Days	PCF	DF
3	2.083	0.48
4	2.664	0.375
5	3.400	0.294
6	4.348	0.230
7	5.552	0.180
8	7.092	0.141
9	9.091	0.110
10	11.63	0.086

Iodine   I123   13.2 hours

Hours	PCF	DF	Hours	PCF	DF
0.25	1.013	0.987	15	2.198	0.455
0.5	1.027	0.974	16	2.317	0.432
0.75	1.04	0.961	17	2.439	0.41
1	1.054	0.949	18	2.573	0.389
2	1.111	0.900	19	2.710	0.369
3	1.171	0.854	20	2.858	0.35
4	1.234	0.810	21	3.012	0.332
5	1.300	0.769	22	3.175	0.315
6	1.370	0.73	23	3.344	0.299
7	1.445	0.692	24	3.526	0.284
8	1.522	0.657	25	3.717	0.269
9	1.605	0.623	26	3.917	0.255
10	1.691	0.591	27	4.132	0.242
11	1.782	0.561	28	4.351	0.23
12	1.878	0.533	29	4.587	0.218
13	1.980	0.505	30	4.832	0.207
14	2.086	0.479			

Iodine   I131   8.05 days or 193.2 hours

Hours	PCF	DF	Days	PCF	DF
1	1.004	0.996	1	1.090	0.917
2	1.007	0.993	2	1.188	0.842
3	1.011	0.989	3	1.295	0.772
4	1.014	0.986	4	1.410	0.709
5	1.018	0.982	5	1.538	0.650
6	1.022	0.979	6	1.678	0.596
12	1.044	0.958	7	1.828	0.547
			8	1.992	0.502
			9	2.169	0.461
			10	2.364	0.423
			11	2.577	0.388
			12	2.809	0.356
			13	3.058	0.327
			14	3.333	0.300

Molybdenum Mo99   2.78 days or 66.7 hours

Pre-Calibration Factors

Hours	PCF		Hours	PCF		Hours	PCF
1	1.010		10	1.111		19	1.221
2	1.021		11	1.122		20	1.234
3	1.032		12	1.134		21	1.247
4	1.043		13	1.146		22	1.260
5	1.054		14	1.158		23	1.273
6	1.065		15	1.170		24	1.287
7	1.076		16	1.183		36	1.459
8	1.088		17	1.195		48	1.656
9	1.099		18	1.208		60	1.878
						72	2.130

Decay Factors

* **Note:** To read this table, select the hours that have elapsed from the left hand column and the hours from the top of the chart. Read across from the left and down from the top. The decay factor appears where the two intersect.

Example: If 15 hours have elapsed since a Mo99 generator was eluted, the decay factor would be 0.856.

Hours	0	1	2	3	4	5	6	7	8	9
0		0.99	0.979	0.969	0.959	0.949	0.94	0.93	0.92	0.911
10	0.901	0.892	0.883	0.874	0.864	0.856	0.847	0.838	0.829	0.821
20	0.812	0.804	0.795	0.787	0.779	0.771	0.763	0.755	0.747	0.74
30	0.732	0.724	0.717	0.709	0.702	0.695	0.688	0.68	0.673	0.666
40	0.66	0.653	0.646	0.639	0.633	0.626	0.62	0.613	0.607	0.6
50	0.594	0.588	0.582	0.576	0.57	0.564	0.558	0.552	0.547	0.541
60	0.536	0.53	0.524	0.519	0.514	0.508	0.503	0.498	0.493	0.488
70	0.483	0.478	0.473	0.468	0.463	0.458	0.453	0.499	0.444	0.44
80	0.435	0.43	0.426	0.422	0.417	0.413	0.409	0.404	0.4	0.396
90	0.392	0.388	0.384	0.38	0.376	0.372	0.368	0.364	0.361	0.357
100	0.353	0.35	0.346	0.346	0.339	0.335	0.332	0.328	0.325	0.322
110	0.318	0.315	0.312	0.309	0.305	0.302	0.299	0.296	0.293	0.29
120	0.287	0.284	0.281	0.278	0.275	0.272	0.27	0.267	0.264	0.261
130	0.258	0.256	0.253	0.25	0.248	0.245	0.243	0.24	0.238	0.235
140	0.233	0.23	0.228	0.226	0.223	0.221	0.219	0.217	0.214	0.212
150	0.21	0.208	0.206	0.203	0.201	0.199	0.197	0.195	0.193	0.191
160	0.189	0.187	0.185	0.183	0.181	0.18	0.178	0.176	0.174	0.172
170	0.17	0.169	0.167	0.165	0.164	0.161	0.16	0.158	0.157	0.155

Nitrogen   N13   9.97 minutes

Minutes	PCF	DF
1	1.072	0.933
2	1.149	0.87
3	1.232	0.812
4	1.321	0.757
5	1.416	0.706
6	1.517	0.659
7	1.627	0.615
8	1.744	0.573

Minutes	PCF	DF
9	1.87	0.535
10	2	0.5
20	4	0.25
30	8.047	0.124
40	16.125	0.062
50	32.31	0.031
60	64.749	0.015

Phophorus   P32   14.28 days

Days	DF
1	0.953
2	0.907
3	0.864
4	0.824
5	0.785
6	0.747
7	0.712
8	0.678
9	0.646

Days	DF
10	0.615
11	0.586
12	0.559
13	0.532
14	0.507
15	0.483
16	0.460
17	0.438
18	0.417

Days	DF
19	0.390
20	0.379
25	0.297
30	0.233
35	0.184
40	0.144
45	0.113
50	0.089
55	0.07

Rubidium   Rb82   1.25 minutes or 75 seconds

＊ Note: As Rb82 is produced by a generator, the decay time begins at time of elution.

Seconds	DF
15	0.871
30	0.758
45	0.660
60	0.574
75	0.500
90	0.435
105	0.379

Seconds	DF
120	0.330
135	0.287
150	0.250
165	0.218
180	0.190
195	0.165
210	0.144

Seconds	DF
225	0.125
240	0.109
255	0.095
270	0.083
285	0.072
300	0.063

Samarium   Sm153   1.93 days or 46.3 hours

Hours	PCF	DF
1	1.02	0.99
2	1.03	0.97
3	1.05	0.96
4	1.06	0.94
6	1.09	0.91
8	1.13	0.89
12	1.20	0.84
16	1.27	0.80
20	1.35	0.74
24	1.43	0.70
36	1.71	0.58
48	2.05	0.49

Strontium   Sr89   50.5 days

Days	PCF	DF	Days	DF
1	1.014	0.986	20	0.760
2	1.028	0.973	30	0.663
3	1.042	0.960	40	0.578
4	1.056	0.947	50	0.504
5	1.071	0.934	60	0.439
6	1.086	0.921	70	0.383
7	1.101	0.908	80	0.334
8	1.116	0.896	90	0.291
9	1.315	0.884	100	0.253
10	1.147	0.872		

Technetium   Tc99m   6.01 hours

> *** Note:** To read these tables select the hours from the left hand column and the minutes from the top of the chart. Read across from the left and down from the top. The pre-calibration factor or decay factor appears where the two intersect.
>
> Example: If 3.5 hours have elapsed since a Tc99m dosage was calibrated, the decay factor would be 0.667.

Pre-Calibration Factors

	Minutes			
Hours	0	15	30	45
0		1.029	1.059	1.09
1	1.122	1.156	1.189	1.224
2	1.259	1.297	1.335	1.374
3	1.414	1.522	1.499	1.543
4	1.587	1.634	1.681	1.733
5	1.779	1.835	1.887	1.946
6	2	2.058	2.119	2.179

Decay Factors

	Minutes											
Hours	0	5	10	15	20	25	30	35	40	45	50	55
0		0.99	0.981	0.972	0.962	0.953	0.944	0.935	0.925	0.917	0.908	0.899
1	0.891	0.882	0.872	0.865	0.857	0.849	0.841	0.833	0.825	0.817	0.809	0.801
2	0.794	0.786	0.778	0.771	0.764	0.756	0.749	0.742	0.735	0.728	0.721	0.714
3	0.707	0.701	0.693	0.657	0.681	0.674	0.667	0.661	0.655	0.648	0.642	0.635
4	0.63	0.624	0.618	0.612	0.606	0.601	0.595	0.589	0.583	0.577	0.572	0.566
5	0.562	0.556	0.55	0.545	0.541	0.535	0.53	0.524	0.519	0.514	0.509	0.504
6	0.5	0.496	0.491	0.486	0.482	0.477	0.472	0.468	0.464	0.459	0.455	0.45
7	0.446	0.442	0.438	0.433	0.429	0.425	0.421	0.417	0.413	0.409	0.405	0.401
8	0.398	0.394	0.39	0.386	0.382	0.379	0.375	0.372	0.368	0.365	0.361	0.358
9	0.354	0.351	0.348	0.344	0.341	0.338	0.334	0.331	0.328	0.325	0.322	0.319
10	0.315	0.313	0.31	0.307	0.304	0.301	0.298	0.295	0.292	0.29	0.287	0.284
11	0.281	0.278	0.276	0.273	0.271	0.268	0.265	0.263	0.26	0.258	0.256	0.253
12	0.25	0.248	0.246	0.244	0.241	0.239	0.236	0.234	0.232	0.23	0.228	0.226

Thallium   Tl201   73.1 hours or 3.04 days

Hours	PCF	DF		Hours	PCF	DF
1	1.010	0.990		15	1.152	0.868
2	1.019	0.981		16	1.164	0.859
3	1.029	0.972		17	1.175	0.851
4	1.038	0.963		18	1.186	0.843
5	1.048	0.954		19	1.198	0.835
6	1.058	0.945		20	1.208	0.828
7	1.068	0.936		21	1.221	0.819
8	1.079	0.927		22	1.232	0.812
9	1.089	0.918		23	1.244	0.804
10	1.099	0.910		24	1.256	0.796
11	1.11	0.901		30	1.327	0.754
12	1.12	0.892		36	1.406	0.711
13	1.13	0.884		42	1.488	0.672
14	1.142	0.876		48	1.578	0.634

Days	PCF	DF
3	1.65	0.505
4	2.488	0.402
5	3.101	0.322
6	3.922	0.255
7	4.926	0.203
8	6.211	0.161
9	7.813	0.128
10	9.804	0.102

Xenon   Xe133   5.24 days or 125.8 hours

Hours	PCF	DF		Days	PCF	DF
1	1.006	0.994		1	1.142	0.876
2	1.011	0.989		2	1.302	0.768
3	1.016	0.984		3	1.488	0.672
4	1.022	0.978		4	1.698	0.589
5	1.028	0.973		5	1.938	0.516
6	1.034	0.968		6	2.212	0.452
7	1.04	0.962		7	2.525	0.396
8	1.045	0.957		8	2.881	0.347
9	1.050	0.952		9	3.289	0.304
10	1.057	0.946		10	3.759	0.266
11	1.063	0.941				
12	1.068	0.936				

Yttrium   Y90   2.67 days or 64.1 hours

Hours	PCF	DF
1	1.011	0.989
2	1.021	0.979
3	1.033	0.968
4	1.044	0.958
5	1.056	0.947
6	1.067	0.937
7	1.079	0.927
8	1.091	0.917
9	1.102	0.907
10	1.114	0.898
11	1.126	0.888
12	1.139	0.878
13	1.151	0.869
14	1.163	0.860
15	1.176	0.851
20	1.241	0.806
25	1.310	0.763

Appendix B. Chi-Square Table

See Instrumentation Section 8 for use of the Chi-Square table.

Values generally useful in clinical nuclear medicine are including in this table. For higher degrees of freedom or lower p-values, refer to any of the numerous web sites that have more expansive chi-square tables.

Degrees of Freedom (N-1)	$P = 0.95$	$P = 0.90$	$P = 0.50$	$P = 0.10$	$P = 0.05$
1	0.004	0.016	0.455	2.706	3.841
2	0.103	0.211	1.386	4.605	5.991
3	0.352	0.584	2.366	6.251	7.815
4	0.711	1.064	3.357	7.779	9.488
5	1.145	1.610	4.352	9.236	11.070
6	1.635	2.204	5.348	10.645	12.592
7	2.167	2.833	6.346	12.017	14.067
8	2.733	3.490	7.344	13.362	15.507
9	3.325	4.168	8.343	14.684	16.919
10	3.940	4.865	9.342	15.987	18.307
11	4.575	5.578	10.341	17.275	19.675
12	5.226	6.304	11.340	18.549	21.026
13	5.892	7.042	12.340	19.812	22.362
14	6.571	7.790	13.339	21.064	23.685
15	7.261	8.547	14.339	22.307	24.996
16	7.962	9.312	15.338	23.542	26.296
17	8.672	10.085	16.338	24.769	27.587
18	9.390	10.865	17.338	25.989	28.869
19	10.117	11.651	18.338	27.204	30.144
20	10.851	12.443	19.337	28.412	31.410

Appendix C. Solutions to Problems

> *** Note:** All answers are rounded according to the criteria described in Basic Math Skills Section 1.

I. Basic Math Skills for Nuclear Medicine Technology

1. Significant figures and rounding of numbers

1.	4	8.	86	15.	2,360
2.	3	9.	10,000	16.	1,230,000
3.	5	10.	0.076	17.	0.0468
4.	1	11.	0.00044	18.	0.000137
5.	2	12.	0.82	19.	1.65
6.	25,000	13.	0.33	20.	18.5
7.	7,900	14.	8.7		

2. Significant figures and mathematical operations

1. 615
2. 0.1
3. 3.96
4. 9,290
5. 0.025
6. 72.2
7. 327
8. 0.00101
9. 0.339
10. 360
11. 35.64 + 74406 = 74441.64. The least accurate number in the operation has no decimal places, so the answer must be rounded as such to 74,442.
12. 6.4163. In this case the two zeros in the number 3.7100 are not just place holders. They represent accurate measurement, therefore the answer should contain decimal four places.
13. 5.2521. The least accurate number in the operation has one decimal place, so the answer must be rounded as such to 5.2.
14. 24.247
15. 240.1
16. 6157.9 – 3.04 = 6154.9
17. 119.07
18. 4293.7
19. 5576.9
20. 21.78

3. Powers and exponents

1. 32
2. 1,000,000
3. 81
4. 5,832

5. 390,625
6. 1
7. 493,039

8. 759,375
9. 100,000,000
10. 1,024

4. Roots

1. 12
2. 15
3. 6
4. 2.9

5. 316
6. 360
7. 38.50

8. 10.4
9. 9.6
10. 29

5. Scientific notation

1. 3.564×10^3
2. 6.1579×10^3
3. 1.203×10^2
4. 2.706325×10^6
5. 4.26×10^2
6. 4.54931×10^4
7. 1.107×10^2
8. 1.001924×10^6
9. 5.5946×10^3
10. 2.73598×10^4
11. 744,000
12. 304
13. 113.3
14. 37,100
15. 1,052,000
16. 2,550
17. 231,400
18. 14,002
19. 1,770

20. 5,574,000
21. 1.63×10^5
22. 2.348×10^5
23. 8.7902×10^{10}
24. 7.74×10^{15}
25. 1.9067427×10^{23}
26. 2.5×10^{-1}
27. 5.0×10^{-3}
28. 1.25×10^{-2}
29. 5.75×10^{-4}
30. 7.5419×10^{-3}
31. 4.69×10^{-2}
32. 3.55×10^{-5}
33. 2.95×10^{-4}
34. 6.06×10^{-1}
35. 1.125×10^{-5}
36. 0.245
37. 0.0000000219

38. 0.0000308
39. 0.00120
40. 0.0532
41. 0.000415
42. 0.116
43. 0.00168
44. 0.0133
45. 0.00000392
46. 2.53×10^{-3}
47. 9.71×10^{-9}
48. 8.54×10^{-20}
49. 1.548×10^{-7}
50. 8.41×10^{-18}
51. 7.99×10^{-6}
52. 3.72×10^{-4}
53. 2.844×10^{-27}
54. 1.76×10^{-10}
55. 8.49×10^{-17}

6. Mathematical operations using exponentials

1. $(2.5 \times 5.0)(10^{-1+(-3)}) = 1.2 \times 10^{-3}$
2. $(1.25 \times 4.69)(10^{2+(-2)}) = 5.86 \times 10^0$; $10^0 = 1$, so the answer is simply written as 5.86.
3. 4.34×10^{-6}
4. 1.05×10^{10}

5. 6.82×10^{-6}

6. 2.45×10^{3}

7. 3.27×10^{2}

8. 4.12×10^{2}

9. 1.653×10^{1}, which is more sensibly written as 16.53.

10. 3.18×10^{2}

11. Convert 3.564×10^{1} to 0.03564×10^{3}

$$\left(0.03564 \times 10^{3}\right) + \left(6.1579 \times 10^{3}\right) = 6.19354 \times 10^{3}$$

Round number to 4 significant figures: 6.194×10^{3}

12. Convert 2.706325×10^{6} to 27063.25×10^{2}

$$\left(1.202 \times 10^{2}\right) + \left(27063.25 \times 10^{2}\right) = 27064.452 \times 10^{2}$$

Round to 4 significant figures and rewrite in scientific notation: 2.706×10^{6}

13. 4.6×10^{4}

14. 1.002×10^{6}

15. 3.2649×10^{4}

16. 7.44×10^{5}

17. 2.58×10^{4}

18. 1.05×10^{6}

19. 2.174×10^{5}

20. 5.57×10^{6}

7. Direct and inverse proportions

1. $(45 \text{ mCi})(0.8 \text{ ml}) = (X \text{ mCi})(2.3 \text{ ml});\ X = \dfrac{(45 \text{ mCi})(0.8 \text{ ml})}{2.3 \text{ ml}} = 16 \text{ mCi}$

2.
$(12,500 \text{ cpm})(X \text{ mCi}) = (500,000 \text{ cpm})(0.51 \text{ mCi});\ X = \dfrac{(500,000 \text{ cpm})(0.51 \text{ mCi})}{12,500 \text{ cpm}} = 20 \text{ mCi}$

3. 0.2 mrem

4. $\dfrac{20,000 \text{ ct}}{3 \text{ min}} = \dfrac{50,000 \text{ ct}}{X \text{ min}};\ X \text{ min} = \dfrac{(50,000 \text{ ct})(3 \text{ min})}{20,000 \text{ ct}} = 8 \text{ min}$

5. $\dfrac{35,000 \text{ cps}}{10 \text{ } \mu\text{Ci}} = \dfrac{X \text{ cps}}{4 \text{ } \mu\text{Ci}};\ X \text{ cps} = \dfrac{(35,000 \text{ cps})(4 \text{ } \mu\text{Ci})}{10 \text{ } \mu\text{Ci}} = 14,000 \text{ cps}$

6. 300 mR

7. 42 mg

8. 600,000 ct

9. 0.8 ml

10. 0.4 ml

11. 100 µCi

12. $\dfrac{(12 \text{ } \mu\text{Ci})(5.0 \text{ ml})}{100 \text{ ml}} = X \text{ } \mu\text{Ci};\ X = 0.6 \text{ } \mu\text{Ci}$

13. $\dfrac{(65{,}000\,\text{cpm})(2.0\,\text{ml})}{420\,\text{cpm}} = X\,\text{ml}$; $X = 309\,\text{ml}$

The answer should be rounded to 2 significant figures, so the correct answer is 310 ml.

14. 89 ml

15. $(4.0\,\text{ml})(15\%) = (50\,\text{ml})(X\,\%)$

$X\,\% = \dfrac{(4.0\,\text{ml})(15\,\%)}{50\,\text{ml}}$; $X = 1.2\,\%$

16. $(2{,}000 \times G)(5\,\text{min}) = (1{,}000 \times G)(X\,\text{min})$; $X = 10\,\text{min}$

17. $(1{,}500 \times G)(15\,\text{min}) = (2{,}000 \times G)(X\,\text{min})$; $X = 11\,\text{min}$

18. $(12{,}600\,\text{counts/ml})(1.0\,\text{ml}) = (63\,\text{counts/ml})(X\,\text{ml})$; $X = 200\,\text{ml}$

19. $(75\,\text{mCi/ml})(1.0\,\text{ml}) = (X\,\text{mCi/ml})(5.0\,\text{ml})$; $X = 15\,\text{mCi/ml}$

20. $(65\,\text{mCi/ml})(2\,\text{ml}) = (X\,\text{mCi/ml})(3.0\,\text{ml})$; $X = 43\,\text{mCi/ml}$

8. Converting within the metric system

1. Inverse proportion method:

Identify powers: $\mu\text{Ci} = 10^{-6}$; $\text{mCi} = 10^{-3}$

Apply inverse proportion equation: $(7.5 \times 10^5)(10^{-6}) = (X)(10^{-3})$;

$X = \dfrac{(7.5 \times 10^5)(10^{-6})}{10^{-3}} = \dfrac{7.5 \times 10^{5+(-6)}}{10^{-3}} = 7.5 \times 10^{-1-(-3)}$; $X = 7.5 \times 10^2$

Quick method:

Calculate Δ: $-6 - (-3) = -3$

Apply Δ to the original exponent: $7.5 \times 10^{5-3} = 7.5 \times 10^2$

> *** Note:** Since the conversion in #1 was from small units to larger ones, the answer should be smaller than the original number, because fewer of the units are needed.

2. Inverse proportion method:

Identify powers: $\text{mCi} = 10^{-3}$; $\mu\text{Ci} = 10^{-6}$

Apply inverse proportion equation: $(8.4 \times 10^7)(10^{-3}) = (X)(10^{-6})$;

$X = \dfrac{(8.4 \times 10^7)(10^{-3})}{10^{-6}} = \dfrac{8.4 \times 10^{7+(-3)}}{10^{-6}} = 8.4 \times 10^{4-(-6)}$; $X = 8.4 \times 10^{10}$

Quick method:

Calculate Δ: $-3 - (-6) = 3$

   Apply Δ to the original exponent: $8.4 \times 10^{7+3} = 8.4 \times 10^{10}$

> *** Note:** Since the conversion in #2 was from large units to smaller ones, the answer should be larger than the original number, because more of the units are needed.

3. 2.5×10^1. Because $10^1 = 10$, it is more practical to write this number as 25.

4. 12.1×10^0. Because $10^0 = 1$, it is more practical to write this number as 12.1.

5. 5.2×10^7

6. 5.0×10^2 or 500

7. 7.5×10^5

8. 2.1×10^3

9. 6.7×10^{-1} or 0.67

10. 10.5×10^9 or 1.05×10^{10}

11. 2,000 µCi

12. 200 µCi

13. 0.075 mCi

14. 1,100 kBq

15. 6,000 kBq; 0.006 GBq

16. 650 µCi

17. 1.076 mCi; 0.001076 Ci or 1.076×10^{-3} Ci

18. 1,300,000 µCi or 1.3×10^6 µCi

19. 2,100 MBq

20. 670 MBq

9.   Converting between curie and becquerel.

Answers are rounded to the appropriate number of significant figures.

1.   (15 µCi)(37 kBq/µCi) = 560 kBq

2.   (0.50 µCi)(37 kBq/µCi)) = 19 kBq

3.   (0.50 mCi)(37 MBq/mCi) = 19 MBq

4.   (25 mCi)(37 MBq/mCi) = 920 MBq

5.   (1.1 mCi)(37 MBq/mCi) = 41 MBq; To convert MBq to GBq, move the decimal point three places to the left: 0.041 GBq (See Basic Math Skills Section 8.)

6.   58,000 kBq or 5.8×10^4 kBq

7.   (752 mCi)(37 MBq/mCi) = 28,00 MBq or 28 GBq

8.   (808 Ci)(37 GBq/Ci) = 30,000 GBq or 30,000,000 MBq or 3×10^7 MBq

9.   9.9 GBq

10. (75 Ci)(37 GBq/Ci) = 2,800 GBq; to convert to kBq, move the decimal six places to the right: 2,800,000,000 kBq or 2.8×10^9 kBq

11. (185 MBq)(27 µCi/MBq) = 5,000 µCi

12. (9.25 MBq)(0.027 mCi/MBq) = 0.25 mCi

13. (7.79 GBq)(27 mCi/GBq) = 210 mCi

14. 16 mCi

15. 110 µCi

16. 670 µCi

17. 0.14 µCi or 1.4×10^{-1} µCi; to convert to Ci move the decimal point 6 places to the right: $1.4 \times 10^{-1+(-6)} = 1.4 \times 10^{-7}$

18. (1687 kBq)(0.027 µCi/kBq) = 46 µCi; to convert µCi to mCi, move the decimal point three places to the left: 0.046 mCi

19. 84 µCi
20. 240 Ci

10. Converting between rad and gray

1. (66 mrad)(0.01 mGy/mrad) = 0.66 mGy; to convert mGy to µGy, move the decimal point three places to the right: 660 µGy
2. (1.8 rad)(0.01 Gy/rad) = 0.018 Gy or 18 mGy
3. 7 mGy
4. 0.039 mGy or 39 µGy
5. (1.5 mGy)(100 mrad/mGy) = 150 mrad
6. (60 mGy)(100 mrad/mGy) = 6,000 mrad; to convert mrad to rad, move the decimal point three places to the left: 6 rad (See Basic Math Skills Section 8.)
7. 75 mrad
8. 300 µrad or 0.3 mrad

11. Converting between rem and sievert

1. (0.1 rem)(0.01 Sv/rem) = 0.001 Sv; to convert Sv to mSv, move the decimal point three places to the right: 1 mSv (See Basic Math Skills Section 8.)
2. (0.5 rem)(0.01 Sv/rem) = 0.005 Sv or 5 mSv
3. 0.5 Sv or 500 mSv
4. 50 mSv
5. 720 mrem: to convert from mrem to rem, move the decimal point three places to the left: 0.72 rem
6. 8 mrem
7. 3 rem
8. 0.5 rem or 500 mrem

12. Converting between pound and kilogram

1. (15.4 lb)(0.45 kg/lb) = 6.9 kg
2. (17 lb)(0.45 kg/lb) = 7.6 kg
3. 61 kg
4. 15 kg
5. 46 kg
6. 20 kg
7. 37 kg
8. 80 kg
9. 92 kg
10. 106 kg
11. (22 kg)(2.2 lb/kg) = 48 lb
12. (96 kg)(2.2 lb/kg) = 211 lb
13. 33 lb
14. 161 lb
15. 20 lb

16. 7 lb
17. 154 lb
18. 95 lb
19. 64 lb
20. 26 lb

13. Logs, natural logs, and antilogs

1.	1.447	11.	34.04	21.	2
2.	2.292	12.	7,551	22.	0.500
3.	3.760	13.	3.526	23.	4.74
4.	−0.408	14.	7.937	24.	0.0446
5.	421.7	15.	−1.022	25.	74
6.	3	16.	1.545	26.	1.594
7.	1,683	17.	8.489	27.	6,438
8.	56.10	18.	3.807	28.	0.227
9.	0.124	19.	6.335	29.	0.0720
10.	0.005321	20.	8.358	30.	0.447

14. Solving equations with an unknown in the exponent

1. $\log 74 = \log 10^{2.37x}$; $1.869 = 2.37x$; $x = \dfrac{1.869}{2.37} = 0.79$

2. Isolate component containing x: $\dfrac{48}{22} = 10^{8.46x}$

    Simplify the side not containing x: $2.18 = 10^{8.46x}$

    Take the log of each side: $\log 2.18 = \log 10^{8.46x}$; $0.338 = 8.46x$

    Isolate and solve for x: $x = \dfrac{0.338}{8.46} = 0.04$

3. Isolate component containing x: $\dfrac{173}{0.6} = 10^{(0.551)\left(\frac{x}{4.1}\right)}$

    Simplify the side not containing x: $288 = 10^{(0.551)\left(\frac{x}{4.1}\right)}$

    Take the log of each side: $\log 288 = \log 10^{(0.551)\left(\frac{x}{4.1}\right)}$; $2.46 = (0.551)\left(\dfrac{x}{4.1}\right)$

    Isolate and solve for x: $x = \dfrac{(2.46)(4.1)}{0.551} = 18$

4. $\ln 1.7 = \ln e^{0.931x}$; $0.531 = 0.931x$; $x = \dfrac{0.531}{0.931} = 0.57$

5. Isolate component containing x and simplify the equation:

$\dfrac{10.5}{8.6} = e^{1.35x}; 1.22 = e^{1.35x}$

Take the ln of each side: $\ln 1.22 = \ln e^{1.35x}; 0.1996 = 1.35x$

Isolate and solve for x: $x = \dfrac{0.1996}{1.35} = 0.15$

6. $\ln \dfrac{110}{12} = \ln\left(e^{(0.443)\left(\frac{x}{0.5}\right)}\right); 2.216 = (0.443)\left(\dfrac{x}{0.5}\right); x = \dfrac{(2.216)(0.5)}{0.443} = 2.5$

7. $\ln \dfrac{0.12}{120} = \ln\left(e^{-(0.693)\left(\frac{x}{0.03}\right)}\right); -6.9078 = -(0.693)\left(\dfrac{x}{0.03}\right); x = \dfrac{(-6.9078)(0.03)}{-0.693} = 0.3$

8. 0.46

9. $\ln \dfrac{7.5}{120} = \ln\left(e^{-(0.693)\left(\frac{0.24}{0x}\right)}\right); -2.772 = -(0.693)\left(\dfrac{0.24}{x}\right); x = \dfrac{(-0.693)(0.24)}{-2.772} = 0.06$

10. $\ln \dfrac{8.6}{25} = \ln\left(e^{-(0.693)\left(\frac{20}{0x}\right)}\right); -1.067 = -(0.693)\left(\dfrac{20}{x}\right); x = \dfrac{(-0.693)(20)}{-1.067} = 13$

11. 67
12. 5.99

15. Graphing on linear and semilog paper

1. 75%
2. 70%
3. semilog
4. 10%
5. 9%
6. semilog
7. 0.54 mCi
8. 0.56 mCi
9. 8,500 cpm
10. 4,000 cpm

11.

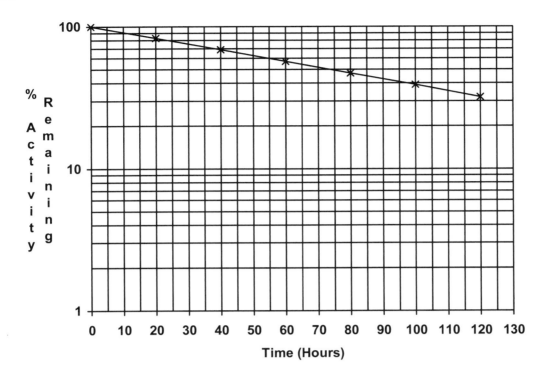

Actual half-life is 73 hours (Tl201).

12.

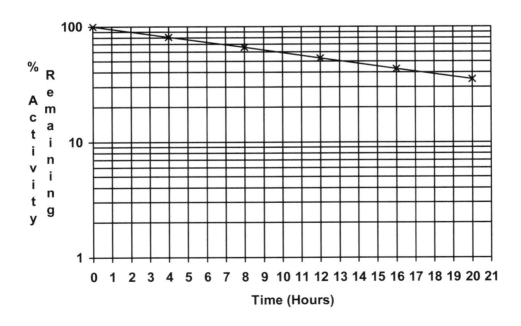

Actual half-life is 13 hours (I123).

13.

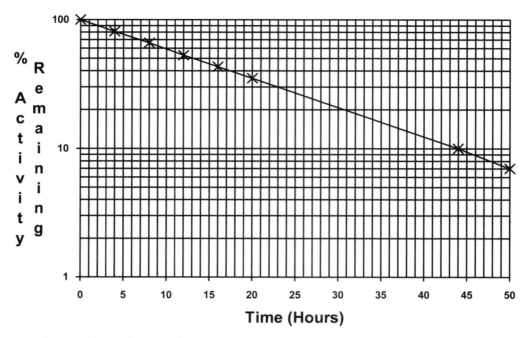

At 44 hours 10% of the activity remains or 90% of the activity has decayed.

14.

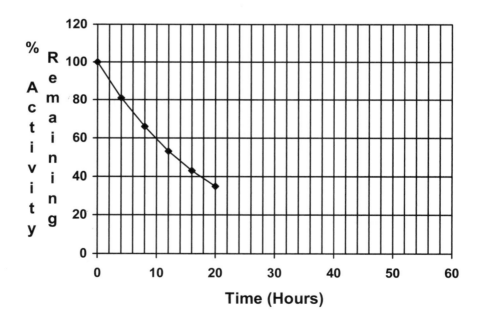

Note that a straight line cannot be extended out from the last point as can be done on the semilog graph. The shape of the curve beyond the last point must be guessed and therefore contains significant error. The answer will vary depending upon the estimated shape of the extended curve.

II. Statistics

1. Percent error or percent difference

1. $\dfrac{25\,\text{mCi} - 21\,\text{mCi}}{25\,\text{mCi}} \times 100\% = \dfrac{4\,\text{mCi}}{25\,\text{mCi}} \times 100\% = 16.0\%$

2. $\dfrac{3.10\,\text{mCi} - 3.42\,\text{mCi}}{3.10\,\text{mCi}} \times 100\% = \dfrac{0.32\,\text{mCi}}{3.10\,\text{mCi}} \times 100\% = 10.3\%$

3. 4.2%
4. 12.0%
5. 8%
6. 5.8%
7. 8.0%
8. 1.6%

---

* Note: In this case the difference is given as part of the problem rather than two values that vary from one another. So instead of performing subtraction in the numerator, the difference (7) is placed there. You are starting one step into the calculation process.

---

9. 13%
10. 27%

2. Count rate determination

1. $\dfrac{74{,}035\,\text{counts}}{2.0\,\text{min}} = 37{,}000\,\text{cpm}$

2. $\dfrac{13{,}952\,\text{counts}}{12.0\,\text{min}} = 1{,}160\,\text{cpm}$

3. 2,500 cpm
4. 190,000 cpm

5. $\dfrac{3{,}291{,}500\,\text{counts}}{(2.0\,\text{h})(60\,\text{min/h})} = 27{,}000\,\text{cpm}$

6. 451 cps

7. $\dfrac{60{,}472\,\text{counts}}{(0.5\,\text{min})(60\,\text{s/min})} = 2{,}000\,\text{cps}$

8. 28 cps
9. 490 cps
10. 580 cps

11. $\dfrac{10{,}000\ \text{counts}}{X\ \text{min}} = 850\ \text{cpm} \qquad X\ \text{min} = \dfrac{10{,}000\ \text{counts}}{850\ \text{cpm}} \approx 12\ \text{min}$

12. 123 minutes or about 2 hours

13. $\dfrac{718{,}500\ \text{counts}}{5.0\ \text{min}} = 140{,}000\ \text{cpm} \qquad \dfrac{2{,}000{,}000\ \text{counts}}{140{,}000\ \text{cpm}} \approx 14\ \text{min}$

3.   Effects of background on counts and count rates

1.   82,977 counts – 509 counts = 82,468 counts; round to 82,500 counts
2.   34,220 counts
3.   95,400 cpm
4.   6,910 cpm
5. $\dfrac{73{,}815\ \text{counts} - 947\ \text{counts}}{3.0\ \text{min}} = 24{,}289\ \text{cpm}$; round to 24,000 cpm
6.   1,300 cpm
7.   4,400 cpm
8.   684 cpm
9.   1,710 cpm
10. 432 cpm
11. 0.5-min count rate = 3,030 cpm; 3-min count rate = 3,390 cpm

$\dfrac{3{,}390\ \text{cpm} - 3{,}030\ \text{cpm}}{3{,}390\ \text{cpm}} \times 100\% = 11\%$ difference

---

* Note: By acquiring about 10,000 counts, you have increased the statistical reliability of your results. A 100-count sampling contains an inherent error of 10%, while a 10,000-count sampling has a 1% inherent error. (See Statistics Section 8.)

---

4.   Mean, median, and mode

1.   mode = 174; median = 174; mean = 167.
2.   mode = 60, median = 60, mean = 57.
3.   no mode; median = 6,855; mean = 6,850.
4.   no mode; median = 57,527; mean = 58,687.
5.   median is half-way between 756 and 903: $\dfrac{756 + 903}{2} = 830$; mean = 771.
6.   median = 10,661; mean = 10,780.
7.   mean = 76,082.

5. Standard deviation of a series of values

1. $\overline{n} = \dfrac{27.2 + 27.6 + 27.9 + 26.8 + 27.4}{5} = 27.38$

$(27.2 - 27.38)^2 = -0.18^2 = 0.0324$

$(27.6 - 27.38)^2 = 0.22^2 = 0.0484$

$(27.9 - 27.38)^2 = 0.52^2 = 0.270$

$(26.8 - 27.38)^2 = -0.58^2 = 0.3364$

$(27.4 - 27.38)^2 = 0.02^2 = 0.0004$

$\sum(n - \overline{n}) = 0.6876 \qquad \sigma = \sqrt{\dfrac{0.6876}{5-1}} = \sqrt{0.1719} = 0.4$

2. $\overline{n} = \dfrac{13{,}967 + 14{,}472 + 14{,}229}{3} = 14{,}223$

$(13{,}967 - 14{,}223)^2 = -256^2 = 65{,}536$

$(14{,}472 - 14{,}223)^2 = 249^2 = 62{,}001$

$(14{,}229 - 14{,}223)^2 = 6^2 = 36$

$\sum(n - \overline{n}) = 127{,}573 \qquad \sigma = \sqrt{\dfrac{127{,}573}{3-1}} = \sqrt{63{,}786} = 252$

3. $\overline{n} = 137$; $\sigma = 16$
4. $\overline{n} = 43.2$; $\sigma = 1.3$
5. $\overline{n} = 10.3$; $\sigma = 0.8$
6. $\overline{n} = 18{,}277$; $\sigma = 364$

6. Confidence intervals and the standard deviation of a single value

1. $\sqrt{10{,}763} = 104$
2. 156
3. 25
4. $2\sqrt{9{,}768} = 198$
5. 243
6. 2,730
7. $3\sqrt{847} = 87$
8. 1,006
9. 760
10. $CI_{68\%} = 100{,}000 \pm \sqrt{100{,}000} = 100{,}000 \pm 316$ so $99{,}684 - 100{,}316$.
11. $CI_{68\%} = 28{,}000 \pm \sqrt{28{,}000} = 28{,}000 \pm 167$ so $27{,}833 - 28{,}167$.
12. $4{,}000 \pm 63$ so $3{,}937 - 4{,}063$.
13. $CI_{95\%} = 11{,}000 \pm 2\sqrt{11{,}000} = 11{,}000 \pm 210$ so $10{,}790 - 11{,}210$.
14. $2{,}600 \pm 102$ so $2{,}498 - 2{,}702$.

15. $48,700 \pm 441$ so $48,259 - 49,141$.

16. $CI_{99\%} = 854,000 \pm 3\sqrt{854,000} = 854,000 \pm 2,772$ so $851,228 - 856,772$.

17. $12,000 \pm 329$ so $11,671 - 12,329$.

18. $CI_{68\%} = 7,882 \text{ ct} \pm \sqrt{7,882} = 7,882 \text{ ct} \pm 89$, so range of values $= 7,793 - 7,971$ counts.

19. $CI_{99\%} = 49,691 \text{ cpm} \pm 3\sqrt{49,691} = 49,691 \text{ cpm} \pm 669$, so the acceptable range is $49,022\text{-}50,360$.

20. $CI_{95\%} = 60,629 \text{ cpm} \pm 492$, so the acceptable range is $60,137 - 61,121$ cpm.

21. $CI_{95\%} = 3,733 \text{ cpm} \pm 122$, so the acceptable range is $3,611 - 3,855$ cpm.

22. $CI_{99\%} = 92,537 \text{ cpm} \pm 912$, so the acceptable range is $91,625 - 93,449$ cpm.

23. $CI_{95\%} = 134 \text{ cpm} \pm 23$, so the acceptable range is $111 - 157$ cpm.

7. Percent error or coefficient of variation for a series of values

1. $\%CV = \dfrac{260}{8,945} \times 100\% = 2.9\%$

2. $\%CV = \dfrac{0.49}{2.89} \times 100\% = 17\%$

3. 3.1%

4. 6.9%

5. 3.5%

6. 2.2%

7. 15%

8. 4.9%; yes, within acceptable limits.

9. $CV_{68} = 4\%$, $CV_{95} = 8\%$, $CV_{99} = 12\%$

8. Error inherent in a single value

1. $\%SD = \dfrac{100\%}{\sqrt{8,000}} = \dfrac{100}{89} = 1.1\%$

2. $\%SD = \dfrac{100\%}{\sqrt{46,500}} = \dfrac{100}{216} = 0.5\%$

3. 0.3%

4. 2.7%

5. $\%SD = \dfrac{(2)(100\%)}{\sqrt{21,750}} = \dfrac{200}{147} = 1.4\%$

6. $\%SD = \dfrac{(2)(100\%)}{\sqrt{6,210}} = \dfrac{200}{79} = 2.5\%$

7. 0.8%

8. 0.4%

9. $\%SD = \dfrac{(3)(100\%)}{\sqrt{5,600}} = \dfrac{300}{75} = 4.0\%$

10. $\%SD = \dfrac{(3)(100\%)}{\sqrt{821}} = \dfrac{300}{28.6} = 10.5\%$

11. 2.9%

12. 1.9%

9.   Determination of counts required for statistical significance

1. $2\% = \dfrac{100\%}{\sqrt{N}} \qquad \sqrt{N} = \dfrac{100}{2} \qquad \sqrt{N} = 50 \qquad \left(\sqrt{N}\right)^2 = 50^2 \qquad N = 2,500$

2.   400

3.   40,000

4. $5\% = \dfrac{(2)(100\%)}{\sqrt{N}} \qquad \sqrt{N} = \dfrac{200}{5} \qquad \left(\sqrt{N}\right)^2 = 40^2 \qquad N = 1,600$

5.   444,444; round to 400,000

6.   81,633; round to 80,000

7. $2\% = \dfrac{(3)(100\%)}{\sqrt{N}} \qquad \sqrt{N} = \dfrac{300}{2} \qquad \left(\sqrt{N}\right)^2 = 150^2 \qquad N = 22,500$, which can be

     rounded to 20,000

8.   90,000

9   360,000; round to 400,000

10.   Standard deviation of a count rate

1. $\dfrac{65,340 \text{ counts}}{5\,\text{min}} = 13,068 \text{ cpm}; \quad \sigma_c = \sqrt{\dfrac{13,068 \text{ cpm}}{5\,\text{min}}} = \sqrt{2,614} = 51$

     so 13,068 cpm $\pm$ 51 or 13,017 $-$ 13,119 cpm.

2. $\dfrac{8,610 \text{ counts}}{10\,\text{min}} = 861 \text{ cpm}; \quad \sigma_c = \sqrt{\dfrac{861 \text{ cpm}}{10\,\text{min}}} = \sqrt{86} = 9$

     so 861 cpm $\pm$ 9 or 852-870 cpm.

3.   36,667 cpm $\pm$ 110 or 36,557 $-$ 36,777 cpm.

4.   479 cpm $\pm$ 6 or 473 $-$ 485 cpm.

5. $\dfrac{35,030 \text{ counts}}{2\,\text{min}} = 17,515 \text{ cpm}; \quad 2\,\sigma_c = 2\sqrt{\dfrac{17,515 \text{ cpm}}{2\,\text{min}}} = 2\sqrt{8,758} = 187$

     so 17,515 cpm $\pm$ 187 or 17,328 $-$ 17,702 cpm.

6. $\dfrac{175,377 \text{ counts}}{15\,\text{min}} = 11,692 \text{ cpm}; \quad 2\,\sigma_c = 2\sqrt{\dfrac{11,692 \text{ cpm}}{15\,\text{min}}} = 2\sqrt{779} = 56$

     so 11,692 cpm $\pm$ 56 or 11,636 $-$ 11,748 cpm.

7.   45,445 cpm $\pm$ 95 or 45,350 $-$ 45,540 cpm

8. 4,137 cpm $\pm$ 74 or 4,063 – 4,211 cpm.

9. $\dfrac{4{,}078 \text{ counts}}{2 \text{ min}} = 2{,}039 \text{ cpm};\quad 3\,\sigma_c = 3\sqrt{\dfrac{2{,}039 \text{ cpm}}{2 \text{ min}}} = 3\sqrt{1{,}020} = 96$

    so 2039 cpm $\pm$ 96 or 1,943 – 2,135 cpm.

10. $\dfrac{395{,}400 \text{ counts}}{12 \text{ min}} = 32{,}950 \text{ cpm};\quad 3\,\sigma_c = 3\sqrt{\dfrac{32{,}950 \text{ cpm}}{12 \text{ min}}} = 3\sqrt{2{,}746} = 157$

    so 32,950 cpm $\pm$ 157 or 32,793 – 33,107 cpm.

11. 1,842 cpm $\pm$ 52 or 1,790 – 1,894 cpm.

12. $3\,\sigma_c = 3\sqrt{5{,}260} = 218$, so 5,260 cpm $\pm$ 218 or 5,042 – 5,478 cpm.

---

* Note: Since 1 is the denominator it can be ignored and the simple equation for the standard deviation of an individual value is used.

---

13. a) 185; 8,341 – 8,711 cpm
    b) 130; 8,396 – 8,656 cpm
    c) 107; 8,419 – 8,633 cpm
    d) 82; 8,444 – 8,608 cpm
    e) 58; 8,468 – 8,584 cpm

11. Propagation of error

1. $\sigma = \sqrt{850{,}200 \text{ cpm} + 2{,}570 \text{ cpm}} = \sqrt{852{,}770} = 923$
2. $\sigma = \sqrt{12{,}500 \text{ cpm} + 480 \text{ cpm}} = \sqrt{12{,}980} = 114$
3. 316
4. 96
5. 245
6. 114
7. 183

III. Radiation Protection

1. Conversion of counts per minute to disintegrations per minute using well counter efficiency

1. $\dfrac{662 \, \text{cpm} - 312 \, \text{cpm}}{0.38} = 921 \, \text{dpm}$

2. $\dfrac{346 \, \text{cpm} - 209 \, \text{cpm}}{0.54} = 254 \, \text{dpm}$

3. 1,968 dpm
4. 3,200 dpm
5. 716 dpm
6. 11,286 dpm
7. 1,812 dpm
8. a. 5,119 dpm
    b. 592 dpm
    c. 6,306 dpm
    d. 2,410 dpm
    e. 288 dpm
    f. 512 dpm

The RSO must be notified immediately concerning wipes a, c, and d.

9. A. 4,479 dpm
    B. 458 dpm
    C. 31,276 dpm

The NRC and the carrier must be notified immediately concerning package C.

10. A. 1,063 dpm
    B. 1,261 dpm
    C. 18,057 dpm

Neither the NRC nor the carrier needs to be notified concerning any of these packages.

2. Exposure rate constants

1. $X \, \text{R/h} = \dfrac{(15 \, \text{mCi})}{(1 \, \text{cm})^2} \times 0.59 \dfrac{\text{R} \cdot \text{cm}^2}{\text{mCi} \cdot \text{h}} = 8.9 \, \text{R/h at 1 cm}$

2. At 10 cm:

$$X \text{ R/h} = \frac{(15 \text{ mCi})}{(10 \text{ cm})^2} \times 0.59 \frac{\text{R} \cdot \text{cm}^2}{\text{mCi} \cdot \text{h}}$$

$$X = \frac{8.85}{100} = 0.089 \text{ R/h or } 89 \text{ mR/ h at } 10 \text{ cm}$$

At 1 m: Change 1 m to 100 cm.

$$X \text{ R/h} = \frac{(15 \text{ mCi})}{(100 \text{ cm})^2} \times 0.59 \frac{\text{R} \cdot \text{cm}^2}{\text{mCi} \cdot \text{h}}$$

$$X = \frac{8.85}{10,000} = 0.00089 \text{ R/h or } 0.89 \text{ mR/ h at } 1 \text{ m}$$

3. 0.084 R/h or 84 mR/h at 4 cm
4. 0.014 R/h or 14 mR/h at 15 cm
5. 0.019 R/h or 19 mR/h at 15 cm

> *** Note:** This is the exposure rate from the gamma photons only.

---

6. 1.8 R/h or 1,800 mR/h at 3 cm

7. 0.00003 R/h or 0.03 mR/h or background at 30 cm
8. 0.0008 R/h or 0.8 mR/h at 15 cm

3. Radiation dose versus time

1. $\left(\dfrac{3.0 \text{ mrem}}{60 \text{ min}}\right)(50 \text{ min}) = 2.5 \text{ mrem}$
2. (0.35 mrem/h)(4 h) = 1.4 mrem
3. (a) $\left(\dfrac{5.8 \text{ mrem}}{60 \text{ min}}\right)(11 \text{ min}) = 1.1 \text{ mrem}$

    (b) $\left(\dfrac{5.8 \text{ mrem}}{60 \text{ min}}\right)(6 \text{ min}) = 0.6 \text{ mrem}$

4. 4.8 mrem
5. 5.8 mrem; 15 mrem
6. $X \text{ mrem} = (16 \,\mu\text{Sv})(2.5 \text{ h}) \quad X = 40 \,\mu\text{Sv}$
7. $\left(\dfrac{85 \,\mu\text{Sv}}{60 \text{ min}}\right)(6 \text{ min}) = 8.5 \,\mu Sv$
8. (a) 12 mrem
    (b) 60 mrem
    (c) 240 mrem

9. (a) Convert the TEDE of 5 rem per year to 5,000 mrem per year.
        240 mrem/month × 12 months = 2,880 mrem/y
        No, the TEDE will not be exceeded.
   (b) Convert the TEDE of 0.5 rem for gestation after declaration to 500 mrem.
        At 60 mrem per week, the TEDE for the fetus will be met in 8 weeks after
        declaration.

4. Radiation dose versus distance from source

1. $(160 \text{ mrem/h})(1 \text{ m})^2 = (x \text{ mrem/h})(3 \text{ m})^2; x = \dfrac{(160 \text{ mrem/h})(1 \text{ m})^2}{(3 \text{ m})^2} = 18 \text{ mrem/h}$

2. $(350 \text{ mrem/h})(3 \text{ in})^2 = (x \text{ mrem/h})(36 \text{ in}); x = \dfrac{(350 \text{ mrem/h})(3 \text{ in})^2}{(36 \text{ in})^2} = 2.4 \text{ mrem/h}$

3. Convert feet to inches; 0.6 mrem/h
4. 36 mrem/h
5.

$$(20 \text{ mrem/h})(1 \text{ ft})^2 = (2 \text{ mrem/h})(x \text{ ft})^2; \quad x^2 = \dfrac{(20 \text{ mrem/h})(1 \text{ ft})^2}{(2 \text{ mrem/h})}$$

$$x^2 = 10; \sqrt{x^2} = \sqrt{10}; \quad x \approx 3 \text{ ft}$$

6.

$$(50 \text{ mrem/h})(3 \text{ in})^2 = (0.5 \text{ mrem/h})(x \text{ in})^2; \quad x^2 = \dfrac{(50 \text{ mrem/h})(3 \text{ in})^2}{(0.5 \text{ mrem/h})}$$

$$x^2 = 900; \sqrt{x^2} = \sqrt{900}; \quad x = 30 \text{ in}$$

7. 95 inches or about 8 feet
8. a) $\dfrac{500 \text{ mrem/y}}{1,960 \text{ h/y}} = 0.26 \text{ mrem/h}$

    b) $(1.5 \text{ mrem/h})(2 \text{ ft})^2 = (0.26 \text{ mrem/h})(x \text{ ft})^2; \quad x^2 = \dfrac{(1.5)(2^2)}{0.26}$

        $x^2 = 23.1; \sqrt{x^2} = \sqrt{23.1}; \quad x = 4.8 \text{ ft}$

9. $(35 \text{ mrem/h})(1 \text{ in})^2 = (x \text{ mrem/h})(12 \text{ in})^2; \quad x = 0.24 \text{ mrem/h}$
10. The generator must be at least 16 inches back from the wall.
11. about 14 in

5. Radiation dose versus shielding

1. 2 HVL decrease original activity to 25%, therefore (0.25)(15 mR/h) = 3.8 mR/h
2. 10 HVL decrease original activity to 0.1%, therefore
    (0.001)(8850 mR/h) = 8.85 mR/hr

3. 6 HVL decrease original activity to 1.6%, therefore (0.016)(0.05 mR/h) = 0.0008 mR/h, which is below the common background reading of 0.01 to 0.03 mR/h. The proper answer should therefore be, "activity was decreased to background levels," because one cannot obtain survey meter readings below background levels.

4.

$$x = (5,300 \text{ mR/h})\left(e^{-(0.693)\left(\frac{0.9 \text{ mm}}{0.27 \text{ mm}}\right)}\right) = (5,300)\left(e^{-(0.693)(3.33)}\right) = (5,300 \text{ mR/h})\left(e^{-(2.31)}\right)$$

$$x = (5,300)(0.099) = 526 \text{ mR/h}$$

5.

$$x = (5,300 \text{ mR/h})\left(e^{-(0.693)\left(\frac{3.8 \text{ mm}}{0.27 \text{ mm}}\right)}\right) = (5,300)\left(e^{-(0.693)(14.07)}\right) = (5,300 \text{ mR/h})\left(e^{-(9.75)}\right)$$

$$x = (5,300)(0.000058) = 0.3 \text{ mR/h}$$

6. 0.23 mR/h

7. 0.012 mR/h or background

8. 0.000002 or 2.0×10^{-6} mR/h or background

9.

$$0.01 \text{ mR/h} = (0.15 \text{ mR/h})\left(e^{-(0.693)\left(\frac{x \text{ mm}}{0.2 \text{ mm}}\right)}\right) \qquad \left(\frac{0.01}{0.15}\right) = e^{-(0.693)\left(\frac{x}{0.2}\right)}$$

$$0.0667 = \left(e^{-(0.693)\left(\frac{x}{0.2}\right)}\right) \qquad \ln 0.0667 = \ln e^{-(0.693)\left(\frac{x}{0.2}\right)} \qquad -2.708 = -(0.693)\left(\frac{x}{0.2}\right)$$

$$x = \frac{(-2.708)(0.2)}{-(0.693)} = 0.78 \text{ mm lead}$$

10.

$$2.0 \text{ mR/h} = (6.4 \text{ mR/h})\left(e^{-(0.693)\left(\frac{x \text{ cm}}{0.7 \text{ cm}}\right)}\right) \qquad \left(\frac{2}{6.4}\right) = e^{-(0.693)\left(\frac{x}{0.7}\right)}$$

$$0.31 = e^{-(0.693)\left(\frac{x}{0.7}\right)} \qquad \ln 0.31 = \ln e^{-(0.693)\left(\frac{x}{0.7}\right)} \qquad -1.17 = -(0.693)\left(\frac{x}{0.7}\right)$$

$$x = \frac{(-1.17)(0.7)}{-(0.693)} = 1.2 \text{ cm lead}$$

11. 2.5 mm lead

6. Effective half-life

1. $T_e = \dfrac{6\,h \times 11\,h}{6\,h + 11\,h} = \dfrac{66}{17} = 4\,h$

2. $T_e = \dfrac{6\,h \times 29\,h}{6\,h + 29\,h} = \dfrac{174}{35} = 5\,h$

3. Convert 10 days to hours: $10\,d \times 24\,h = 240\,h$; $T_e = 56\,h$

    OR convert 73 hours to 3 days; $T_e = 2.3\,d$ or 56 h

4. For 17%: 22 h

    For 83%: Convert 25 days to hours: $25\,d \times 24\,h = 600\,h$; $T_e = 69\,h$

5. Convert 5.3 days to minutes: $5.3\,d \times 24\,h \times 60\,min = 7{,}632\,min$

    $T_e = 0.37\,min$

6. 11 days

7. 3.7 days

IV. Instrumentation.

1. Calculation of acceptable ranges for dose calibrator accuracy and constancy

1.   1.34 mCi ± 0.13 = 1.21 to 1.47 mCi
2.   195 μCi ± 19.5 = 176 to 214 μCi
3.   62.6 μCi ± 6.3 = 56.3 to 68.9 μCi
4.   81.3 μCi ± 8.1 = 73.2 to 89.4 μCi
5.   (260 μCi)(0.05) = 13 μCi; 260 μCi ± 13 = 247 to 273 μCi
6.   148 μCi ± 7.4 = 141 to 155 μCi
7.   90.4 μCi ± 4.5 = 85.9 to 94.9 μCi
8.   76.2 μCi ± 3.8 = 72.4 to 80.0 μCi
9.   2-year decay factor = 0.878; (153 μCi)(0.878) = 134 μCi on June 1, 1997;
     134 μCi ± 13.4 = 121 to 147 μCi
10. 30-day decay factor = 0.926; (76.0 μCi)(0.926) = 70.4 μCi on May 31;
     (70.4 μCi)(0.05) = 3.5 μCi; 70.4 μCi ± 3.5 = 66.9 to 73.9 μCi
11. 8-year decay factor = 0.831; (63.8 μCi)(0.831) = 53.0 μCi on March 1, 1996;
     53.0 μCi ± 5.3 = 47.7 to 58.3 μCi
12. 90-day decay factor = 0.794; (122 μCi)(0.794) = 96.9 μCi expected activity at 90
     days; 96.9 μCi ± 9.7 = 87.2 to 107 μCi, so 90.2 μCi is acceptable.
13. 8-year decay factor = 0.594; (96.2 μCi)(0.594) = 57.1 μCi expected activity at 8
     years; 57.1 μCi ± 5.7 = 51.4 to 62.8 μCi, so 49.9 μCi is not acceptable.

2. Percent error for dose calibrator accuracy and constancy

1. $\dfrac{198\,\mu Ci - 187\,\mu Ci}{198\,\mu Ci} \times 100\% = 5.6\%$; yes.

2. $\dfrac{0.96\,mCi - 1.03\,mCi}{0.96\,mCi} \times 100\% = 7.3\%$; yes.

3.   9.9%; yes.
4.   3%; yes.
5.   11.0%; no.
6.   5.9%; no.
7. $A = A_0 e^{(-0.693)(t/T_p)}$; $A = (126\,\mu Ci)e^{(-0.693)(4\,y/30\,y)} = (126\,\mu Ci)(0.912) = 114.9\,\mu Ci$ or use

     decay factor: 4 y DF = 0.912; (126 μCi)(0.912) = 114.9 μCi;

     $\dfrac{114.9\,\mu Ci - 116.3\,\mu Ci}{114.9\,\mu Ci} \times 100\% = 1.2\%$; yes.

8.   Calculate 15-year activity using half-life of 10.66 years:
     $A = (154\,\mu Ci)e^{(-0.693)(15\,y/10.66\,y)} = (154\,\mu Ci)(0.377) = 58.0\,\mu Ci$
     Calculate % error: 5.6%; meets standards.

9. Calculate 2.25-year activity using half-life of 5.26 years:

    $A = (80.2 \, \mu Ci)e^{(-0.693)(2.25 \, y/5.26 \, y)} = (80.2 \, \mu Ci)(0.743) = 59.6 \, \mu Ci$

    Calculate % error: 10.7%; does not meet standards.

10. Calculate 18.3-year activity using half-life of 30.0 years:

    $A = (85.2 \, \mu Ci)e^{(-0.693)(18.3 \, y/30.0 \, y)} = (85.2 \, \mu Ci)(0.655) = 55.8 \, \mu Ci$

    Calculate % error: 4.3%; meets standards.

3. Dose calibrator geometry and percent error for syringes

1. Calculate expected activity: 94.5 mCi - 71.7 mCi = 22.8 mCi; calculate percent

    error: $\dfrac{22.8 \, mCi - 21.6 \, mCi}{22.8 \, mCi} \times 100\% = 5.3\%$

2. Expected activity = 10.4 mCi; % error = 6.7%; no correction factor needed.
3. Expected activity = 22.2 mCi; % error = 13.1%; yes, correction factor needed.
4. Expected activity = 9.5 mCi; % error = 11.6%; yes, correction factor needed.
5. Expected activity = 5.3 mCi; % error = 3.8%; no correction factor needed.
6. Expected activity = 45.6 mCi; % error = 1.5%; no correction factor needed.

4. Dose calibrator geometry and percent error for vials

1. $\dfrac{2.63 \, mCi - 2.34 \, mCi}{2.63 \, mCi} \times 100\% = 11.0\%$; need to use a correction factor.

2. $\dfrac{1.94 \, mCi - 1.89 \, mCi}{1.94 \, mCi} \times 100\% = 2.6\%$; no correction factor needed.

3. 4%; no correction factor needed.
4. 10.7%; must use a correction factor.
5. 7%; no correction factor needed.
6. 2.3%; no correction factor needed.
7. 8.8%; yes, acceptable
8. 6%; no correction factor needed.

5. Dose calibrator linearity of response and percent error

1. $\dfrac{37.2 \, mCi - 37.6 \, mCi}{37.2 \, mCi} \times 100\% = 1.1\%$

2. $\dfrac{45.3 \, mCi - 40.1 \, mCi}{45.3 \, mCi} \times 100\% = 11.5\%$; a correction factor would be needed.

3. 7%; no correction factor is needed.
4. 10.6%; correction factor needed.
5. 1.5%; no correction factor is needed.
6. DF = 0.125; (3.28 mCi)(0.125) = 0.410 mCi or 410 μCi

    $\dfrac{410 \, \mu Ci - 375 \, \mu Ci}{410 \, \mu Ci} \times 100\% = 8.5\%$

7. PCF = 2; (2.85 mCi)(2) = 5.70 mCi expected activity
    $$\frac{5.70\,\text{mCi} - 5.45\,\text{mCi}}{5.70\,\text{mCi}} \times 100\% = 4.4\%$$

8. Monday 8:00 am is 30 hours before reference, so PCF = 32
    (4.72 mCi)(32) = 151.0 mCi expected activity;
    $$\frac{151.0\,\text{mCi} - 154.2\,\text{mCi}}{151.0\,\text{mCi}} \times 100\% = 2.1\%$$

9. Tuesday 1:00 pm is 24 hours before reference, so PCF = 16;
    expected activity = 27.8 mCi; 3.6% error; no correction factor needed.

6. Calculation and use of correction factors for dose calibrator geometry and linearity

1. $\dfrac{8.04\,\mu\text{Ci}}{9.83\,\mu\text{Ci}} = 0.82$

2. $\dfrac{0.39\,\mu\text{Ci}}{0.35\,\mu\text{Ci}} = 1.1$

3. 0.904

4. 1.13

5. (522 μCi)(0.89) = 464 μCi

6. (76.8 μCi)(1.16) = 89.1 μCi

7. 38 μCi

8. 9.63 mCi

9. (120.8 mCi)(1.19) = 143.8 mCi

10. (206 μCi)(0.87) = 179 μCi; does not meet minimum, may decrease the quality of the study.

7. Energy resolution

1. $\dfrac{689\,\text{keV} - 635\,\text{keV}}{662\,\text{keV}} \times 100\% = 8.2\%$; acceptable

2. $\dfrac{713\,\text{keV} - 611\,\text{keV}}{662\,\text{keV}} \times 100\% = 15.4\%$; unacceptable

3. 9.7%; acceptable

---

* Note: Differences in individual readings of the practice graphs will cause some variations in the results for problems 4 through 6. Do not be concerned if your answer is slightly different from the author's. Reading small reproductions of graphs can be difficult.

---

4. half-maximum = 7,400 ct; 685 keV–637 keV = 48 keV spread; 7.2%; unacceptable

5. half-maximum = 5,000 ct; 708 keV–617 keV = 91 keV spread; 13.7%; unacceptable

6. half-maximum = 6,000 ct; 696 keV–622 keV = 74 keV spread; 11.2%; acceptable

8. Well counter or uptake probe constancy (precision) using chi-square

1.

	η	$\eta - \bar{\eta}$	$\left(\eta - \bar{\eta}\right)^2$
1	13,777	127	16,129
2	13,765	115	13,225
3	13,575	−75	5,625
4	13,511	−139	19,321
5	13,615	-35	1,225
6	13,715	65	4,225
7	13,529	−121	14,641
8	13,557	−93	8,649
9	13,783	133	17,689
10	13,678	28	784

$\Sigma \eta = 136{,}505$ $\qquad \Sigma\left(\eta - \bar{\eta}\right)^2 = 101{,}513$

$$\bar{\eta} = \frac{136{,}505}{10} = 13{,}650 \qquad x^2 = \frac{\sum\left(\eta - \bar{\eta}\right)^2}{\bar{\eta}} = \frac{101{,}513}{13{,}650} = 7.4368$$

OR

$$(9)\frac{(106.20)^2}{13{,}650} = 7.4366$$

Degrees of Freedom = 9; acceptable.

2.

	η	$\eta - \bar{\eta}$	$\left(\eta - \bar{\eta}\right)^2$
1	11,553	-38	1,444
2	11,721	130	16,900
3	11,773	182	33,124
4	11,628	37	1,369
5	11,580	−11	121
6	11,610	19	361
7	11,412	−179	32,041
8	11,569	−22	484
9	11,395	−196	38,416
10	11,672	81	6,561

$\Sigma \eta = 115{,}913$ $\qquad \Sigma\left(\eta - \bar{\eta}\right)^2 = 130{,}821$

$$\bar{\eta} = \frac{115{,}913}{10} = 11{,}591 \qquad x^2 = \frac{\sum\left(\eta - \bar{\eta}\right)^2}{\bar{\eta}} = \frac{13{,}0821}{11{,}591} = 11.2864$$

OR

$$(9)\frac{(120.56)^2}{11{,}591} = 11.2864$$

Degrees of Freedom = 9; acceptable.

3. $\Sigma\,\eta = 137{,}925$; $\overline{\eta} = 13{,}792$; $\Sigma\left(\eta - \overline{\eta}\right)^2 = 5{,}549$; $x^2 = 0.4023$; OR $(9)\dfrac{(24.82)^2}{13{,}792} = 0.4022$;

 not acceptable.

4. $\Sigma\,\eta = 102{,}993$; $\overline{\eta} = 10{,}299$; $\Sigma\left(\eta - \overline{\eta}\right)^2 = 968{,}117$; $x^2 = 94.0010$; OR

 $(9)\dfrac{(327.98)^2}{10{,}299} = 94.001$; not acceptable.

5. $\Sigma\,\eta = 111{,}872$; $\overline{\eta} = 11{,}187$; $\Sigma\left(\eta - \overline{\eta}\right)^2 = 56{,}674$; $x^2 = 5.0660$; OR

 $(9)\dfrac{(79.35)^2}{11{,}187} = 5.0660$; acceptable.

9. Well counter efficiency

1. $\dfrac{294{,}000\ \text{cpm}}{(0.3\ \mu\text{Ci})(2{,}220{,}000\ \text{dpm})(0.85)} \times 100\% = 52\%$

2. $\dfrac{664{,}000\ \text{cpm}}{(1.6\ \mu\text{Ci})(2{,}220{,}000\ \text{dpm})(0.85)} \times 100\% = 22\%$

3. $\dfrac{240{,}000\ \text{cpm}}{(0.41\ \mu\text{Ci})(2{,}220{,}000\ \text{dpm})(0.85)} \times 100\% = 31\%$

4. 79%

5. 60%

6. 47%

7. 40%

10. Window calculations: Centerline plus percent window

1. 140 keV ±10 = 130 to 150 keV

2. 296 keV ±30 = 266 to 326 keV

3. 93 keV ±9 = 84 to 102 keV; 185 keV ±18 = 167 to 203 keV

4. 30% window: 364 keV ±55 = 309 to 419 keV; 20% window: 364 keV ±36 = 328 to 400 keV; 10% window: 364 keV ±18 = 346 to 382 keV.

5. upper level of 171 keV peak: 171 keV + 17 = 188 keV
 lower level of 245 keV peak: 245 keV – 24 = 221 keV; no overlap.

---

* Note: Although the windows do not overlap, there will be spill down of the attenuated 245-keV photons into the 171-keV window. Simply using a lower window does not eliminate the effects of higher energy photons. However, lower energy photons can be eliminated by window selection when selecting for higher energy photons, if the photopeaks are sufficiently separated.

---

6. 140 keV – 18 = 122 keV; no.

7. 171 keV ± 17 = 154 to 188 keV; yes.

11. Window calculations: Upper and lower discriminators

1. 159 keV ± 8; LLD = 151 keV; ULD = 167 keV.
2. 662 keV ± 10; LLD = 652 keV; ULD = 672 keV.
3. 122 keV ± 6; LLD = 116 keV; ULD = 128 keV.
4. 662 keV ± 33; threshold = 629 keV; window = 66 keV.
5. threshold = 146 keV; 172 keV to 146 keV = 26 keV, so window = 26 keV.
6. 122 keV ± 6; threshold = 116 keV; window = 12 keV.
7. 364 keV ± 36; threshold = 328 keV; window = 72 keV.
8. threshold = 618 keV; 90 keV window; $\dfrac{708\,keV - 618\,keV}{662\,keV} \times 100\% = 14\%$ window
9. $\dfrac{130\,keV - 110\,keV}{122\,keV} \times 100\% = 16\%$ window

---

* Note: Differences in individual readings of the practice graphs will cause some variations in the results for problems 10 through 12. Do not be concerned if your answer is slightly different from the author's. Reading small reproductions of graphs can be difficult.

---

10. maximum = 11,600 ct; (11,600)(0.25) = 2,900 ct; $\dfrac{383\,keV - 261\,keV}{320\,keV} \times 100\% = 38\%$

11. maximum = 15,200 ct; (15,200)(0.25) = 3,800 ct; $\dfrac{879\,keV - 752\,keV}{810\,keV} \times 100\% = 16\%$

12. maximum = 16,000 ct; (16,000)(0.25) = 4,000 ct; $\dfrac{360\,keV - 275\,keV}{320\,keV} \times 100\% = 26\%$

12. Camera sensitivity

1. $\dfrac{57,508\,cpm - 850\,cpm}{185\,\mu Ci} = 306$ cpm/μCi
2. 232 cpm/μCi
3. 403 cpm/μCi
4. 342 cpm/μCi
5. 404 cpm/μCi
6. May 1   289 cpm/μCi; calculate acceptable level: 10% of 289 = 29;
     289 – 29 = 260 cpm/μCi; results should be reported when they fall below this value.
     May 2   281 cpm/μCi
     May 3   282 cpm/μCi
     May 4   275 cpm/μCi
     May 5   256 cpm/μCi; results are below 260 cpm/μCi, so they should be reported.

7.   Week Sensitivity
        1   396
        2   412
        3   388
        4   409
        5   391
        6   414
        7   383
        8   395

$$\text{mean} = \frac{3,188 \text{ cpm}/\mu\text{Ci}}{8} = 398 \text{ cpm}/\mu\text{Ci} \; ; \; 398 \text{ cpm}/\mu\text{Ci} - 40 = 358 \text{ cpm}/\mu\text{Ci}$$

acceptable sensitivity.

13. Acquisition time and counts per projection for SPECT studies

1.   total counts: (30 stops)(56,000 ct/stop) = 1,700,000 ct
      acquisition time: (30 s)(30 stops) = 900 s or 15 min
2.   acquisition time: (62 stops)(20 s/stop) = 1,240 s or ≈ 21 min
      total counts: (62 stops)(74,000 ct/stop) = 4,600,000 ct
3.   acquisition time: $\dfrac{3,000,000 \text{ ct}}{260,000 \text{ cpm}} = 11.5$ min

      time per stop: $\dfrac{11.5 \text{ min}}{32 \text{ stops}} = 0.36$ min/stop or 22 s/stop

      counts per stop: (260,000 cpm)(0.36 min/stop) = 94,000 ct/stop
4.   acquisition time: (30 s/stop)(60 stops) = 1,800 s or 30 min
      counts per stop: (73,000 cpm)(0.5 min/stop) = 370,000 ct/stop
      total counts: (37,000 ct/stop)(60 stops) = 2,200,000 ct
5.   total acquisition time: $\dfrac{1,000,000 \text{ ct}}{49,000 \text{ cpm}} = 20$ min

      acquisition time per frame: $\dfrac{20 \text{ min}}{64 \text{ frames}} = 0.31$ min/frame or 19 s/frame
6.   counts per stop: Convert 20 s to 0.33 min; (240,000 cpm)(0.33 min/stop) = 80,000 ct/stop
      total counts: (80,000 ct/stop)(64 stops) = 5,100,000 ct
      acquisition time: (20 s/stop)(64 stops) = 1,280 s or 21 min
7.   counts/stop at 20 s/stop: (82,000 cpm)(0.33 min/stop) ≈ 27,000 ct/stop
      counts/stop at 30 s/stop: (82,000 cpm)(0.5 min/stop) = 41,000 ct/stop
      total counts at 20 s/stop: (27,000 ct/stop)(64 stops) ≈ 1,700,00 ct
      total counts at 30 s/stop: (41,000 ct/stop)(64 stops) = 2,600,00 ct
      total acquisition time at 20 s/stop: (20 s/stop)(64 stop) = 1,280 s or ≈21 min
      total acquisition time at 30 s/stop: (30 s/stop)(64 stop) = 1,920 s or 32 min

14. Obtaining desired flood or phantom fill activities

1.

$$\frac{720 \text{ cpm}}{6 \text{ μCi}} = \frac{15,000 \text{ cpm}}{X \text{ μCi}} \quad \text{Cross - multiply and isolate } X.$$

$$X \text{ μCi} = \frac{(15,000 \text{ cpm})(6 \text{ μCi})}{720 \text{ cpm}} = 125 \text{ μCi}$$

2. $X \text{ mCi} = \dfrac{(30,000 \text{ cpm})(1.2 \text{ mCi})}{1,800 \text{ cpm}}; X = 20 \text{ mCi}$

3. 1,190 μCi or ≈1.2 mCi

4. 626 μCi

5.

$$X \text{ ml} = \frac{(30,000 \text{ cpm})(0.2 \text{ ml})}{1,820 \text{ cpm}}; X = 3.3 \text{ ml}$$

6. 1.9 ml

7. Calculate counts per min: $\dfrac{80,000 \text{ ct}}{3 \text{ min}} = 26,700 \text{ cpm}$

$$X \text{ ml} = \frac{(26,700 \text{ cpm})(1 \text{ ml})}{7,340 \text{ cpm}}; X = 3.6 \text{ ml}$$

15. Total pixels by matrix size

1. (64 pixels)(64 pixels) = 4,096 pixels

2. $\dfrac{(256 \text{ pixels})(256 \text{ pixels})}{(64 \text{ pixels})(64 \text{ pixels})} = 16 \text{ frames}$

3. 65,536 pixels

4. 4 frames

5. 1,024 pixels

6. 64 frames

16. Computer memory requirements based on matrix size and storage mode

1. (32)(32)(60) = 61,440 bytes

2. $\dfrac{61,440}{2} = 30,720 \text{ words}$

3. 491,520 words

4. 983,040 bytes

5. 5,898,240 words

6. 1,048,576 bytes or about 1 MB

7. (64 stops)(64 × 64)(9 bins) = 2,359,296 bytes or about 2.4 MB

8. stress study: (64 stops)(64 × 64)(9 bins) = 2,359,296 bytes
    rest study: (64 stops)(64 × 64) = 262,144 bytes
    2,359,296 + 262,144 bytes = 2,621,440 bytes per patient or 2.6 MB per patient
    $$\frac{700 \text{ MB}}{2.6 \text{ MB/patient}} \approx 269 \text{ patients}$$

17. Pixel calibration

1. $\dfrac{25 \text{ cm}}{40 \text{ pixels}} = 0.625 \text{ cm / pixel or } 6.25 \text{ mm / pixel}$

2. $\dfrac{30 \text{ cm}}{47 \text{ pixels}} = 0.638 \text{ cm / pixel or } 6.38 \text{ mm / pixel}$

3. 0.305 cm/pixel or 3.05 mm/pixel

4. 0.312 cm/pixel or 3.12 mm/pixel

5. 0.319 cm/pixel or 3.19 mm/pixel

6. x-axis: $\dfrac{25 \text{ cm}}{42 \text{ pixels}} = 0.595 \text{ cm / pixel}$ y-axis: $\dfrac{25 \text{ cm}}{45 \text{ pixels}} = 0.556 \text{ cm / pixel}$

    0.595 cm − 0.556 cm = 0.039 cm; yes, within 0.05 of one another

7. x-axis: $\dfrac{30 \text{ cm}}{101 \text{ pixels}} = 0.297 \text{ cm / pixel}$ y-axis: $\dfrac{30 \text{ cm}}{97 \text{ pixels}} = 0.309 \text{ cm / pixel}$

    0.309 cm − 0.297 cm = 0.012 cm; yes, within 0.05 of one another

V. Radiopharmacy

1. Decay calculations using half-life

1. $A = 432\,\text{mCi} \times e^{-0.693 \times (8\,\text{h}/6.01\,\text{h})} = 432\,\text{mCi} \times e^{-0.922} = 432\,\text{mCi} \times 0.398 = 172\,\text{mCi}$
2. $A = 12.8\,\text{mCi} \times e^{-0.693 \times (25\,\text{h}/73.1\,\text{h})} = 12.8\,\text{mCi} \times e^{-0.237} = 12.8\,\text{mCi} \times 0.790 = 10.1\,\text{mCi}$
3. 7.5 days elapsed; 8.2 mCi remain.
4. 13 days elapsed; 2.4 mCi remain.
5. 0.03 µCi/ml
6. 69 hours elapsed; 1.1 Ci remain
7. 504 hours elapsed; 0.0084 Ci or 8.4 mCi remain.
8.

$$120\,\text{mCi} = X\,\text{mCi} \times e^{-0.693 \times 5\,\text{h}/6.01\,\text{h}}$$

$$120\,\text{mCi} = X\,\text{mCi} \times e^{-0.58}$$

$$120\,\text{mCi} = X\,\text{mCi} \times 0.56$$

$$\frac{120\,\text{mCi}}{0.56} = X \qquad X = 214\,\text{mCi}$$

9.

$$1.2\,\text{Ci} = X\,\text{Ci} \times e^{-0.693 \times (41\,\text{h}/66.6\,\text{h})}$$

$$1.2\,\text{Ci} = X\,\text{Ci} \times e^{-0.43}$$

$$1.2\,\text{Ci} = X\,\text{Ci} \times 0.65$$

$$\frac{1.2\,\text{Ci}}{0.65} = X \qquad X = 1.8\,\text{Ci}$$

10. I123 activity at 24 hours equals 90.8 µCi
    I124 activity at 24 hours equals 4.2 µCi

    At calibration time: $\dfrac{5\,\mu\text{Ci}}{320\,\mu\text{Ci} + 5\,\mu Ci} \times 100 = 1.5\%\ \text{I124 contamination}$

    24 hours later: $\dfrac{4.2\,\mu\text{Ci}}{90.8\,\mu\text{Ci} + 4.2\,\mu Ci} \times 100 = 4.4\%\ \text{I124 contamination}$

11. No, the activity will only be 48 µCi.

2. Decay calculation using decay charts

1. 2 hours and 45 minutes elapsed; DF = 0.728; 54.7 mCi × 0.728 = 39.8 mCi remain.
2. 2 hours elapsed; DF = 0.794; 492 mCi remain.
3. 24 hours elapsed; DF = 0.796; 2.0 mCi remain.
4. 4 days or 96 hours elapsed; DF = 0.427; 5.1 mCi remain.
5. 30-day DF = 0.233, so 60-day DF = 0.234 × 0.234 = 0.055; 1.4 mCi remain.
6. 70-day DF = 0.446 and 5-day DF = 0.944, so 75-day DF = 0.446 × 0.944 = 0.420; 126 µCi remain.
7. 15 days elapsed; DF = 0.275; 33 mCi remain.

8. 200-day DF = 0.598, 60-day DF = 0.857, 2-day DF = 0.995
    so 262-day DF = (0.598)(0.857)(0.995) = 0.51; 118 μCi remain.
9. 3-hour DF = 0.707, so 21.8 mCi remain.
10. 6-hour DF = 0.73, so 184 μCi remain.

3. Pre-calibration factors

1. 3 hours pre-calibration; factor = 1.414; 10 mCi × 1.414 = 14 mCi needed.
2. 22 hours pre-calibration; factor = 1.232; 148 mCi needed.
3. 2 hours pre-calibration; factor = 1.259; 5.0 mCi needed.
4. 3 days pre-calibration; factor = 1.295; 194 mCi needed.
5. 48 hours pre-calibration; DF = 0.654; 8.0 mCi ÷ 0.654 = 12 mCi needed.
6. 24 hours pre-calibration; DF = 0.284; 704 μCi needed.
7. 6 days pre-calibration; DF = 0.596; 11.7 mCi needed.
8. 14 days pre-calibration; pre-calibration factor calculation: 7 day factor = 1.828, so
    1.828 × 1.828 = 3.342; 300 mCi × 3.342 = 1,003 mCi or 1 Ci needed.
9. 7-day pre-calibration = 2.525; 20 mCi × 2.525 = 50 mCi needed.
10. 3-day or 72-hour PCF = 2.130; 2.130 × 2.0 Ci = 4.3 Ci

4. Specific concentration

1. $\dfrac{368 \text{ mCi}}{5 \text{ ml}} = 73.6 \text{ mCi / ml}$

2. 2. $\dfrac{198 \text{ mCi}}{7.6 \text{ ml}} = 26.0 \text{ mCi / ml}$

3. 3.1 mCi/ml

4. 2 hours elapsed; DF = 0.794; $\dfrac{63.2 \text{ mCi}}{5.0 \text{ ml}} \times 0.794 = 10.0 \text{ mCi/ml}$

5. 1.5 hours elapsed; DF = 0.841; concentration = 43.4 mCi/ml.
6. 2 hours and 15 minutes elapsed; DF = 0.771; concentration = 8.4 mCi/ml.
7. 4 hours and 20 minutes elapsed; DF = 0.606; concentration = 26.7 mCi/ml.
8. 1 hour and 35 minutes elapsed; DF = 0.833; concentration = 54.7 mCi/ml.

5. Dose volume calculations

1. $\dfrac{135 \text{ mCi}}{1.2 \text{ ml}} = 112.5 \text{ mCi / ml}$ $\dfrac{45 \text{ mCi}}{112.5 \text{ mCi / ml}} = 0.4 \text{ ml}.$

2. concentration = 13.0 mCi/ml; volume needed = 0.3 ml.
3. concentration = 38.0 mCi/ml; volume needed = 2.6 ml.
4. concentration = 13.6 mCi/ml; volume needed = 0.7 ml.
1. concentration = 2.5 mCi/ml; volume needed = 1.2 ml.
2. concentration = 9.8 mCi/ml; volume needed = 0.3 ml.
7. 4 hours elapsed; DF = 0.63; activity at 7:00 pm = 202 mCi; concentration at
    7:00 pm = 72 mCi/ml; volume needed = 0.6 ml.

8. 1 hour elapsed; DF = 0.891; activity at 9:30 am = 110 mCi; concentration at 9:30 am = 48 mCi/ml; volume needed = 0.8 ml.

9. 1 1/2 hours elapsed; DF = 0.841; activity at 3:00 pm = 241 mCi; concentration at 9:30 am = 46 mCi/ml; volume needed = 0.4 ml.

10. 9 hours & 45 minutes elapsed; DF = 0.325; activity at 4:45 pm = 138 mCi; concentration at 4:45 pm = 13.8 mCi/ml; volume needed = 2.9 ml.

11. 4 hours & 20 minutes elapsed; DF = 0.606; activity at 9:00 am = 193 mCi; concentration at 9:00 am = 46 mCi/ml; volume needed = 1.1 ml.

12. 10:00 am calculations:
    45 minutes elapsed; DF = 0.917; activity at 10:00 am = 159 mCi; concentration at 10:00 am = 50 mCi/ml; volume needed = 0.4 ml.

    Calculate activity and volume remaining in vial after dose withdrawn:
    159 mCi – 20 mCi = 139 mCi.
    3.2 ml – 0.4 ml = 2.8 ml.

    11:00 am calculations:
    1 hour elapsed; DF = 0.891
    Calculate activity at 11:00 am: 139 mCi × 0.891 = 124 mCi.
    Calculate activity remaining after 20 mCi dose is removed:
    124 mCi – 20 mCi = 104 mCi.

13. 9 hr DF = 0.923; 25.8 mCi × 0.923 = 23.8 mCi; concentration = 8 mCi/ml; volume needed + 1 ml.

14. Concentration = 36 mCi/ml; volume used = 0.6 ml.

15. Original concentration = 14.5 mCi/ml; volume needed = 0.3 ml
    Activity and volume remaining after dose is drawn: 27 mCi in 1.9 ml.

    3 1/2 hours later:
    DF = 0.667; activity: 27 mCi × 0.667 = 18.0 mCi
    concentration: $\dfrac{18.9 \text{ mCi}}{1.9 \text{ ml}} = 9.5 \text{ mCi / ml}$; volume needed = 0.5 ml.
    Activity and volume remaining after dose is drawn: 18 mCi – 5 mCi = 13 mCi in 1.4 ml.

    4 3/4 hours later:
    DF = 0.577; activity: (13 mCi × 0.577) = 7.5 mCi
    Yes, there is enough for another 5 mCi dose.

---

* Note: To determine the activity remaining after a dose is withdrawn, subtract the dose from the activity in the vial at the time the dose was drawn, NOT from the original activity prior to application of the necessary decay factor. In this problem, the first 20-mCi dose must be subtracted from 159 mCi NOT 173 mCi, because at the time the dose was withdrawn the vial actually contained only 159 mCi.

16. Concentration = 83 mCi/ml
    MDP kit: 2.4 ml needed; activity & volume remaining: 628 mCi in 7.6 ml.
    DTPA kit: 1.8 ml needed; activity & volume remaining: 478 mCi in 5.8 ml.
    MAA kit: 0.7 ml needed; activity & volume remaining: 418 mCi in 5.1 ml.

6. Calculation of total activity to provide given number of kits or doses

1.

Time	Elapsed Time	Pre-Calibration Factor	Activity at Calibration	Activity Needed for Preparation
9:00 am	2 h	1.259	40 mCi	50.4 mCi
10:00 am	3 h	1.414	20 mCi	28.3 mCi
10:00 am	3 h	1.414	8 mCi	11.3 mCi
11:00 am	4 h	1.587	40 mCi	63.5 mCi

Total = 153.5 mCi or 154 mCi

* Note: The answer is a minimum activity to be added. Since a larger activity will actually be used, it is both convenient and reasonable to work with rounded numbers and not bother with the decimal places in these calculations.

2.

Time	Elapsed Time	Pre-Calibration Factor	Activity at Calibration	Activity Needed for Preparation
10:00 am	2 h	1.259	4 mCi	5 mCi
11:00 am	3 h	1.414	4 mCi	6 mCi
2:00 pm	6 h	2	4 mCi	8 mCi
3:00 pm	7 h	2.244	4 mCi	9 mCi

Total = 28 mCi

3.

Time	Elapsed Time	Pre-Calibration Factor	Activity at Calibration	Activity Needed for Preparation
8:00 am	1 h	1.122	2 × 22 mCi	49 mCi
9:00 am	2 h	1.259	2 × 22 mCi	55 mCi
10:00 am	3 hr	1.414	2 × 22 mCi	62 mCi

Total = 166 mCi

4.

Time	Elapsed Time	Pre-Calibration Factor	Activity at Calibration	Activity Needed for Preparation
10:00 am	3 h	0.707	10 mCi	14 mCi
12:00 pm	5 h	0.562	10 mCi	18 mCi
2:00 pm	7 h	0.446	10 mCi	22 mCi

Total = 54 mCi

5.

Time	Elapsed Time	Decay Factor	Activity at Calibration	Activity Needed for Preparation
Mon. 12:00 pm	8 h	0.932	6 mCi	6 mCi
Tues 7:00 pm	27 h	0.787	6 mCi	8 mCi
Wed. 12 pm	56 h	0.609	4 mCi	7 mCi
				Total = 21 mCi

6.

Time	Elapsed Time	Decay Factor	Activity at Calibration	Activity Needed for Preparation
10:00 am	2 h	0.794	15 mCi	19 mCi
11:30 am	3.5 h	0.667	15 mCi	23 mCi
1:30 pm	5.5 h	0.53	15 mCi	28 mCi
				Total = 70 mCi

7.

Time	Elapsed Time	Decay Factor	Activity at Calibration	Activity Needed for Preparation
9:00 am	0.5 h	0.944	20 mCi	21 mCi
9:30 am	1 h	0.891	20 mCi	22 mCi
11:30 am	3 h	0.707	20 mCi	28 mCi
1:30 pm	5 h	0.562	8 mCi	14 mCi
2:00 pm	5.5 h	0.53	15 mCi	28 mCi
				Total = 113 mCi

8.

Time	Elapsed Time	Decay Factor	Activity at Calibration	Activity Needed for Preparation
9:00 am	4 h	0.810	200 μCi	247 μCi
11:00 am	6 h	0.73	50 μCi	68 μCi
3:00 pm	10 h	0.591	300 μCi	508 μCi
				Total = 823 μCi

7. **Total volume to be added to kit considering volume limits and desired concentration**

1. concentration = 83 mCi/ml; 0.6 ml eluate needed; yes, at least 1.4 ml saline must be added.
2. concentration = 58 mCi/ml; 0.9 ml eluate needed; yes, at least 1.1 ml saline must be added.
3. concentration = 55 mCi/ml; 0.5 ml eluate needed; 4.5 ml saline must be added.
4. concentration = 57 mCi/ml; 1.4 ml eluate needed; at least 2.6 ml saline must be added.
5. concentration = 78 mCi/ml; 2.3 ml eluate needed; at least 0.7 ml saline must be added.

6.

Time	Elapsed Time	Decay Factor	Activity at Calibration	Activity Needed for Preparation
9:30 am	1.5 h	0.841	20 mCi	24 mCi
10:30 am	2.5 h	0.749	40 mCi	53 mCi
12:30 pm	4.5 h	0.595	40 mCi	67 mCi
1:00 pm	5 h	0.562	20 mCi	36 mCi

Total = 180 mCi

No, a second kit must be used to prepare the 1:00 pm dose.

7.

Time	Elapsed Time	Decay Factor	Activity at Calibration	Activity Needed for Preparation
10:00 am	2 h	1.259	20 mCi	25 mCi
11:00 am	3 h	1.414	20 mCi	28 mCi
12:00 pm	4 h	1.587	20 mCi	32 mCi
1:00 pm	5 h	1.779	20 mCi	36 mCi

Total = 121 mCi

Yes, the four doses can be obtained from one kit.

8.

Time	Elapsed Time	Decay Factor	Activity at Calibration	Activity Needed for Preparation
9:00 am	1 h	1.122	2 × 20 mCi	45 mCi
10:00 am	2 h	1.259	2 × 20 mCi	50 mCi
11:00 am	3 h	1.414	1 × 10 mCi	14 mCi
12:00 pm	4 h	1.587	2 × 20 mCi	63 mCi
1:00 pm	5 h	1.779	2 × 20 mCi	71 mCi

Total = 243 mCi

No, the 1:00 doses must come from a second kit.

9.

Time	Elapsed Time	Decay Factor	Activity at Calibration	Activity Needed for Preparation
10:00 am	1 h	1.122	10 mCi	11 mCi
11:00 am	2 h	1.259	5 mCi	6 mCi
12:00 pm	3 h	1.414	10 mCi	14 mCi
1:00 pm	4 h	1.587	5 mCi	8 mCi
2:00 pm	5 h	1.779	10 mCi	18 mCi

Total = 57 mCi

Yes, the five doses can be obtained from one kit.

8. Dose calculation based on activity per unit weight

1. $(40 \text{ lb})(25 \ \mu\text{Ci/lb}) = 1,000 \ \mu\text{Ci or } 1.0 \text{ mCi}$
2. 18 mg
3. 42.5 kg
4. 10,400 μCi or 10.4 mCi

5. Convert 185 lb to kg: (185 lb)(0.45 kg/lb) = 83 kg. Administer 47 mg.
6. Convert 138 lb to 62 kg. Administer 1.2 μg.
7. Convert 12 kg to 26 lb. Administer 650 μCi.
8. Convert 220 lb to 99 kg. Administer 3,960 mcg or 4 mg (rounded).
9. Convert 167 lb to 75 kg. (140 mcg)(75 kg)(6 min)= 63,000 mcg or 63 mg.

9. Unit dose adjustments

1. Concentration = 2.7 mCi/ml; volume to be retained = 0.9 ml; volume to be discarded = 0.3 ml.
2. Concentration = 3.8 mCi/ml; volume to be retained = 2.6 ml; volume to be discarded = 0.8 ml.
3. 4 hour pre-calibration factor = 1.587; activity at 10:00 am = 31.7 mCi; concentration at 10:00 am = 26.4 mCi/ml; volume to be retained = 0.8 ml; volume to be discarded = 0.4 ml.
4. 2 hours elapsed; DF = 0.794; activity at 3:00 pm = 19.8 mCi; concentration at 3:00 pm = 13.2 mCi/ml; volume to be retained = 1.2 ml; volume to be discarded = 0.3 ml.
5. 1 hour and 10 minutes elapsed; DF = 0.872; activity at 11:10 pm = 34.9 mCi; concentration at 11:10 PM = 11.6 mCi/ml; volume to be retained = 2.6 ml; volume to be discarded = 0.4 ml.
6. 1 hour and 20 minutes elapsed; DF = 0.857; activity at 9:20 am = 25.7 mCi; concentration at 9:20 am = 12.9 mCi/ml; volume to be retained = 1.6 ml; volume to be discarded = 0.4 ml.
7. 96-hour DF = 0.427; activity at 96 hours = 3.4 mCi; concentration at 96 hours = 1.5 mCi/ml; volume to be retained = 1.3 ml; volume to be discarded = 1.0 ml
8. 2-hour pre-calibration factor = 1.259; activity at 12:00 noon = 25.2 mCi; concentration at 12:00 noon = 50 mCi/ml; volume to be retained = 0.2 ml; volume to be discarded = 0.3 ml.
9. 20 hours elapsed; DF = 0.828; activity at 10:00 am = 1.5 mCi/ml; volume to be retained = 0.7 ml; volume to be discarded = 0.5 ml.
10. 72 hours elapsed; DF = 0.529; activity in each syringe on Thursday = 3.2 mCi; concentration on Thursday = 1.6 mCi/ml; total volume needed = 3.1 ml. Therefore use all 2 ml in one syringe and 1.1 ml from the second. 0.9 ml would be discarded from the second syringe before use.
11. 5 hours elapsed; DF = 0.562; activity in each syringe at 1:00 pm = 11.2 mCi; concentration at 1:00 pm = 28 mCi/ml; total volume needed = 0.7 ml. Therefore use 0.4 ml from one syringe and 0.3 ml from the second. 0.1 ml would be discarded from the second syringe before use.

10. Pediatric dose calculations using Clark's formula

1. $$\frac{(90 \text{ lb})(20 \text{ mCi})}{150 \text{ lb}} = 12 \text{ mCi}$$

2. $$\frac{(120 \text{ lb})(6 \text{ mCi})}{150 \text{ lb}} = 4.8 \text{ mCi}$$

3. 6.0 mCi
4. 7.3 mCi
5. 10 mCi
6. 19 mCi
7. 1.1 mCi
8. 120 μCi
9. Convert 32 kg to lb: (32 kg)(2.2 lb/kg) = 70 lb. 1.9 mCi dose needed; concentration = 2.1 mCi/ml; 0.9 ml to be administered.
10. 7.1 mCi dose needed; 2 1/2 hours elapsed; DF = 0.749; activity at 4:30 = 69.5 mCi; concentration = 14.8 mCi/ml; 0.5 ml to be administered.
11. Convert 36 kg to 79 lb. 5.3 mCi dose needed; 1 hour and 45 minutes elapsed; DF = 0.817; activity at 1 hour and 45 minutes = 43.3 mCi; concentration = 10.3 mCi/ml; 0.5 ml to be administered.

11. Pediatric dose calculations using body surface area

1. fraction of adult dose: 0.18; (20 mCi)(0.18) = 3.6 mCi to be administered.
2. fraction of adult dose: 0.62; 5.0 mCi to be administered.
3. fraction of adult dose: 0.11; 0.55 mCi or 550 μCi to be administered.
4. estimate fraction of adult dose: 0.70; 14 mCi to be administered OR

$$\frac{(42\,kg)^{0.7}}{11 \times 1.779} = 0.70 \qquad (20\,mCi)(0.70) = 14\,mCi$$

5. estimate fraction of adult dose: 0.65; 3.9 mCi to be administered OR

$$\frac{(37\,kg)^{0.7}}{11 \times 1.779} = 0.64 \qquad (6\,mCi)(0.64) = 3.8\,mCi$$

---

* Note: The difference between 3.9 mCi and 3.8 mCi is not significant, so either method is valid.

---

6. fraction of adult dose: 0.13; 39 μCi to be administered.
7. fraction of adult dose: 0.27; 3.2 mCi to be administered.
8. estimate or calculate fraction of adult dose: 0.81; 8.1 mCi to be administered.
9. fraction of adult dose: about 0.70; 14 mCi to be administered.
10. fraction of adult dose: about 0.83; 5 mCi to be administered.
11. fraction of adult dose: 0.43; 8.4 mCi to be administered.
12. fraction of adult dose: about 0.46; 10 mCi to be administered.
13. fraction of adult dose: about 0.61; 12 mCi to be administered.
14. fraction of adult dose: about 0.94; 19 mCi to be administered.
15. fraction of adult dose: 0.24; 1.9 mCi to be administered.
16. fraction of adult dose: about 0.52; 156 μCi to be administered.

12. Pediatric dose calculations using Talbot's nomogram

1. 78% of adult dose; 0.78×20 mCi = 16 mCi; Clark's formula called for a 12-mCi dose.

---

* **Note:** Because body mass measurements were used to create Talbot's nomogram, the higher organ to body mass ratio was taken in to account. For this reason Talbot's nomogram calls for a higher dose than Clark's formula, which is strictly weight dependent.

---

2. 92% of adult dose; 0.92×6 mCi = 6 mCi. This is 1.2 mCi greater than the 4.8-mCi dose calculated by Clark's formula or 20% greater.

---

* **Note:** This is the adult dose. A child who is close to standard adult weight will be receiving the same dose as a adult according to body mass calculations.

---

3. 45% of adult dose = 9 mCi, which is 3 mCi greater than Clark's calculation or 33% greater.
4. 49% of adult dose = 11 mCi.
5. 68% of adult dose = 14 mCi.
6. 100% of adult dose or 20 mCi.
7. 26% of adult dose = 2.1 mCi.
8. 57% of adult dose = 171 μCi.
9. Convert 4.5 kg to lb: (4.5 kg)(2.2 kg/lb) = 10 lb. 14% of adult dose = 2.8 mCi
10. 46% of adult dose = 4.6 mCi
11. Convert 9 kg to 20 lb. 26% of adult dose = 1.3 mCi
12. 64% of adult dose = 3.8 mCi
13. Convert 45 kg to 99 lb. 82% of adult dose = 16 mCi
14. 35% of adult dose = 1.4 mCi
15. Convert 50 kg to 110 lb. 88% of adult dose = 3.5 mCi;
    $$\frac{42 \text{ mCi}}{3.8 \text{ ml}} = 11 \text{ mCi / ml}; \quad \frac{3.5 \text{ mCi}}{11 \text{ mCi / ml}} = 0.3 \text{ ml}$$
16. 20% of adult dose = 1 mCi; $\dfrac{25 \text{ mCi}}{5.2 \text{ ml}} = 4.8 \text{ mCi / ml}; \quad \dfrac{1 \text{ mCi}}{4.8 \text{ mCi / ml}} = 0.2 \text{ ml}$
17. Convert 18 kg to 40 lb. 43% of adult dose = 8.6 mCi;
    $$\frac{20 \text{ mCi}}{1.4 \text{ ml}} = 14 \text{ mCi / ml}; \quad \frac{8.6 \text{ mCi}}{14 \text{ mCi / ml}} = 0.6 \text{ ml}$$
18. 57% of adult dose = 12 mCi; $\dfrac{22 \text{ mCi}}{0.8 \text{ ml}} = 28$ mCi/ml at 9:00 am;

    2-hour DF=0.794; 28 mCi/ml $\times$ 0.794 = 22 mCi/ml at 11:00 am;
    $$\frac{12 \text{ mCi}}{22 \text{ mCi / ml}} = 0.5 \text{ ml to be retained; so discard } 0.3 \text{ ml}.$$

13. Minimum and maximum pediatric doses

1. BSA fraction = 0.11; 0.11 × 10 mCi = 1.1 mCi; exceeds minimum dose of 1.0 mCi so 1.1 mCi is used.
2. 10 lb is about half way between 8.8 and 11 lbs on BSA chart, so estimated fraction = 0.14; 0.14 × 3 mCi = 0.42 mCi or 420 μCi; so must use minimum of 500 μCi.
3. BSA fraction = 0.27; 0.27 × 10 mCi = 2.7 mCi; so must use minimum of 3 mCi.
4. BSA fraction = 0.18; 0.18 × 5 mCi = 0.9 mCi or 900 μCi; exceeds minimum dose of 500 μCi so 900 μCi is used.
5. BSA fraction = 0.11; 0.11 × 4 mCi = 0.44 mCi or 440 μCi; so must use minimum of 500 μCi.
6. BSA fraction = 0.18; 0.18 × 200 μCi = 36 μCi; exceeds minimum dose of 30 μCi so 36 μCi is used.
7. Calculated pediatric dose: 24,500 μCi or 24.5 mCi; exceeds maximum dose of 20 mCi, so 20 mCi must be administered.
8. Calculated pediatric dose: 25,500 μCi or 25.5 mCi; exceeds maximum dose of 20 mCi, so 20 mCi must be administered.
9. Calculate pediatric dose: 5,500 μCi or 5.5 mCi; does not exceed maximum dose of 15 mCi, so 5.5 mCi can be administered.
10. Calculated pediatric dose: 22,000 μCi or 22 mCi; exceeds maximum dose of 15 mCi, so 15 mCi must be administered.
11. Convert 18 kg to 40 lb. Calculated pediatric dose: 25 μCi/lb × 40 lb = 1,000 μCi or 1 mCi; does not exceed maximum dose of 2 mCi, so 1 mCi can be administered.
12. Convert 10 kg to 22 lb. Calculate pediatric dose: 100 μCi/lb × 22 lb = 2,200 μCi or 2.2 mCi; so must use minimum of 2.5 mCi.
13. Calculate pediatric dose: 25 μCi/lb × 32 lb = 800 μCi; exceeds minimum of 500 μCi so 800 μCi is used.
14. Convert 33 lb to 15 kg. Calculate pediatric dose: 50 μCi/kg × 15 kg = 750 μCi or 0.75 mCi; so must use minimum of 1 mCi.

14. Lung perfusion radiopharmaceutical particle calculations

1. $\dfrac{14{,}000{,}000 \text{ particles}}{5 \text{ ml}} = 2{,}800{,}000 \text{ particles} / \text{ml}$

2. $\dfrac{8{,}000{,}000 \text{ particles}}{6 \text{ ml}} = 1{,}333{,}000 \text{ particles} / \text{ml}$

3. (0.3 ml)(800,000 particle/ml) = 240,000 particles
4. (0.7 ml)(500,000 particles/ml) = 350,000 particles

5.   Calculate particle concentration: $\dfrac{5,500,000 \text{ particles}}{6 \text{ ml}} = 920,000 \text{ particles / ml}$

Calculate specific concentration: $\dfrac{40 \text{ mCi}}{6 \text{ ml}} = 6.6 \text{ mCi}$

Calculate dose volume: $\dfrac{4 \text{ mCi}}{6.6 \text{ mCi / ml}} = 0.6 \text{ ml}$

Determine particle concentration: (0.6 ml)(920,000 particles/ml) = 552,000 particles.

6.   Particle concentration = 1,500,000 particles/ml; specific concentration = 10 mCi/ml; dose volume = 0.3 ml; particles in dose = 450,000 particles.

7.   Particle concentration = 1,600,000 particles/ml; specific concentration = 8 mCi/ml; dose volume = 0.5 ml; particles in dose = 800,000 particles.

8.   3-hour DF = 0.707; 8 mCi/ml)(0.707) = 5.6 mCi/ml; dose volume = 0.7 ml; particles in dose = 1,120,000 particles.

9.   4-hour DF = 0.63; current activity = 57 mCi; specific activity = 11.3 mCi/ml; dose volume = 0.4 ml; particle concentration = 2,400,000 particles/ml; particles in dose = 960,000 particles.

10. $\dfrac{0.5 \text{ ml}}{400,000 \text{ particles}} = \dfrac{X \text{ ml}}{5,000,000 \text{ particles}};\ X = 6.3 \text{ ml}$

11. $\dfrac{0.4 \text{ ml}}{300,000 \text{ particles}} = \dfrac{X \text{ ml}}{8,000,000 \text{ particles}};\ X = 10.7 \text{ ml}$

12. $\dfrac{1.0 \text{ ml}}{1,200,000 \text{ particles}} = \dfrac{X \text{ ml}}{2,500,000 \text{ particles}};\ X = 2.1 \text{ ml}$

15. Generator yield based on efficiency

1. $\dfrac{550 \text{ mCi}}{600 \text{ mCi}} \times 100 = 92\%$

2. $\dfrac{830 \text{ mCi}}{1000 \text{ mCi}} \times 100 = 83\%$

3.   78%

4.   72%

5.   88%

6.   (880 mCi)(0.87) = 766 mCi

7.   (1,200 mCi)(0.82) = 984 mCi

8.   231 mCi

9.   502 mCi

16. Generator yield based on decay

1.   60 hours elapsed time; Mo99 DF = 0.536; Tc/Mo ratio = 0.944; (6.6 Ci)(0.536)(0.944) = 3.3 Ci.

2.   6 hours elapsed time; Mo99 DF = 0.94; Tc/Mo ratio = 0.441; (610 mCi)(0.94)(0.441) = 253 mCi.

3. 16 hours elapsed time; Mo99 DF = 0.847; Tc/Mo ratio = 0.769;
    (495 mCi)(0.847)(0.769) = 322 mCi.
4. 24 hours elapsed time; Mo99 DF = 0.779; Tc/Mo ratio = 0.870;
    (1.2 Ci)(0.779)(0.870) = 0.813 Ci or 813 mCi.
5. 7 hours elapsed time; Mo99 DF = 0.93; Tc/Mo ratio = 0.492;
    (270 mCi)(0.93)(0.492) = 124 mCi.
6. 18 hours elapsed time; Mo99 DF = 0.829; Tc/Mo ratio = 0.803; efficiency = 80%;
    (315 mCi)(0.829)(0.803)(0.80) = 168 mCi.
7. 3 hours elapsed time; Mo99 DF = 0.969; Tc/Mo ratio = 0.255; efficiency = 87%;
    (720 mCi)(0.969)(0.255)(0.87) = 155 mCi.
8. 22 hours elapsed time; Mo99 DF = 0.795; Tc/Mo ratio = 0.852; efficiency = 80%;
    (690 mCi)(0.0.795)(0.852)(0.80) = 373 mCi.
9. 25 hours elapsed time; Mo99 DF = 0.771; Tc/Mo ratio = 0.877; efficiency = 80%;
    (690 mCi)(0.771)(0.877)(0.80) = 373 mCi.
10. 32 hours elapsed time; Mo99 DF = 0.717; Tc/Mo ratio = 0.913; efficiency = 80%;
    (690 mCi)(0.717)(0.913)(0.80) = 361 mCi.
11. 3 hours elapsed time; Mo99 DF = 0.969; Tc/Mo ratio = 0.255; efficiency = 80%;
    (1540 mCi)(0.969)(0.255)(0.80) = 304 mCi.
12. 5 hours elapsed time; Mo99 DF = 0.949; Tc/Mo ratio = 0.386; efficiency = 80%;
    (1540 mCi)(0.949)(0.386)(0.80) = 451 mCi.
13. 7 hours elapsed time; Mo99 DF = 0.93; Tc/Mo ratio = 0.492; efficiency = 80%;
    (1540 mCi)(0.93)(0.492)(0.80) = 564 mCi.

17. Allowable Mo99 content in generator eluate

1. (0.15 µCi/mCi)(748 mCi) = 112 µCi
2. (0.15 µCi/mCi)(237 mCi) = 36 µCi
3. 187 µCi
4. 13 µCi
5. 77 µCi
6. 20 µCi
7. 123 µCi
8. $\dfrac{93\,\mu Ci\,Mo99}{727\,mCi\,Tc99m} = 0.13\,\mu Ci\,Mo99/\,mCi\,Tc99m$; Yes.
9. $\dfrac{182\,\mu Ci\,Mo99}{916\,mCi\,Tc99m} = 0.20\,\mu Ci\,Mo99/\,mCi\,Tc99m$; No.
10. 0.12 µCi Mo99.mCi Tc99m; Acceptable.
11. 0.08 µCi Mo99.mCi Tc99m; Yes.
12. 0.14 µCi Mo99.mCi Tc99m; Yes, within acceptable limits.
13. 0.11 µCi Mo99.mCi Tc99m; Yes.

14. 4 hours elapsed

Calculate activity of Tc99m remaining: DF = 0.63; (380 mCi)(0.63) = 239 mCi

Calculate activity of Mo99 remaining: DF = 0.959; (53 µCi)(0.959) = 50.8 µCi

Determine Mo/Tc ratio: $\dfrac{50.8\,\mu\text{Ci Mo99}}{239\,\text{mCi Tc99m}} = 0.21\,\mu\text{Ci Mo99/ mCi Tc99m}$

No, eluate exceeds limits.

15. 6 hours elapsed

Calculate activity of Tc99m remaining: DF = 0.5; (189 mCi)(0.5) = 94.5 mCi

Calculate activity of Mo99 remaining: DF = 0.94; (13 µCi)(0.94) = 12.2 µCi

Determine Mo/Tc ratio: $\dfrac{12.2\,\mu\text{Ci Mo99}}{94.5\,\text{mCi Tc99m}} = 0.13\,\mu\text{Ci Mo99/ mCi Tc99m}$

Yes, solution can be used.

16. 3 hours elapsed

Calculate activity of Tc99m remaining: DF = 0.707; (65 mCi)(0.707) = 46 mCi

Calculate activity of Mo99 remaining: DF = 0.969; (9.0 µCi)(0.969) = 8.7 µCi

Determine Mo/Tc ratio: $\dfrac{8.7\,\mu\text{Ci Mo99}}{46\,\text{mCi Tc99m}} = 0.19\,\mu\text{Ci Mo99 / mCi Tc99m}$

No, eluate is not usable.

18. Eluate expiration time based on Mo99 content

1. $\dfrac{-\ln(74\,\mu\text{Ci}/573\,\text{mCi})}{0.1052} - 18.03 = \dfrac{2.0468}{0.1052} - 18.03 = 1.4\,\text{hours}$, or about 1 hour and 25 minutes.

2. $\dfrac{-\ln(12\,\mu\text{Ci}/188\,\text{mCi})}{0.1052} - 18.03 = \dfrac{2.7515}{0.1052} - 18.03 = 8.1\,\text{hours}$, or about 8 hours and 5 minutes.

3. $\dfrac{-\ln(6\,\mu\text{Ci}/130\,\text{mCi})}{0.1052} - 18.03 = \dfrac{3.0768}{0.1052} - 18.03 = 11.2\,\text{hours}$, or about 11 hours and 10 minutes.

4. Expiration time: 12:00 noon plus 3 hours and 35 minutes = 3:35 pm.

5. Expiration time: 5:30 pm plus 5 hours and 30 minutes = 11:00 pm.

6. Expiration time: 2:15 pm plus 30 minutes = 2:45 pm.

7. Expiration time: 7:30 am plus 2 hours and 20 minutes = 9:50 pm; Eluate cannot be used at 10:00 am.

8. Expiration time: 1:00 pm plus 7 hours = 8:00 pm; Eluate cannot be used at 9:00 pm.

9. Expiration time: 4:00 pm plus 1 hour and 40 minutes = 5:40 pm; Eluate can be used at 5:15 pm.

10. Expiration time: 10:30 am plus 3 hours and 15 minutes = 1:45 pm; Eluate can be used at 1:30 pm.

19. Chromatography calculations

1. $\dfrac{49{,}270\,\text{cpm} - 102\,\text{cpm}}{(525\,\text{cpmv}102\,\text{cpm}) + (49{,}270\,\text{cpm} - 102\,\text{cpm})} \times 100 = 99.1\%$

2. $\dfrac{87{,}920\,\text{cpm} - 620\,\text{cpm}}{(87{,}920\,\text{cpm} - 620\,\text{cpm}) + (2{,}450\,\text{cpm} - 620\,\text{cpm})} \times 100 = 97.9\%$

3. $\dfrac{125{,}000\,\text{cpm} - 135\,\text{cpm}}{(2{,}246\,\text{cpm} - 135\,\text{cpm}) + (125{,}000\,\text{cpm} - 135\,\text{cpm})} \times 100 = 98.3\%$

4. 99.6%

5. 2.3% free Tc

6. 2.6% HR-Tc

7. 6.5% HR-Tc

8. 15.6% free Tc

9. Free Tc impurity: $\dfrac{23.9\,\text{mCi}}{253\,\text{mCi} + 23.9\,\text{mCi}} \times 100 = 8.6\%$

   HR-Tc impurity: $\dfrac{6.4\,\text{mCi}}{147\,\text{mCi} + 6.4\,\text{mCi}} \times 100 = 4.2\%$

   Percent purity = 100% − 8.6% − 4.2% = 87.2%

10. Free Tc impurity = 7.8%

    HR-Tc impurity = 5.0%

    Percent purity = 100% − 7.8% − 5.0% = 87.2%

VI. Clinical Procedures

1. Left ventricle ejection fraction

1. $\dfrac{69{,}510 \text{ counts} - 30{,}700 \text{ counts}}{69{,}510 \text{ counts}} \times 100\% = 56\%$

2. $\dfrac{28{,}900 \text{ counts} - 20{,}170 \text{ counts}}{28{,}900 \text{ counts}} \times 100\% = 30\%$

3. 65%
4. 40%
5. 43%
6. 71%

7. $\text{net ES counts} = 29{,}300 \text{ counts} - \left(\dfrac{1{,}220 \text{ counts}}{46 \text{ pixels}} \times 520 \text{ pixels} \right) = 15{,}510 \text{ counts}$

   $\text{net ED counts} = 34{,}570 \text{ counts} - \left(\dfrac{1{,}220 \text{ counts}}{46 \text{ pixels}} \times 612 \text{ pixels} \right) = 18{,}340 \text{ counts}$

   $\dfrac{18{,}340 \text{ counts} - 15{,}510 \text{ counts}}{18{,}340} \times 100\% = 15\%$

8. $\text{net ES counts} = 23{,}610 \text{ counts} - \left(\dfrac{2{,}180 \text{ counts}}{114 \text{ pixels}} \times 237 \text{ pixels} \right) = 19{,}080 \text{ counts}$

   $\text{net ED counts} = 50{,}140 \text{ counts} - \left(\dfrac{2{,}180 \text{ counts}}{114 \text{ pixels}} \times 449 \text{ pixels} \right) = 41{,}550 \text{ counts}$

   $\dfrac{41{,}550 \text{ counts} - 19{,}080 \text{ counts}}{41{,}550} \times 100\% = 54\%$

9. correct background

   $\text{net ES counts} = 25{,}170 \text{ counts} - \left(\dfrac{1{,}800 \text{ counts}}{60 \text{ pixels}} \times 360 \text{ pixels} \right) = 14{,}370 \text{ counts}$

   $\text{net ED counts} = 48{,}630 \text{ counts} - \left(\dfrac{1{,}800 \text{ counts}}{60 \text{ pixels}} \times 596 \text{ pixels} \right) = 30{,}750 \text{ counts}$

   $\dfrac{30{,}750 \text{ counts} - 14{,}370 \text{ counts}}{30{,}750} \times 100\% = 53\%$

   background region including portion of spleen

   $\text{net ES counts} = 25{,}170 \text{ counts} - \left(\dfrac{2{,}900 \text{ counts}}{60 \text{ pixels}} \times 360 \text{ pixels} \right) = 7{,}770 \text{ counts}$

   $\text{net ED counts} = 48{,}630 \text{ counts} - \left(\dfrac{2{,}900 \text{ counts}}{60 \text{ pixels}} \times 596 \text{ pixels} \right) = 19{,}820 \text{ counts}$

   $\dfrac{19{,}820 \text{ counts} - 7{,}770 \text{ counts}}{19{,}820} \times 100\% = 61\%$

9. (continued)
    background region extending outside the body margin

$$\text{net ES counts} = 25{,}170 \text{ counts} - \left(\frac{120 \text{ counts}}{60 \text{ pixels}} \times 360 \text{ pixels} \right) = 24{,}450 \text{ counts}$$

$$\text{net ED counts} = 48{,}630 \text{ counts} - \left(\frac{120 \text{ counts}}{60 \text{ pixels}} \times 596 \text{ pixels} \right) = 47{,}440 \text{ counts}$$

$$\frac{47{,}440 \text{ counts} - 24{,}450 \text{ counts}}{47{,}440 \text{ counts}} \times 100\% = 48\%$$

As background counts/pixel increase, the EF erroneously increases.
As background counts/pixel decrease, the EF erroneously decreases.

10. correct end diastole region: $\dfrac{47{,}130 \text{ counts} - 23{,}670 \text{ counts}}{47{,}130 \text{ counts}} \times 100\% = 50\%$

    end diastole region drawn too large: $\dfrac{50{,}130 \text{ counts} - 23{,}670 \text{ counts}}{50{,}130 \text{ counts}} \times 100\% = 53\%$

    end diastole region drawn too small: $\dfrac{43{,}130 \text{ counts} - 23{,}670 \text{ counts}}{43{,}130 \text{ counts}} \times 100\% = 45\%$

As the ED region size and counts increase, the EF erroneously increases.
As the ED region size and counts decrease, the EF erroneously decreases.

11. correct end systole region: $\dfrac{47{,}130 \text{ counts} - 23{,}670 \text{ counts}}{47{,}130 \text{ counts}} \times 100\% = 50\%$

    end systole region drawn too large: $\dfrac{47{,}130 \text{ counts} - 26{,}670 \text{ counts}}{47{,}130 \text{ counts}} \times 100\% = 43\%$

    end systole region drawn too small: $\dfrac{47{,}130 \text{ counts} - 20{,}670 \text{ counts}}{47{,}130 \text{ counts}} \times 100\% = 56\%$

As the ES region size and counts increase, the EF erroneously decreases.
As the ES region size and counts decrease, the EF erroneously increases.

2. Cardiac output and stroke volume

1. 108 ml – 39 ml = 69 ml; (69 ml)(60 bpm) = 4140 ml/min or 4.1 L/min
2. 127 ml – 42 ml = 85 ml; (85 ml)(65 bpm) = 5525 ml/min or 5.5 L/min
3. 93 ml; 5,115 ml/min or 5.1 L/min
4. 58 ml; 4,350 ml/min or 4.4 L/min
5. 52 ml; 3,640 ml/min or 3.6 L/min

6. 74 ml; 5,550 ml/min or 5.6 L/min

7. 69 ml; $\dfrac{108\ ml - 39\ ml}{108\ ml} \times 100\% = 64\%$; 5,382 ml/min or 5.4 L/min

8. 36 ml; $\dfrac{55\ ml - 19\ ml}{55\ ml} \times 100\% = 65\%$; 3,312 ml/min or 3.3 L/min

9. 32 ml; 16%; 2,240 ml/min or 2.2 L/min

10. 59 ml; 42%; 4,779 ml/min or 4.8 L/min

3. Gall bladder ejection fraction

1. $\dfrac{235,000\ counts - 174,000\ counts}{235,000\ counts} \times 100\% = 26\%$

2. $\dfrac{142,800\ counts - 84,310\ counts}{142,800\ counts} \times 100\% = 41\%$

3. 25%

4. 81%

5. 40%

6. 31%

7. 26%

8. 75%

9.

$$\text{net maximum GB counts} = 268,000\ counts - \left(\dfrac{14,000\ counts}{191\ pixels} \times 269\ pixels \right) = 248,000\ counts$$

$$\text{net minimum GB counts} = 193,000\ counts - \left(\dfrac{4,100\ counts}{102\ pixels} \times 186\ pixels \right) = 186,000\ counts$$

$$\dfrac{248,000\ counts - 186,000\ counts}{248,000\ counts} \times 100\% = 25\%$$

10.

$$\text{net maximum GB counts} = 84,320\ counts - \left(\dfrac{5,760\ counts}{96\ pixels} \times 284\ pixels \right) = 67,280\ counts$$

$$\text{net minimum GB counts} = 53,140\ counts - \left(\dfrac{1,420\ counts}{79\ pixels} \times 220\ pixels \right) = 49,190\ counts$$

$$\dfrac{67,280\ counts - 49,190\ counts}{67,280\ counts} \times 100\% = 27\%$$

11. net maximum GB counts = 181,000
    net minimum GB counts = 109,000
    GBEF = 40%

3. Gastroesophageal reflux

1. $\dfrac{1,090 \text{ counts} - 110 \text{ counts}}{18,300 \text{ counts}} \times 100\% = 5.4\%$

2. $\dfrac{984 \text{ counts} - 44 \text{ counts}}{32,800 \text{ counts}} \times 100\% = 2.9\%$

3. 1.5%

4.
Pressure	Reflux Index
20	0.8%
40	0.9%
60	2.6%
80	5.5%

---

* Note: The maximum stomach ROI counts (22,847) are used for each calculation as required by the equation.

---

5. Before therapy: 8.9%
    After therapy: 4.6%

---

* Note: Because two separate studies are performed and therefore, two separate doses administered, the stomach ROI counts obtained in each study are used in the calculation.

---

6. Upright: 2.9%
    Supine: 6.7%
    The patient is experiencing positional reflux.

4. Gastric emptying

1. $\dfrac{\sqrt{(43,200 \text{ cpm})(40,800 \text{ cpm})}}{\sqrt{(59,300 \text{ cpm})(57,900 \text{ cpm})} \times 0.944} \times 100\% = 76\%$

2. $\dfrac{\sqrt{(23,500 \text{ cpm})(19,600 \text{ cpm})}}{\sqrt{(41,600 \text{ cpm})(37,100 \text{ cpm})} \times 0.917} \times 100\% = 60\%$

3. $\dfrac{\sqrt{(33,600 \text{ cpm})(30,200 \text{ cpm})}}{\sqrt{(78,400 \text{ cpm})(73,300 \text{ cpm})} \times 0.841} \times 100\% = 50\%$

4. 82%

5.

Time	Geometric Mean	% Remaining	Time	Geometric Mean	% Remaining
0	62,700		60	39,900	71
15	55,400	91	90	24,600	47
30	50,100	85	120	10,300	21

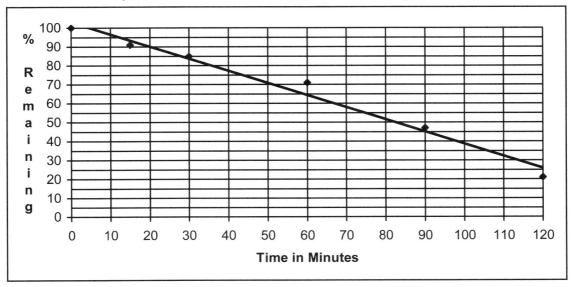

Half emptying time about 80 to 85 minutes

6.

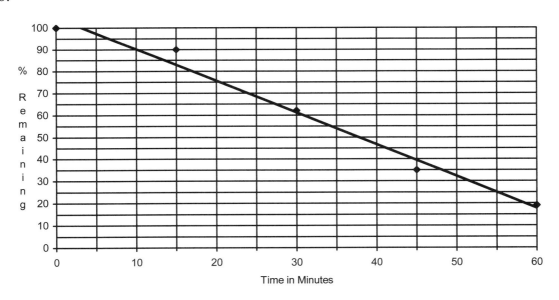

Half emptying time is about 35 to 40 minutes

7.

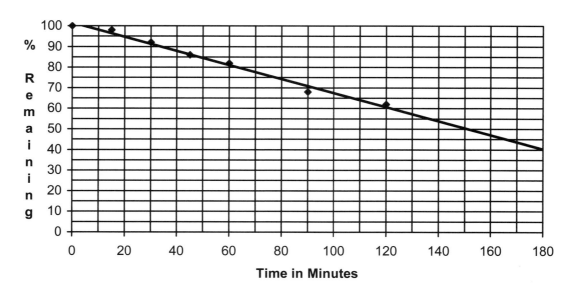

Estimated half emptying time about 150 to 160 minutes

8. | Time | Geometric Mean | Time 0 Mean Corrected for Decay |
      |------|----------------|--------------------------------|
      | 0 | 78,400 | |
      | 2 | 43,700 | 62,200 |

$$\frac{62,200 - 43700}{62,200} \times 100\% = 30\% \text{ emptied}$$

9. | Time | Geometric Mean | Percent Emptying |
      |------|----------------|------------------|
      | 0 | 14,500 | |
      | 1 | 3,100 | 79 |

10. | Time | Geometric Mean | Time 0 Mean Corrected for Decay | Percent Emptying |
      |------|----------------|--------------------------------|------------------|
      | 0 | 64,500 | | |
      | 2 | 25,200 | 51,200 | 51 |

11. | Time | Geometric Mean | Time 0 Mean Corrected for Decay | Percent Emptying |
      |------|----------------|--------------------------------|------------------|
      | 0 | 44,400 | | |
      | 1 | 12,300 | 39,600 | 69 |
      | 2 | 9,800 | 35,200 | 72 |

5. Calculation of expected bladder capacity for voiding cystogram

1.   240 ml
2.   90 ml
3.   180 ml
4.   150 ml
5.   no, expected bladder capacity is 300 ml

6. Quantitation of residual bladder volume and reflux with a voiding cystogram

1. 29 ml
2. 21 ml

3. $(3826 \text{ ct})\left(\dfrac{180 \text{ ml}}{96,244 \text{ ct}}\right) = 7.2 \text{ ml}$

4. initial volume = 285 ml – 260 ml = 25 ml
    bladder volume at reflux = 25 ml + 240 ml = 265 ml

5. $\text{residual volume} = \dfrac{(132 \text{ ml})(24,451 \text{ counts})}{121,903 \text{ counts} - 24,451 \text{ counts}} = 33 \text{ ml}$

    total volume = 132 ml + 33 ml = 165 ml

    $\text{reflux volume right kidney} = 6,850 \text{ counts} \times \dfrac{165 \text{ ml}}{121,903 \text{ counts}} = 9.3 \text{ ml}$

    $\text{reflux volume left kidney} = 1,372 \text{ counts} \times \dfrac{165 \text{ ml}}{121,903 \text{ counts}} = 1.8 \text{ ml}$

6. $\text{residual volume} = \dfrac{(110 \text{ ml})(70,347 \text{ counts})}{164,368 \text{ counts} - 70,347 \text{ counts}} = 82 \text{ ml}$

    total volume = 110 ml + 78 ml = 188 ml
    initial volume = 188 ml – 170 ml = 18 ml
    reflux bladder volume = 18 ml + 105 ml = 123 ml

    $\text{reflux volume} = 9,880 \text{ counts} \times \dfrac{188 \text{ ml}}{164,368 \text{ counts}} = 11 \text{ ml}$

7. residual volume = 50 ml
    total volume = 240 ml
    initial volume = 5 ml
    reflux bladder volume = 195 ml
    reflux volume right kidney = 2.7 ml
    reflux volume left kidney = 6.3 ml

8. residual volume = 93 ml; no, condition has not improved.

7. Lung quantitation

1. right lung   38%
    left lung   62%
2. right apical lobe   17%
    right middle lobe   15%
    right basal lobe   27%
    left apical lobe   16%
    left basal lobe   24%

---

* Note: The total percentage does not add up to 100% due to rounding off of individual numbers.

3. 44%
4. ~5%
5. right lung   35%
    left lung 65%
6. right upper segment   6%
    right middle segment   17%
    right lower segment   9%
    left upper segment   18%
    left middle segment   37%
    left lower segment   13%

8. Thyroid uptake with and without decayed standard

1. $\dfrac{245,000\,\text{cpm} - 1,200\,\text{cpm}}{1,142,000\,\text{cpm} - 56\,\text{cpm}} \times 100\% = 21\%$

2. $\dfrac{376,750\,\text{cpm} - 436\,\text{cpm}}{755,060\,\text{cpm} - 121\,\text{cpm}} \times 100\% = 50\%$

3. 2%
4. 6%
5. 18%
6. 30%
7. 25%

8. $\dfrac{29,760\,\text{cpm} - 683\,\text{cpm}}{(734,915\,\text{cpm} - 103\,\text{cpm})(0.810)} \times 100\% = 4.8\%\,;\ \text{round to } 5\%$

9. $\dfrac{52,905\,\text{cpm} - 438\,\text{cpm}}{(805,312\,\text{cpm} - 65\,\text{cpm})(0.73)} \times 100\% = 8.9\%\,;\ \text{round to } 9\%$

10. $\dfrac{167,136\,\text{cpm} - 374\,\text{cpm}}{(969,140\,\text{cpm} - 87\,\text{cpm})(0.284)} \times 100\% = 60\%$

11. 32%
12. 58%; yes
13. 14%

9. Calculation of concentration of a solution

1. $\dfrac{50\,\mu\text{Ci}}{10\,\text{ml}} = 5\,\mu\text{Ci/ml}$

2. $\dfrac{12.5\,\mu\text{Ci}}{50\,\text{ml}} = 0.25\,\mu\text{Ci/ml}$

3. 0.01 µCi/ml
4. 4 µCi/ml
5. 5 µCi/ml

6. $\dfrac{5\,\mu\text{Ci}}{0.1\,\mu\text{Ci/ml}} = 50\,\text{ml}$ OR $0.1\,\mu\text{Ci/ml} = \dfrac{5\,\mu\text{Ci}}{X\,\text{ml}}\,;\ \text{Isolate and solve for } X$

7. $\dfrac{20\,\mu Ci}{0.5\,\mu Ci/ml} = 40$ ml OR $0.5\,\mu Ci/ml = \dfrac{20\,\mu Ci}{X\ ml}$; Isolate and solve for X

8. 500 ml

9. $(10\,\mu Ci/ml)(100\ ml) = 1{,}000\,\mu Ci$ OR $10\,\mu Ci/ml = \dfrac{X\,\mu Ci}{100\ ml}$; Isolate and solve for X

10. $(0.02\,\mu Ci/ml)(50\ ml) = 1\mu Ci$ OR $0.02\,\mu Ci/ml = \dfrac{X\,\mu Ci}{50\ ml}$; Isolate and solve for X

11. 2 μCi

10. Preparing standards from bulk solution (dilutions)

1. $(10\%)(X\ ml) = (1\%)(100\ ml)$; $X\ ml = \dfrac{(1\%)(100\ ml)}{10\%} = 10$ ml

2. $(10\%)(X\ ml) = (0.5\%)(100\ ml)$; $X\ ml = \dfrac{(0.5\%)(100\ ml)}{10\%} = 5$ ml

3. Convert 1 liter to 1,000 ml.
    $(25\%)(X\ ml) = (1\%)(1{,}000\ ml)$; $X = 40$ ml

4. 10 ml

5. 25 ml

6. 250 ml

7. $(0.5\ \%)(10\ ml) = (X\%)(50\ ml)$; $X\ ml = \dfrac{(0.5\%)(10\ ml)}{50\ ml} = 0.1\%$

8. $(0.25\ \%)(10\ ml) = (X\%)(50\ ml)$; $X\ ml = \dfrac{(0.25\%)(10\ ml)}{50\ ml} = 0.05\%$

9. 2%

10. 0.1%

11. $(20\%)(10\ ml) = (2\%)(X\ ml)$; $X = 100$ ml

12. $(5\%)(5\ ml) = (0.1\%)(X\ ml)$; $X = 250$ ml

13. 1,000 ml or 1 liter

14. Do not be distracted by the 200 μCi. This number is not used in the calculations.
    If a given activity or dose is diluted to 100 ml, then each ml contains 1% of the dose:
    $1\ ml \div 100\ ml = 0.01$ or 1%.
    $(1\ \%)(1\ ml) = (X\ \%)(100\ ml)$; $X = 0.01\%$

15. If a given activity is diluted to 50 ml, then each ml contains 2% of the dose:
    $1\ ml \div 50\ ml = 0.02$ or 2%.
    $(2\ \%)(1\ ml) = (X\ \%)(100\ ml)$; $X = 0.02\%$

16. If a given activity is diluted to 100 ml, then each ml contains 1% of the dose as
    shown in problem #14.
    $(1\%)(10\ ml) = (X\%)(100\ ml)$; $X = 0.1\%$
    $(1\%)(10\ ml) = (X\%)(50\ ml)$; $X = 0.2\%$
    $(1\%)(50\ ml) = (X\%)(100\ ml)$; $X = 0.5\%$

11. Plasma volume

1. $\dfrac{(1{,}490 \text{ cpm/ml})(4{,}000)(1 \text{ ml})}{3{,}221 \text{ cpm/ml}} = 1{,}850 \text{ ml}$

2. $\dfrac{(2{,}946 \text{ cpm/ml})(1{,}000)(2 \text{ ml})}{2{,}343 \text{ cpm/ml}} = 2{,}515 \text{ ml}$

3. $\dfrac{(390 \text{ cpm/ml})(4{,}000)(1 \text{ ml})}{891 \text{ cpm/ml}} = 1{,}751 \text{ ml}$

4. Convert counts per 5 minutes to cpm, then apply values to equation.
$\dfrac{(10{,}467 \text{ cpm/ml})(1{,}000)(1 \text{ ml})}{3{,}642 \text{ cpm/ml}} = 2{,}874 \text{ ml}$

5. Convert counts per 3 minutes to cpm, then apply values to equation.
$\dfrac{(6{,}256 \text{ cpm/ml})(1{,}000)(2 \text{ ml})}{4{,}108 \text{ cpm/ml}} = 3{,}046 \text{ ml}$

6. Average the counts, then apply the values to the equation.
$\dfrac{(3{,}608 \text{ cpm/ml})(1{,}000)(1 \text{ ml})}{1{,}618 \text{ cpm/ml}} = 2{,}230 \text{ ml}$

7. Average the counts, then apply the values to the equation.
$\dfrac{(16{,}717 \text{ cpm/ml})(4{,}000)(1 \text{ ml})}{15{,}863 \text{ cpm/ml}} = 4{,}215 \text{ ml}$

8. Average the counts, then apply the values to the equation.
$\dfrac{(4{,}740 \text{ cpm/ml})(4{,}000)(1 \text{ ml})}{4{,}751 \text{ cpm/ml}} = 3{,}990 \text{ ml}$

9. Average the counts, then apply the values to the equation.
$\dfrac{(10{,}517 \text{ cpm/ml})(4{,}000)(1 \text{ ml})}{16{,}779 \text{ cpm/ml}} = 2{,}504 \text{ ml}$

12. Red cell mass

1. Std Pct: $1 - 0.27 = 0.73$
Patient Pct: $1 - 0.47 = 0.53$
$\text{RCV} = \dfrac{[(10{,}055 \text{ cpm} \times 100) - (312 \text{ cpm} \times 0.73)](10 \text{ ml})}{2{,}098 \text{ cpm} - (436 \text{ cpm} \times 0.53)} \times 0.47 = 2{,}531 \text{ ml}$

2. Std Pct: $1 - 0.26 = 0.74$
Patient Pct: $1 - 0.43 = 0.57$
$\text{RCV} = \dfrac{[(4{,}498 \text{ cpm} \times 100) - (360 \text{ cpm} \times 0.74)](10 \text{ ml})}{970 \text{ cpm} - (63 \text{ cpm} \times 0.57)} \times 0.43 = 2{,}069 \text{ ml}$

3. Std Pct: $1 - 0.30 = 0.70$
Patient Pct: $1 - 0.54 = 0.46$
$\text{RCV} = \dfrac{[(15{,}352 \text{ cpm} \times 100) - (498 \text{ cpm} \times 0.70)](10 \text{ ml})}{3{,}035 \text{ cpm} - (233 \text{ cpm} \times 0.46)} \times 0.54 = 2{,}831 \text{ ml}$

4. Std Pct: $1 - 0.28 = 0.72$
    Patient Pct: $1 - 0.51 = 0.49$

$$RCV = \frac{[(7,686\,cpm \times 100) - (280\,cpm \times 0.72)](10\,ml)}{1,689\,cpm - (148\,cpm \times 0.49)} \times 0.51 = 2,424\,ml$$

5. Std Pct: $1 - 0.29 = 0.71$
    Patient Pct: $1 - 0.56 = 0.44$

$$RCV = \frac{[(9,657\,cpm \times 100) - (347\,cpm \times 0.71)](10\,ml)}{1,822\,cpm - (185\,cpm \times 0.44)} \times 0.56 = 3,105\,ml$$

6. Std Pct: $1 - 0.26 = 0.74$
    Patient Pct: $1 - 0.49 = 0.51$

$$RCV = \frac{[(14,991\,cpm \times 100) - (1,027\,cpm \times 0.74)](10\,ml)}{3,881\,cpm - (252\,cpm \times 0.51)} \times 0.49 = 1,957\,ml$$

7. Std Pct: $1 - 0.30 = 0.70$
    Patient Pct: $1 - 0.52 = 0.48$

$$RCV = \frac{[(11,456\,cpm \times 100) - (526\,cpm \times 0.70)](10\,ml)}{1,918\,cpm - (422\,cpm \times 0.48)} \times 0.52 = 3,470\,ml$$

13. Total blood volume with dual nuclide method

1. 4,161 ml
2. 3,645 ml
3. 6,211 ml

References

Adenoscan® adenosine injection package insert. Deerfield, IL: Astellas Pharma US Inc.; 2005.

Balon HR, Brill DR, Fink-Bennett DM, et al. *Procedure guideline for hepatobiliary scintigraphy.* Version 3.0. Society of Nuclear Medicine. June 23, 2001.

Balon HR, Silberstein EB, Meier DA, et al. *Procedure guideline for thyroid uptake measurement.* Version 3.0. Society of Nuclear Medicine. September 5, 2006.

Ceretec™ Kit for the Preparation of Technetium Tc99m Exametazime Injection package insert. Arlington Heights, IL: GE Healthcare; 2006.

Chandra R. *Nuclear medicine physics: the basics.* 6th ed. Philadelphia, PA: Lippincott Williams & Wilkins; 2004.

Cherry SR, Sorensen JA, Phelps ME. *Physics in nuclear medicine.* 3rd ed. St. Louis, MO: Mosby; 2003.

Chilton HM, Witkofski RL. *Nuclear pharmacy: an introduction to the clinical application of radiopharmaceuticals.* Philadelphia, PA: Lea & Febiger; 1986.

Christian PE, Waterstram-Rich K, eds. *Nuclear medicine & PET/CT technology and techniques.* 6th ed. St. Louis, MO: Mosby; 2007.

Crawford ES, Husain SS. *Nuclear cardiac imaging: terminology and technical aspects.* Reston, VA: Society of Nuclear Medicine; 2003.

Dipyridamole Injection USP package insert. Bedford, OH: Bedford Laboratories; 2007.

Donohoe KJ, Maurer AH, Ziessman HA, et al. *Procedure guideline for adult solid-meal gastric-emptying study.* Version 3.0. Society of Nuclear Medicine. February 8, 2009.

DraxImage™ MAA Kit for Preparation of Technetium Tc99m Albumin Aggregated Injection package insert. Kirkland, Quebec, Canada: Draximage, Inc.; 1997.

Early PJ, Sodee DB. *Principles and Practice of Nuclear Medicine.* 2nd ed. St. Louis, MO: Mosby-Year Book Inc.; 1995.

Faber TL, Cooke CD, Folks RD, et al. Left ventricular function and perfusion from gated SPECT perfusion images: an integrated method. *J Nucl Med.* 1999;40:650–659.

Harbert J, da Rocha AFG. *Textbook of nuclear medicine: volume I. Basic science.* 2nd ed. Philadelphia, PA: Lea & Febiger; 1984.

Harbert J, da Rocha AFG. *Textbook of nuclear medicine: volume II. Clinical procedures.* 2nd ed. Philadelphia, PA: Lea & Febiger; 1984.

Institute for Safe Medication Practices. *List of error-prone abbreviations, symbols, and dose designations.* 2010. https://www.ismp.org/tools/abbreviations/. Accessed March 13, 2010.

International Atomic Energy Agency. *Nuclear medicine resources manual.* Vienna, Austria: International Atomic Energy Agency; 2006.

International Committee for Standardization of Haematology. Recommended methods for measurement of red-cell and plasma volume. *J Nucl Med*. 1980;21:793–800.

Itturalde MP. *Dictionary and handbook of nuclear medicine and clinical imaging*. Boca Raton, FL: CRC; 1990.

Kinevac® Sincalide for Injection package insert. Princeton, NJ: Bracco Diagnostics Inc; 1994.

Kowalsky RJ, Fallon SW. *Radiopharmaceuticals in nuclear medicine and nuclear pharmacy*. 2nd ed. Washington, DC: American Pharmacists Assoc; 2004.

Mettler Fa, Guiberteau MJ. *Essentials of nuclear medicine imaging*. 5th ed. Philadelphia, PA: W.B. Saunders; 2005.

O'Connor MK, ed. *The Mayo Clinic manual of nuclear medicine*. NYC: Churchill Livingstone; 1996.

Palmer EL, Scott JA, Strauss HW. *Practical nuclear medicine*. Philadelphia, PA: W.B. Saunders; 1992.

Poswer RA, Powsner ER. *Essentials of nuclear medicine physics*. 2nd ed. Malden, MA: Blackwell Science; 2006.

Pulmolite® Kit for the Preparation of Technetium Tc99m Albumin Aggregated Injection(MAA) package insert. Bedford, MA: Pharmalucence. www.pharmlucence.com. Accessed March 3, 2010.

Saha GB. *Fundamentals of nuclear pharmacy*. 4th ed. NY: Springer-Verlag; 1998.

Scheiner J, Sinusas A, Wittry M, et al. *Procedure guideline for gated equilibrium radionuclide ventriculography*. Version 3.0. Society of Nuclear Medicine. June 15, 2002.

Steves AM, Wells PC. *Review of nuclear medicine technology*. 3rd ed. Reston, VA: Society of Nuclear Medicine; 2004.

Talbot N, Richie R. The advantages of surface area of the body as a basis for calculating pediatric dosages. *Pediatrics* 1959;24:495–498.

The Joint Commission. *The official "do not use" list of abbreviations*. December 29, 2009. http://www.jointcommission.org/PatientSafety/DoNotUseList/. Accessed March 13, 2010.

United States Department of Transportation. *Federal Regulations*. Annual ed. Title 49, Chapter 1, Part 173. Washington, DC: GPO; October 1, 2008.

United States Nuclear Regulatory Commission. *Federal Regulations*. Annual ed. Title 10, Chapter 1, Part 20. Washington, DC: GPO; January 1, 2009.

—. *Federal Regulations*. Annual ed. Title 10, Chapter 1, Energy, Part 35. Washington, DC: GPO; January 1, 2009.

—. *Consolidated Guidance About Materials Licenses: Program- Specific Guidance About Medical Use Licenses, Final Report*. NUREG-1556, Vol 9, Revision 2. January 2008. http://www.nrc.gov/reading-room/doc-collections/nuregs/staff/sr1556/. Accessed March 13, 2010.

Venes D. *Tabor's cyclopedic medical dictionary*. 21st ed. Philadelphia, PA: F.A. Davis; 2009.

INDEX